Mental Health in Primary Care

Mental Health in Primary Care—a new approach

Edited by

Andrew Elder
General Practitioner and Honorary Consultant in General Practice and Primary Care, The Tavistock and Portman NHS Trust, London

and

Jeremy Holmes
Consultant Psychotherapist and Senior lecturer in Psychotherapy, University of Exeter

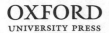

OXFORD
UNIVERSITY PRESS

OXFORD
UNIVERSITY PRESS

Great Clarendon Street, Oxford OX2 6DP

Oxford University Press is a department of the University of Oxford.
It furthers the University's objective of excellence in research, scholarship,
and education by publishing worldwide in

Oxford New York

Auckland Bangkok Buenos Aires Cape Town Chennai
Dar es Salaam Delhi Hong Kong Istanbul Karachi Kolkata
Kuala Lumpur Madrid Melbourne Mexico City Mumbai Nairobi
São Paulo Shanghai Taipei Tokyo Toronto

Oxford is a registered trade mark of Oxford University Press
in the UK and in certain other countries

Published in the United States
by Oxford University Press Inc., New York

© Oxford University Press 2002

The moral rights of the author have been asserted

Database right Oxford University Press (maker)

First published 2002

A catalogue record for this title is available from the British Library

Library of Congress Cataloging in Publication Data

Mental health in primary care, a new approach/edited by Andrew Elder
and Jeremy Holmes.
    Includes bibliographical references and index.
    1. Psychiatry.   2. Primary care (Medicine)   3. Psychotherapy.
    4. Patients—Mental health.   I. Elder, Andrew, 1945–   II. Holmes, Jeremy.

    RC454.4 .M4585 2002   616.89—dc21   2002074297

ISBN 0 19 850894 8 (alk. paper: Pbk.)

10 9 8 7 6 5 4 3 2 1

Typeset in India by Integra Software Services Pvt. Ltd, Pondicherry, India
www.integra-india.com
Printed in Great Britain
on acid-free paper by
T.J. International Ltd, Padstow

Contents

List of contributors

Gwen Adshead,
Consultant Adult Psychiatrist,
Traumatic Stress Clinic, 73 Charlotte
Street, London W1P 1LB.

Eia Asen,
Consultant Child Psychiatrist and
Family Therapist, Marlborough
Family Service, 38 Marlborough
Place, London NW8 0PJ.

Mary Burd,
Joint Head of Psychology and
Counselling Services,
Tower Hamlets PCT/ELCMHT
(Tower Hamlets Locality),
Steels Lane Health Centre,
384 Commercial Rd, London E1 0LR.

Tom Burns,
Professor of Social and Community
Psychiatry, St George's Hospital
Medical School, Jenner Wing,
Cranmer Terrace, London SW17 0RE.

John Cape,
Head of Psychology and
Psychotherapy Services,
Camden and Islington Mental
Health NHS Trust, St Pancras
Hospital, 4 St Pancras Way,
London NW1 0PE.

Peter J. Cooper,
Professor of Psychology,
Winnicott Research Unit, 3 Earley
Gate, Whiteknights, PO Box 238,
Reading RG6 6AL.

Ilana Crome,
Professor of Addictions,
Addictive Behaviour Centre,

120-122 Corporation Street,
Birmingham B4 6SX.

Ed Day,
Specialist Registrar in
Addiction Psychiatry,
Addictive Behaviour Centre,
120-122 Corporation Street,
Birmingham B4 6SX.

Maret Dymond,
Research Student,
Department of Psychology,
Winnicott Research Unit,
3 Earley Gate, PO Box 238,
Reading RG6 6AL.

Andrew Elder,
General Practitioner,
Paddington Green Health Centre,
4 Princess Louise Close,
London W2 1LQ
Hon Consultant in General Practice
and Primary Care, Tavistock Centre,
London NW3 5BA.

Jonathan Evans,
Senior Lecturer,
Division of Psychiatry, University of
Bristol, Cotham House, Cotham Hill,
Bristol BS6 6JL.

Adrian Feeney,
Specialist Registrar in Forensic
Psychiatry, Froneside Clinic,
Manor Road, Bristol BS16 2EW.

Hilary Graham,
General Practitioner (ret'd) and
Family Therapist, 29 Benhall Green,
Benhall, Saxmundham,
Suffolk IP17 1HL.

Iona Heath,
General Practitioner, Caversham
Practice, 4 Peckwater Street,
Kentish Town, London NW5 2UP.

Jeremy Holmes,
Consultant Psychiatrist and
Psychotherapist, North Devon
District Hospital, Raleigh Park,
Barnstaple, Devon EX31 4JB.

Brian Hurwitz,
Part-time GP Principal, London.
Professor of Medicine and the Arts,
King's College London, Strand,
London WC2R 2LS.

John Launer,
General Practitioner, Senior Clinical
Lecturer in General Practice and
Primary Care, Tavistock Clinic, 120
Belsize Lane, London NW3 5BA.

Robert Mayer,
General Practitioner,
Highgate Group Practice, 44 North
Hill, Highgate, London N6 4QA.

Jane Milton,
Psychiatrist and Psychoanalyst,
6 Narcissus Road, London NW6 1TH.

Lynne Murray,
Professor, Winnicott Research Unit,
Department of Psychology,
The University of Reading,
3 Earley Gate, Whiteknights,
PO Box 238, Reading,
Berkshire RG6 6AL.

David Nutt,
Professor of Psychopharmacology,
University of Bristol, School of
Medical Sciences, University Walk,
Bristol BS8 1TD.

Glenys Parry,
Professor of Health Care Psychology,
Director of Sheffield Health and
Social Research Consortium,
Fulwood House, Old Fulwood
Road, Sheffield, F10 3TH.

Paul Sackin,
General Practitioner and VTS
Course Organiser,
12 Stukeley Park, Chestnut Grove,
Great Stukeley, Huntingdon,
Cambs PE 28 4AD.

Ulrike Schmidt,
Senior Lecturer of Eating Disorders
Research Unit, Institute of
Psychiatry, De Crespigny Park,
Denmark Hill, London SE5 8AZ.

Sam Smith,
General Practitioner,
1 Landscape Dene, Helsby,
Frodsham, Cheshire WA6 9LG.

Richard Westcott,
General Practitioner,
East Street Surgery, South Molton,
North Devon, EX36 4BU.

Jan Wiener,
Jungian Analyst and Senior Adult
Psychotherapist (Thorpe Coombe
Hospital), 24 Dyne Road,
London NW6 7XE.

Christine Wright,
Consultant Psychiatrist and
Honorary Senior Lecturer,
Social and Community Psychiatry,
Department of Community
Psychiatry, St George's Hospital
Medical School, Jenner Wing,
Cranmer Terrace, London
SW17 0RE.

Introduction: the need for a new approach

Andrew Elder and Jeremy Holmes

It is paradoxical that family doctors—who conduct more psychiatric consultations than any other group of professionals in the Health Service—are often not considered 'mental health' practitioners. In our view a new approach is needed to mental health thinking, which places primary care—with its accompanying differences in emphasis and philosophy—as the base from which to build a fully integrated Mental Health Service. At least 30 per cent of consultations with general practitioners have a direct psychological component and the figure far higher if indirect psychological aspects are included. The vast majority of this distress is contained within the general practitioner's setting: no more than 10 per cent of such patients are ever referred on to specialist services. Despite this—recent shift in Government policy notwithstanding—there is a continuing tendency among policy makers, researchers, and writers to adopt the paradigms, perspectives, and classificatory systems of the secondary services when considering primary care.

The precursors of established psychiatric disorders are sought, and diagnostic and treatment approaches are transposed from the secondary setting to primary care, rather than focusing on the ways in which psychological distress arises and subsides in the general practice setting, and the factors that enable such distress to be contained without recourse to specialist referral. The extent to which practices are able to perform this *containing* function remains largely unstudied. What factors sustain it? Which undermine it? How might Primary Care Trusts seek to enhance this aspect of primary care in the future? These considerations not only have a significant bearing on the welfare of patients, but on the shape and effectiveness of the surrounding secondary services as well.

There is an implicit, but largely unexamined value system operating here:

- severity (as defined by secondary services) is seen as more important than frequency; established disease is more significant than undifferentiated distress;
- diagnosis ('medical model' or 'one-person' thinking) more important than relationship (or inter-personal thinking);

- a focus on episode rather than the evolution of complex narrative;
- additionally, there is a barely noticed discounting of the body (and the links between mind and body) in favour of a view derived from a specialized and exclusively 'mental' health approach.

The *experience* of an encounter with psychological pain is down-played or avoided, together with its uncertainties, emotional components for both sufferer and doctor, time course, decision points, and place within the spectrum of the general practitioner's work.

Patients often develop deep and dependent relationships with their doctors (and 'the practice'), which have the effect of amplifying the significance and, therefore, the impact of the mental health work that is done in a primary care team. A practice becomes a *secure base* to which patients attach themselves in a variety of characteristic and complex ways over the years, and understanding these processes can enhance the effectiveness of primary care mental health work.

An analogy can be drawn between the ways in which psychological pain is represented within the individual psyche and its representation in general practice. There is increasing evidence that the capacity to symbolize and think about emotional distress is a significant protective factor in maintaining psychological health (Fonagy *et al.* 1995). This 'narrative competence', arising out of parental capacity to see children as sentient beings, able to feel pain and needing to be soothed, acts as a buffer against the vicissitudes of life. The enhancement of *reflective function* is a key component of psychological therapies. The parent or therapist starts as an observing and listening 'other', but as development proceeds, this reflective function becomes internalized as a part of the self that protects against further distress, and may prevent or slow down the development of frank psychological illness.

Just as the healthy mind—developing at first from the sensitive care of the infant's body—provides a mental 'space' in which feelings can be represented and thought about, so primary care—in the general practitioner's surgery—can provide a place, time, and an *actively listening* ear, which can help individuals and families to feel held, understood, and helped. One of the general practitioner's tasks is to be midwife to transient or vaguely formed feelings of distress (often experienced and presented through physical illness), and to help them emerge into the light of care and containment, so that they can be examined for what they are. The fate of these now crystallized stories and symptoms will then be determined by the collaborative relationship between practitioner and patient. Many will remain held within the doctor–patient relationship, some will need help from other members of the primary care team, a few will be referred on to secondary services, and yet others shared between the different agencies. This process through which illness becomes 'organized' to a greater or lesser extent (Balint 1957), or is 'constructed' through the interaction and susceptibilities of patient and doctor together is a much under-estimated factor in mental health thinking, and plays a large part in the genesis, course, and outcome of mental distress, as well as to the degree of stigma which is often attached to it.

In addition to this capacity for the representation of distress as it arises, primary care has unique access to two other dimensions of the life cycle of psychological illness. First is an intimate knowledge of the *psychosocial context* in which distress and illnesses occur—the neighbourhood in both its physical and social aspects, the house or flat in which the patient lives, employment patterns, and the family ramifications of which the patient is but a part. Secondly, the general practitioner has a privileged relationship to his patients over *time*, often knowing individuals and their families over several decades, thus acquiring a deep knowledge of the ebb and flow, and patterns of psychological distress, and the strengths and weaknesses of his patients as they encounter life's difficulties. Patients often present to their general practitioners at a *time of need*, which intensifies the potential therapeutic effect of their relationship. Psychological conflicts often present with bodily ills, and may remain expressed through physical symptoms and the need for medical care for some time, just as physical illness itself and its accompanying loss of function is one of the factors that can give rise to significant psychological distress. Thus, general practice straddles the *mind–body* divide in such a way that no distinction need be made between the two as symptoms and suffering pass from one arena to another. This, in turn, has a significant impact on the general practitioner's capacity to respond to mental illness and the means through which he can do so.

These three aspects—representation, context, and time—underpin the *illness narrative*, or story of which general practitioners are the guardian and whose many strands they hold in trust for their patients. This narrative always arises from an inter-personal relationship—an interaction between two people, in which the view of one is inescapably derived from the viewpoint of the other. One doctor's response to a patient or an illness is never the same as another's. Each patient—to a certain extent—becomes a different patient with every different doctor. In truth, GPs (and all clinicians to a certain extent) are not only the custodians of illness narrative, but its co-authors too. It is perhaps easy to slide past a word such as 'inter-personal', assuming no more than a familiar shorthand reference to the well-documented need for doctors to be better trained in communication skills. Our intention is to signal something deeper— not new, but, once accepted, radical in the extent it alters our understanding of the underlying determinants and possible outcomes of clinical activity. This inter-personal and narrative-based medicine is the counterpart to the evidence-based approach, which has become such an important focal point for contemporary medical thinking (Hurwitz and Greenlaugh 1998).

The philosophy underlying this book asserts the importance of this narrative-based approach, and indicates the need to explore the ways in which it interweaves with scientific evidence, without, we trust, confusing the provenance and applicability of either. Our aim is to provide the best available framework for understanding how patients with psychological illness in primary care can be helped, and at the same time indicate directions for further research, development, and training. Mental health thinking, particularly in primary care, is unlikely to flourish until these different (but equally necessary) modes of thought are brought more closely together. One of the many arts of general practice is to be able to apply knowledge derived from general categories—medical evidence—to the life situations of individual patients. However good the evidence is for one course of action as opposed to another, the GP (or other clinician) still has to apply it within the context of a particular relationship and, for this, she may need access to evidence derived from the clinical narrative as well. It is the attempted integration of these two sources of information that matters, not only in clinical work, but also within the structures of a more fully integrated Mental Health Service as a whole.

At least two aspects of current government policy make this an opportune time for such an exploration. First, the shift of health commissioning and management towards primary and away from secondary services opens new possibilities for conceptualization and treatment of mental illness in the community. For the first time GPs will be in a position to shape the pattern of services their patients need. In the UK there is an opportunity for Primary Care Trusts to adopt a distinctively primary care-based approach to the commissioning and development of mental health services, and to think more ecologically about the mental health needs of their particular populations, rather than either relying on unsubstantiated individual whim, or on statistical generalities that lack personal or local meaning, based on diagnostic categories derived from secondary care. Secondly, a new approach to community care for the mentally ill— a 'third way' between the stasis of incarceration and the chaos of community neglect—is being developed by secondary services in which general practitioners have a vital part to play. In addition, there is an opportunity for the implications of recent research linking early experience of infants and later mental illness to inform a longer-term and preventative approach to mental illness in the community (see Chapter 11).

The structure of our book is itself designed to reflect our ideal of a patient-centred, interpersonally-focused, general practice-based, mental health service. It falls into four parts, with the reader being able to start in the GP's surgery in Part I, and there encounter psychological distress and mental illness described through the language, concepts, priorities, and perspectives that belong to that setting. Here, there are large numbers of patients with a wide range and variety of problems associated with the vicissitudes of ordinary living—some will have established mental illness, others transient symptoms that are part of current distress.

Part II stays in general practice, but focuses more on the implications of the inter-personal nature of a GP's clinical work, and uses this to examine more deeply such questions as morale, motivation, burn-out, and what makes a patient 'difficult'; through accepting the value of the subjective in interactions with patients, we argue for more appropriate forms of training and supervision for GPs.

A genuinely primary care-based Mental Health Service must first give attention to strengthening the mental health work undertaken by primary care teams; recognizing its nature and value, reflecting on its complexity, and investing in forms of training (undergraduate level onwards) and team development that hearten the practicing professionals and not (as is so easy via an imported specialist approach) undermine them.

The question then arises as to how best to incorporate other mental health workers in the surgery. Part III examines this and discusses the complex inter-relationship of disciplines that attends this move, indicating a process of mutual change—with psychologists and therapists adapting to the rhythms of primary care, and GPs learning to accommodate more specialized mental health professionals within the surgery, or indeed, initiating a more specialist service themselves (e.g. in family thinking), but doing so in a way best suited to primary care. Again, these developments need to augment and build on the character of the existing GP practice, rather than be seen as a foreign body. If this can be achieved, accessible psychological help can be provided for patients in a way that is often more acceptable to them than attending (or failing to attend) secondary services; less 'other', less stigmatizing, and better able to take therapeutic advantage from the pre-existing (and after-existing) relationship that the patient has with the practice. There are many unresearched aspects of such arrangements, but one stands out. Over 40 per cent of practices now have attached therapists (Mellor Clarke 2000) for their adult patients, practically none have for children. Children are the adult patients of the future.

Part IV moves on from the relative fluidity of the general practitioner's role, through different models of outreach and collaboration between primary and secondary services—described principally in relation to the management of serious mental illness and substance misuse—and comprises chapters written from the more defined perspectives (and diagnostic frames) of specialists, to whom the general practitioner might need to refer and who, in turn, need to adapt their thinking to the needs of primary care.

Thus, the book encompasses the full spectrum of mental health and psychiatric care, but is centred on the needs of a reader (of whatever discipline) working in general practice. Although our emphasis is focused mainly on doctors, mental health work is undertaken as much or more by non-medical workers (indeed, we believe that every member of a primary care team, including reception staff, contributes to its mental health work), and in our emphasis on the multi-disciplinary teams and contributions from psychologists and psychotherapists we recognize the spirit (and regrettably, to a lesser extent the letter) of this precept. For in primary care the lines of clinical narrative often reside not in individuals alone, but in the many different members of a primary care team, and are by their nature often disturbing, hidden and fragmented. Patterns may only begin to emerge if there is a commitment to meet as a team and discuss work with patients together. Only then will the elements of a complex story begin to reassemble through being brought to life by the various members of the practice 'family' itself, through shared discussion.

In assembling this book we have been forcibly struck by the contrast between the two 'ends' of the book. The GP perspective, with which we start, is personal, subjective, experience-based, poetic at times, philosophical, and discursive. The tone emanating from the right-hand end or 'back' of the book written by workers in secondary or tertiary care feels utterly different: cool, objective, structured, somewhat detached, and, as the current jargon has it, evidence-based. Our editorial stance arises out of a commitment to bringing these two 'ends' closer together, and we have tried to persuade our contributors to think and write along similar lines. We want to assert the importance of narrative experience as 'evidence' no less important than that provided by biomedical science. Equally, we want subjective impressions to be held up to critical scrutiny. In the end, however, perhaps there is a partially irreconcilable tension between the two perspectives that simply has to be lived with—as it does every day for the working general practitioner (Balint *et al.* 1993). Perhaps we might hope, at least, that within the organization of a more fully integrated Mental Health Service, recognition is given to the inter-dependence of these two strands of clinical work, and that the relative weight given to one conceptual stance or the other, changes as attention moves from the starting point in primary care, where the predominance is with narrative—towards the more specialized perspectives on mental health and psychiatric thinking, where the predominance is with medical evidence.

This brings us, finally, to our title. In what sense can we claim our approach to be 'new'? The term might at first sight seem ironic, given the fact that both of us are reaching the end of our careers and have held the basis of these views for many years. We would justify the word 'new' in three ways at least. First, with the shift of resources away from secondary care there are suddenly new opportunities for developing a primary care-based approach to mental health that, as it evolves, will inevitably produce services that look very different to those that are currently available. If our approach informs Primary Care Trusts in the commissioning process—for example, through investment in time for reflection and staff support—then 'new' patterns of service provision will appear. Secondly, academic medicine has at last begun to think about the mental health needs of populations as a whole, to promote 'early intervention' strategies in the prevention of entrenched psychiatric illness (which inevitably means a primary care perspective), and develop treatment methods (often forms of psychological therapy) that can be practiced in the primary care setting. Thirdly, although this is perhaps new in the sense of old wine in new bottles, the insights, experience, commitments, and epistemology of general practice are—through its more narrative approach and the consequent development of qualitative research strategies to articulate this—at last beginning to influence the mainstream of medical discourse.

The paradox referred to at the beginning of this introduction—the work of GPs is somehow invisible when it comes to mental health, and yet they are responsible for nine-tenths of provision—arises from two main sources. First, the predominance given in our culture to positivist knowledge, to the 'naming of things', which in medicine tends to lead to the comforts (and value) of specialist knowledge, and to the relative discounting of attitudes of enquiry that lead to awareness of the connections between them, which in medicine is the particular provenance of the generalist. Secondly, to the marked and persistent degree to which the disciplines of mind and body remain separate. If 'mental health' is regarded solely from within the institutions of the mind—psychology, psychiatry, psychotherapy—then the world of primary care (including the patients whose illnesses are contained there) largely disappears in a hemianopia wrought by this split. These phenomena, if they continue largely unrecognized (or worsen) will have a deleterious effect on the development of better integrated mental health services. Recognition of the importance of holding and containment, toleration of uncertainty, the value of not organizing too quickly into 'illness', and the therapeutic (or counter-therapeutic) impact of the relationship between patient and professional, underpin the 'new' approach we advocate. Without this foundation there is a danger that the split will deepen, 'mental' health becoming ever more the province of psychiatrists (whether provided in secondary or primary care), and GPs retreating to being 'physical' health doctors. Patients—who loose out when their care is divided in this way—will suffer. If, however, GPs remain firm in their commitment to an approach that is narrative, generalist, inter-personal, and undivided between body and mind, then the exercise of these skills becomes the centre, the core component of a GP's work, affecting all aspects of general practice care and benefiting, potentially, the mental health of all patients.

We stick, therefore, unashamedly with 'new' in our hopes for mental health practice in primary care and hope our readers—of a book that is primarily practical in its aspiration—will agree.

Part I
In the consulting room

1 In the consulting room

Sam Smith

My first significant encounter with mental illness was during my student days working as a volunteer in a large mental hospital. Most of the patients with whom I came in contact had been there many, many years. Some seemed to suffer greatly, others not at all. Some appeared to be incarcerated in a mental space devoid of emotional life, endlessly wandering the long corridors in search of cigarette-ends, little if any vestige of former existence or personality remaining. All had at one time been ascribed a diagnosis which the attrition of time, the effects of institutionalization and long-term medication had rendered both indistinguishable and irrelevant. Certainly, whatever they suffered and felt seemed at some remove from the mental and emotional distress of the people I was to encounter later as a general practitioner. Such large institutions are now a thing of the past. Taken as a whole, however, mental illness remains a problem, not simply in terms of its diagnosis and treatment, but also in terms of how we conceptualize and seek to define it. Only recently I returned to this hospital to find it had been converted into up-market homes for the up and coming.

My intention in this chapter is to explore something of the experience of mental illness within the primary care consultation. Consultations with emotionally or psychologically distressed and disturbed people can be both distressing and disturbing. How we cope with such consultations as clinicians depends on many things; for example, on our own personal strengths and susceptibilities, on our beliefs, how we value others, on our training, and not least upon a social and cultural context we cannot escape. That we recognize patients as mentally ill depends on an interactive amalgam of the nature of their suffering and our responses to it, together with the influences that guide those responses. Because of this essentially inter-personal and social nature, mental illness cannot easily be accommodated within a medical model of disease. It is perhaps not surprising, therefore, that there is some confusion and inconsistency in our attempts to define exactly what mental illness is.

The statistics of mental illness form part of an evidence-base that informs the construction of mental health programmes and underpins clinical practice. However, this evidence-based, statistical view is necessarily concerned with cases, rather than individuals. The scientific gaze objectifies and reifies mental illness divorcing it from the individual details of human lives. We say 'it' of mental illness as if it might exist as a thing in itself, independent of the actual person to whom it attaches or the context in which, somehow, it is made manifest. The general practitioner in the consulting room deals with people before they become cases. In this setting, therefore, a more personal, idiographic and phenomenological account of mental and emotional suffering is more helpful. Such an account is based on an individual story told in the context of an inter-personal engagement, which can become intense. In the telling of this story it is precisely the details that matter.

Interaction

When asked, patients often say that what mattered above all in the course of their clinical management, whatever the nature of their complaint, was that they were (or were not) properly *listened* to. The clinical transaction, wherever it occurs, offers a space in which we have an opportunity to listen to and explore, elaborate and help give shape to our patients' problems. Because dependent on interaction, both parties contribute to whatever emerges and it is by no means assured that underlying reasons for a problem will be productively revealed. Indeed, they may be driven further into obscurity and the problem exacerbated. The potential creativity of this space is therefore limited by the extent to which we are able to develop, share and communicate a common understanding.

Although an interchange between individuals, a consultation is embedded within a rich and complex context, an interactive hierarchy of systems—lay and professional, social and societal. This complexity is fully present in every clinical transaction since both patient and doctor inevitably import into this system, influences deriving from all the other systems of which they are or have previously been members (Norton and Smith 1994). Each system has a language attuned to its own goals and purposes, and finding a common language in which to share understanding is often far from straightforward. The task may be all the more difficult because the details of personal suffering may not readily find expression in words. They are neither easily told nor comfortably attended to.

The concept of the consultation as a *creative space* is not simply metaphorical since the human relationship must evolve within a variety of settings. Health Centre buildings and waiting areas are more or less comfortable and welcoming, and consulting rooms can be forbiddingly clinical or more personally expressive of the clinicians inhabiting them. Furthermore, access to the inner sanctum is often obstructed by the need to negotiate appointment systems and the reception staff who manage them. Inevitably, buildings and people reflect the endemic ambivalence of the system as a whole—'we would like to help—but we must not be overwhelmed'. Every point of contact, human, or material, communicates something to patients with the potential to influence significantly the telling of their stories.

From the complexity of this meeting with our patients, something recognizable as mental illness may emerge (almost always, but not necessarily, attaching to the patient). Perhaps more accurately, what is first recognized is not a 'thing' called mental illness, but rather a certain quality of interaction with the patient. This quality cannot solely be located in the patient because it is something felt and experienced by the clinician. It may, for instance, be a familiar empathic pang of emotion. We hear of loss or injustice and feel the prick of tears or a sudden surge of anger, or somehow sense the unleavened weight of depression. However, on occasion the experience is more that of being drawn into a world where landmarks have lost their usual familiarity. I remember going out to visit a young man in the early hours of the morning. Neatly dressed and standing relaxed against a kitchen counter, he casually told me how, some years ago, he had been assaulted and raped, and that he was now planning revenge. He had insisted on the visit so that he could let somebody know. The harrowing content of his story was so at odds with its matter-of-fact telling that I felt a distinct frisson of madness and danger.

As primary care clinicians we cannot escape becoming participating witnesses in the unfolding of distressed and distressing, confused, and confusing personal narratives. We both explore and play a part in the human relationships that structure the form and content of those narratives, investing them with their emotional significance. We become involved. Yet simultaneously, as professionals, we strive to retain a certain detachment hoping, thereby, to apply our professional knowledge and skills appropriately. The impetus of that professional role, moulded by culture and society, and years of training, is towards defining and diagnosing illness. However, in the primary care setting much of our experience will be of distress or suffering that is self-limiting and frequently evades a meaningful diagnostic label. After all, stress, anxiety, depression, and grief are normal conse-quences of the vicissitudes of human life and are not illnesses—certainly not diseases—in quite the same way as measles or rheumatoid arthritis.

To complicate matters, mental illness need not manifest itself as suffering, but become apparent, for example, in perceived oddities of dress or manner, or through the nature and quality of behaviour and relationships. If so, can we trust ourselves to draw a line between individual quirkiness and significant psychopathology? If not mentally ill, some patients will risk being considered and labelled difficult. Only a few will evoke that eerie, sometimes frightening sense of something sufficiently alien to be called madness. However, perhaps still more confusing is the fact that most kinds of mental or psychological suffering are, often primarily, expressed bodily (see next chapter). In the face of physical symptoms our diagnostic routines are legitimately invoked and it can be difficult to avoid the practice of making diagnoses.

Three patients

In my earlier days as a GP I visited a young woman who complained of a headache that, worsening as the day went on, had become severe enough for her husband to call for a visit after surgery hours. I could discover no obvious explanation for her headache, but what made the encounter memorable was a moment during the taking of her medical history. In some distress, she related that she had had a miscarriage 6 weeks previously, an event of which I had been completely ignorant.

My confused reaction of sympathy and embarrassment must have been obvious because she responded, in turn, by extending a hand towards me saying it was all right, she was feeling much better and it was just her headache that was bothering her.

More recently, a well-dressed man in his late thirties attended surgery. After a brief interchange during which he seemed to be weighing me up, he hunched forward over his knees and, looking at his feet, began to describe a series of symptoms. He was always tired, irritable, slept poorly, and was suffering uncharacteristically from headaches. He had lost weight and was distressed by a complete loss of interest in sex. Relationships with his wife and children were strained and each morning he had to drag himself out of bed to face a day's work he was beginning to dread. He felt depressed and, researching via the Internet, concluded with his wife that his symptoms were of depressive illness. Could I prescribe a SSRI (an antidepressant) and provide a note for some time off work as he had also read that the medication might take some time to take effect?

Until an untimely and unanticipated death from a heart attack not so long ago, I had been seeing a middle-aged professional woman at frequent, mostly regular and pre-arranged intervals of 2 or 3 weeks. Her main complaint was of recurrent abdominal pain and erratic bowel habit. She felt exhausted and barely able to manage her work and household chores, and in the end had retired on medical grounds. Her problems, she explained, were of deliberate poisoning, via the domestic water supply, by an unnamed conspiracy of executives employed by the Water Company supplying the town where she had lived at the time her symptoms started. Since then she had taken a daily array of minerals and vitamins to counteract the effects of the poison. Innumerable investigations, medical, surgical, and psychiatric consultations and two spells of hospital admission, when she had become acutely psychotic, had revealed no organic cause of her bowel symptoms. Her husband had remained loyal in spite of her quite frequent verbal and physical violence towards him. Our appointments were spent reviewing her symptoms and ruminating over the details of the poisoning which had ruined her life. Incidentally, she also suffered from asthma for which she took conventional medication, managing the condition well without fuss or concern.

The first encounter above brought home to me how rapid and powerful is the interaction between patient and doctor at an emotional level. Furthermore, it made it obvious that this is very much a two-way process. As clinicians we are never merely health technicians. Our own personal responses, as well as those of our patients, significantly affect the course of the clinical transactions in which we engage. Attributes of style and manner, as well as the moment-to-moment reactions to what we hear, see, touch, or smell all communicate something. For each clinician and patient, an amalgam of such qualities and responses shapes a richly contoured surface capable, perhaps with some adjustment, of fitting more or less well with the other. In primary care particularly, patients and doctors have an extended opportunity to select each other depending on this fit—some prefer a close fit, others actively avoid it. A good fit, however, is not necessarily productive. In this first encounter, the young woman, seeing the distress in my face, sought to comfort me, but in that moment, the grief she felt seemed to recede. My pained reaction to her loss and her reassuring response, although closely matched, distanced us both from the emotional core of her own distress. Her headache may well have been a manifestation of that grief, but the opportunity to explore the emotional origin of her symptoms was lost. As far as I am aware she did not later pursue help for this with any of us in the practice.

The young man with depression might at first sight seem to be an ideal patient. He attended with an accurate diagnosis, supported by his history and demeanour, and a clear idea about the treatment he wanted, which was probably appropriate. Furthermore, he left the consulting room within the allotted 10 minutes. In spite of this (or perhaps because of it), he posed a more difficult problem, at the time, than had the young woman's headache. Gone was the security of the more paternalistic, doctor-centred consultation. Here, instead, was a truly clinical transaction—an engagement of equals (if, indeed, I was an equal). There was no need to persuade this man that his physical symptoms were those of depression or convince him of the benefits of medication. Neither was there any opportunity to explore why he had become so overwhelmed at this point in his life; he offered no window for empathy, no personally compatible, interlocking surface. My role was merely that of health technician—to confirm the diagnosis for certification purposes and prescribe the appropriate treatment. He did not wish for counselling with me or anyone else. I felt a little taken aback after his departure, a little irritated that he seemed to take what I had to offer so much for granted. Perhaps, in retrospect, I might have gained more control of the consultation had I withheld the note and prescription until he had completed a Hospital Anxiety and Depression Questionnaire or Beck's Depression Inventory.

Whereas the self-directed surfer above might be described as a case of mild to moderate mental illness and, despite my feeling of being uncomfortably mismatched, did very well on medication, the illness of my last patient was severe (at least at times) and enduring. Although consultations were frequent and often overlong, by the time she died I had come to hold her in great affection. Despite her unnerving madness, which would at times strike me with an alien intensity, she retained the capacity to recognize the difficulties she caused her husband,

and to appreciate my efforts to monitor and contain her illness. For most of the time she refused neuroleptic medication and seemed to maintain a reasonable level of functioning. All I had to do was be willing to prescribe something for abdominal pain and spend time listening to her grievances. I had to take care to signal my absences from work well in advance—one of her admissions with psychosis occurred whilst I was away on holiday. My liking for her surprised me, for she held sometimes offensively right-wing views, which she expounded at length, especially when castigating her poisoners. My reaction, as she related how she had suffered at their hands and what she would like to do to them, was to feel an almost irresistible urge to fall asleep.

My management of all these patients, such as it was, certainly depended on my medical training. The confidence to exclude a significant medical cause for the young woman's headache, to diagnose and prescribe appropriately for depressive illness, and to arrange acute admission to a psychiatric bed are all part of routine clinical practice. However, what to me is of more interest are those aspects of each encounter that seemed to fall outside, or at least stretch and question the knowledge and skills that that medical training provided. Why did the young woman seek to comfort me and deny her grief? Why did I let her? What was the source of my irritation and discomfort with the Internetist? I have, after all, searched the web for answers myself. Why should I so consistently struggle against sleep in the face of paranoia? Answers to these questions seem to have escaped the pages of my medical textbooks.

Diagnosis

Increasingly, perhaps, patients recognize that their bodily symptoms are a manifestation of anxiety, stress, or some other form of emotional and psychological suffering. In spite of this, our first assumption as patients or clinicians is most commonly that physical symptoms indicate physical illness or disease. The intensity of the young woman's headache made her fearful of some immediate physical threat and my first task was to reassure her that this was not so. Confronted with physical symptoms, the pursuit of a diagnosis seems quite straightforward initially and, I suspect like most doctors, I find a certain satisfaction in medical detective work. There is a simple pleasure to be taken in the exercise of medical skills. As soon as the clues dry up, however, or seem to be leading nowhere, the whole encounter can become more burdensome. It is neither easy nor satisfying to leave questions unanswered and simple reassurance that nothing serious is wrong often fails in the face of the pressing nature of symptoms.

A diagnosis of mental illness can be stigmatizing. Even to be deemed to be suffering from anxiety, stress, or other emotional disorder can be taken to impute some form of personal inadequacy or deficiency. Frequently, patients only attend at the behest of partners or spouses, as if seeking to distance themselves from an admission of such frailty. They may describe the impatience, even intolerance, of work-mates, parents, or other family members towards this perceived weakness. It is not surprising, therefore, that intimations of emotional suffering are often resisted by both patient and clinician. Pursuing them at any length and to any depth can be distressing for both and so they may, by tacit agreement, be dealt with perfunctorily or even ignored altogether. The line of least resistance can be to medicalize the problem, even to the point of organizing (and submitting to) perhaps unnecessary investigations or referrals. If so, the result may well be the *somatic fixation* of symptoms described by Grol (1981). Such a process may also account in part for reports that depression, for example, has hitherto been under-diagnosed in primary care (Department of Health 1999a; see Chapter 14).

In any event, meaningful diagnosis or otherwise, we are still faced with the altogether more demanding business of situating the problem within the personal context of a patient's life and circumstances (Gannik 1995). Whenever we suspect and opt to pursue the emotional or psychological origin of symptoms, however, the main task is arguably one of translation, rather than diagnosis. If patients are to be convinced that they are 'mentally' ill, we must somehow enable them to locate their symptoms in the immediate and felt reality of emotional suffering. Nausea and vomiting may, perhaps, indicate a patient sick with worry or chest pains reveal the anguish of a broken heart. It is precisely here, in opening up this alternative reality, that the full range of our personal and emotional responses to the patient's predicament must inform our professional engagement. Without this empathic level of engagement it is unlikely that the patient's story will emerge. In our efforts to understand and to communicate that understanding, we must rely on our own personal experiences of suffering to guide us. It may, however, be as difficult for us as it is for our patients to be open and attentive to this aspect of ourselves. In such a situation, whilst recognizing the necessity of holding on to professional objectivity, applying the robust framework of the medical model too assiduously can hinder, rather than help.

The construction of symptoms

Emotional or psychological suffering thus often finds signification in the language of the body more readily than in words (Broom 1997). Somatization is both common and confusing. It may even be true that certain symptom complexes, perhaps anorexia or bulimia, can symbolize a particular emotional conflict that, once understood, becomes amenable to therapeutic interpretation (Farrell 1995; for further discussion, see Chapter 12). The concept of a 'language of the body' is surely metaphorical, but as with all illness, 'mental' illness is embodied. Even the self-diagnosing Internetist was not *just* describing a mood or the nature of his thoughts. He sat hunched with eyes averted. He felt physically fatigued and was aware of the failures of his body—his lost appetite for food and for sex—as well as his joylessness. Nor is illness confined to our personal bodies. It is also embodied within the activities of day-to-day living, both reflecting and affecting relationships with those around us.

However, what exactly are symptoms? To the diagnostician they may be clues to a differential diagnosis, but to the patient they are an inextricable amalgam of sensation and cognition demanding explanation. They may begin as feelings or perceptions experienced as somehow alien and worrying, which demand a more or less conscious, more or less urgent effort to make sense of and manage them. That effort extends to our immediate community where, usually, we seek explanation and support from those about us. When such self-perceptions and experiences defy explanation or are for some other reason unacceptable, they crystallize as symptoms. That is at least part of what it is to be ill.

Symptoms are difficult to locate because they not only confound the Cartesian dichotomy of mind and body, but also blur the distinction between individual and community. Within families, for example, there may or may not be immediate agreement that a feeling or the perception of disturbance or loss of bodily function experienced by one of them is a symptom that demands attention. The rest of the family may judge it to be normal, to have little or no significance, to be merely attention seeking, or perhaps even downright manipulative. So might their doctor. On the other hand, whilst an individual may regard feelings and actions as both explicable and acceptable, for example, the behaviour and dress of adolescence, they may seem alien—symptomatic—when considered from a parental perspective. Perhaps more significantly, differences in race and culture may prompt similar reactions. Of course, we as clinicians, by virtue of our race or stage of parenthood, are by no means immune to such reactions. Finally, symptoms may be obvious to others, but denied by or beyond the awareness of the individual.

At their inception, therefore, symptoms are not fixed and stable entities. They are shaped both individually and collectively from feelings, perceptions, and actions. When they can no longer be contained and managed within the person and his or her social system, help is sought either by or on behalf of the sufferer. Such an account implies that 'symptoms', as such, are socially constructed and that a diagnosis of mental illness is but a further step in this process in which doctors are assigned a particular and defining role. According to this view, diagnosis depends not so much on the objective reality of specific symptoms corresponding to a particular illness as on the limits of the discourse within which the account of illness is framed. The terms, definitions, and objectives of the medical scientific discourse, which as clinicians we may find impossible to escape, are not necessarily congruent with those of the social discourse of the patient. For example, women and black people are over-represented within certain diagnostic categories of mental illness (Parker *et al.*, 1995). A medical view would claim that such a finding is based on accurate clinical diagnosis, and is thus both explicable and acceptable within its terms. Such an explanation would certainly not be acceptable in terms of an alternative understanding of prejudice, oppression, and deprivation (see Chapter 4).

The interests enshrined in professional, political, and lay discourse are partisan and often conflict (Williamson 1992). Even when caught up in the process of a consultation with an individual patient, our thinking and understanding of the problem presented to us is a product of the interplay of these influences. Nevertheless, to the extent that we are aware of the limits they impose we can at least attempt to set them to one side and rethink them within an alternative framework, in an effort to better understand our patients and their problems.

The patient as 'other'

These contrasting medical and constructionist models (in the sense that our understanding is shaped by social forces as much as by biomedical 'facts') provide different, perhaps conflicting accounts of the purpose, function, and process of the consultation, and of the diverse ailments addressed therein. Neither approach describes adequately the inter-personal dynamics of doctor and patient, and the effect their interaction has on process and outcome, although it is true that psychodynamic theories derived from psycho-analysis often provide a valuable perspective. To the extent that any such theoretical model or framework is held in common it permits a shared understanding of the phenomena it seeks to explain. It is quite likely, however, that despite the increasing availability of medical information, lay and professional models of understanding will be quite different. We are likely to be faced in the consultation, therefore, with the task of first exploring openly our patients' understanding and then finding common ground upon which mutual understanding can be built. This experience of discovering and sharing (rather than imposing) understanding can itself be both rewarding and therapeutic.

In none of the three patients described above, however, did this happen very easily or productively. With the young woman a deeper understanding was prevented by our embarrassment, which we chose to deal with, rather than addressing the underlying problem. The depressed man came with his understanding ready to hand and needing only to be rubber-stamped. No opportunity was afforded to explore the more personal details of his depression. The third patient's understanding of her illness was so at odds with my own that there was little possibility of sharing it. It could be that her delusions symbolized some internal conflict open to interpretation. I am not sure. What we did share was a mutual warmth and trust by virtue of which I believe, for the most part, I was able to help contain and ameliorate her illness.

Important as sharing is, consultations grant us another opportunity and that is to recognize our patients as truly other than ourselves. It is the experience of this moment of recognition upon which respect for our patients ultimately depends. The moral philosopher Emmanuel Levinas calls the moment of recognition an epiphany (Levinas 1969; Smith, 1999). It is by virtue of the recognition of the 'patient-as-other' that respect for our patient becomes alive and real. To my mind, this experience—humbling, eerie, and fleeting—defies adequate description. However, it is our respect for the patient-as-other that grants us the capacity to bear witness to our patients' suffering. This mute necessity must come before suffering is given voice, codified, and confined within the bounds of common understanding. Too easily, our socially appointed role as clinicians and the impetus of our training can lead us away from the obligation to bear witness. We are more likely to take up the task of fixing and stabilizing symptoms, framing personal narratives within a more or less rigid matrix of medical understanding, a task that, if successful, ascribes a diagnosis and confers social legitimacy to the patient's nascent illness. This is also a task, despite its mutual undertaking, which is prone to unrecognized misunderstandings and the insidious intrusion of paternalism. The moment of epiphany, if experienced at all, then becomes but a faint reminder that something more is demanded of us.

Somewhat paradoxically it is the symptom itself, whether it be a communication, a social construction or an indicator of disease, which alerts us to the other. By its nature the symptom is alien and demands attention. By making us sit up and take notice, the otherness of the symptom reminds us of the otherness of the patient. However, symptoms are also distracting. The otherness of psychotic symptoms, for example, can be so alarming that our attention is forced away from the patient as a person. Fuelled by anxiety, the effort instead becomes one of containing symptoms within the realm of the understandable, of finding a place for them, whether it is within the spectrum of medically defined disease or at the intersection of conflicting discourses. Using the terminology of the former, but taking the perspective of the latter, I shall now consider the impact of psychosis and personality disorder as they present in general practice.

Facing psychosis

Useful as they are, our models of understanding only afford partial protection against the feelings we experience when consulting. Psychodynamic therapy obviously depends on this fact, for it is in part through the thoughtful awareness of our feelings that we come to understand our patient's predicament. Although medical and constructionist models contribute understanding, neither goes very far towards illuminating the actual experience of confronting a clearly distressed, irrational, or threatening patient and the inter-personal dynamics at work. Here, the problem is one of recognizing and managing feelings, in ourselves as well as our patients, of understanding and acknowledging destructive ways of relating, which may often be hidden, but no less powerful for that. In the face of these sometimes intense emotions, the problem becomes one of preserving our ability to provide practical help.

The effort to listen, perhaps to understand and certainly to bear witness, is itself likely to be therapeutic, and may even be all that is needed. That effort, on occasion, can also be exhausting, and leaves little mental and emotional energy for the remaining patients on a surgery list. The most severe forms of distress or psychotic illness are encountered relatively less frequently in general practice, but clinicians can find the experience traumatizing, even overwhelming, especially if faced alone. Usually, however, acute and severe illness of this sort erupts outside the consulting room and others, such as family, social services or the police, will already be involved before the GP is called. In such situations there may be little opportunity for any meaningful exploration of personal narratives and, perforce, clinicians may have to depend on practices that are not tailored to the individual.

Of course, psychotic illness does not necessarily erupt in such a florid way. Especially in young people, illness may be slow to develop and symptoms emerge only fleetingly, perhaps to be discounted as part of normal adolescent development (McGlashan, 1998). Many years ago I was involved with a teenage boy who came to see me of his own accord. He was distressed by his body odour, which he found offensive and which he felt was drastically affecting his ability to make relationships with his peers. At first, discussion and reassurance seemed to help, but as time went on he found that he was washing himself over and over again with an increasingly compulsive anxiety. The family became involved, and we all made heroic efforts to contain and normalize his behaviour which continued to deteriorate. In the end, after much intense and distressing debate, I agreed with the parents, but against the boy's wishes, to ask a psychiatrist to see him at home.

In retrospect it was clear that this boy's illness had become psychotic, but at exactly what point the transition occurred was hard to say. I met him a year or so later, whilst he was out shopping with his mother. She told me he was very much better. Indeed, he was, but I was distressed by the obvious effect on his personality of the powerful medication he was taking. Often parents or teachers are first to voice concerns that something odd, but indefinable is wrong. It is particularly important to listen to their concerns and investigate the possibility of serious illness, since early treatment may prevent or ameliorate the chronic disability that the progression of such illness often represents (McGlashan 1998; Birchwood et al. 1998; see Chapter 13). At such an important transitional stage in life the implications of making a diagnosis are enormous. The consequences of not making one, however, can be disastrous.

When patients who suffer psychotic illness are seen in the consulting room they are most often either on powerful medication, or their illness is not so disruptive or severe. The quality of interaction can nonetheless be rather disturbing and can make the pursuit of other medical concerns more difficult. In my engagement with the poisoned woman described earlier, the consultation was marked by episodes of seeming normality when symptoms and treatment were discussed. If, however, I offered a routine medical explanation of her bowel symptoms her gaze would become more fixed, and she would launch into a ruminative account of the poison and its effects. This was usually followed by a vitriolic tirade directed against those she held responsible. She would proceed to an explanation of their motivation for singling her out to be eliminated. There was nothing disordered about her thinking and the account she gave was seductively rational. At times, I would be drawn into this world and find myself questioning her about details as though I believed it all to be true. Were I to do so, however, she would become more and more agitated, and I would start to feel uneasily that she might spiral out of control. To my relief, she never did in the consulting room. If I managed to resist being drawn in, and merely nodded and made appropriate noises, I found my eyelids drooping and my concentration wandering. This was not simply due to boredom. The level of affect was too intense for that. It seemed to me more an involuntary shutting down of my own thinking and feeling because it could make no meaningful connection with hers.

In spite of her madness, I gradually learned about her life beyond the capsule of her delusions. Well educated and financially secure, she had children, grandchildren, a loving husband, and no indication from the glimpses into this other life of any cause for her psychosis. She did not speak of her childhood or parents, and I did not ask her about them. She was obviously capable of loving and being loved, and showed little of the disintegration of thinking and personality that is so often attendant upon psychotic illness. Unblunted by medication, her affect was lively to say the least and she had been protected from the effects of long-term institutionalization, social isolation, and exclusion. She presented a far from typical case of psychotic or, to use more contemporary terminology, severe and enduring mental illness. Perhaps a diagnosis such as paranoia would alert us to this distinction, but not necessarily to the experience of being with her that had such a powerful effect. Furthermore, as I have already mentioned, when dealing with her asthma there was no hint of this alternative mode of thinking, feeling and acting.

Among the lessons that my involvement with this extraordinary woman taught me was that being with patients of this kind can be draining. Support is needed from somewhere and, in the increasingly frenetic world of modern primary care, this can be difficult to find. Not only might we need to off-load some of the feelings such involvement can generate, but we may also need help in understanding what they signify. There may well be a need for someone who can ensure that over-involvement does not lead the clinical management of the patient too far off the beaten track. In these situations, I envy the formalized supervision that counsellors and psycho-therapists enjoy (this theme is taken up in Chapters 6, 7, 8, and 10). A second and equally important lesson is that however ill our patients might be, however bizarre or frightening their thinking or behaviour, we must always seek to address and relate to each one as a person. As I have intimated above, I believe that effort communicates itself beyond the boundaries of language. We should also endeavour not to let a diagnosis of mental illness become a stigmatizing label that places the patient beyond our help.

Personality disorder

Far more common in primary care are those patients variously described as difficult, heart-sink, fat-folder, frequent-attender, or by some other similar and usually pejorative label (Schrire 1986; O'Dowd 1988; see Chapter 5). By no means all such patients, if any, suffer from an easily definable mental illness or personality disorder. They may simply be awkward, quirky or eccentric—but then so may their doctors or nurses. The labelling process is stigmatizing, and when institutionalized, within primary or secondary care, can be a very effective barrier to meaningful communication (Norton and Smith 1994; Smith and Norton 1999). Suffice it to say here, that the process of labelling is an interactive one, and many of the problems encountered are more productively understood as deriving from the interaction of patient and professional, rather than residing in either person alone.

Processes of transference and counter-transference work in both directions, and in the heat of a difficult encounter a diagnostic label of mental illness may not always be applied with the patient's best interests at heart. There is even a risk that our application of such a diagnosis will have a subconsciously punitive motivation. The diagnosis of mental illness is not only stigmatizing, but more seriously, may be taken to signify mental incompetence, with the potential loss of autonomy or even civil liberty that this implies. Nor is it simply the interaction of individuals that is important in these respects. Each of the participants brings with them something of the attitudes, prejudices, and objectives of their social or professional group, a way of understanding and speaking about the world and each person's place in it—in other words, a discourse. If such discourses clash or are incommensurable, then the other may be perceived to be awkward, stupid, mad, or bad. The outcome may then depend on issues of power, personal, or institutional, rather than of truth and reality, let alone any altruistic desire to be of service.

Personality disorders find definition within the Diagnostic and Statistical Manual of Mental Disorders (DSM) and the International Classification of Diseases (ICD), but often resist ready and consistent diagnosis, and are notoriously difficult to treat (Lewis and Appleby 1988). They sit very uncomfortably within a medical model of illness. What seems more important from my own clinical experience is that my interaction with some people seems to lack something, some vital connection or window for empathy, rather as I felt with the depressed man described earlier. It is as though the narrative they relate not only obscures, but is also somehow disconnected from the true cause of their suffering. Perhaps a similar lack or absence made it difficult for me to engage with the Internetist. It was as if the concern and care that I usually have no difficulty in feeling for most of my patients, finding no echo or resonance, had become muted. The process of the consultation became an effort, partly due to the need to disguise the irritation I was feeling. I could find no reflection of myself as a healer, bountiful provider, competent diagnostician, or anything other than a mechanical conduit. He expressed no gratitude and I felt rebuffed. It was not merely that he came armed with words from the web; patients are increasingly doing so. Although reciprocity should not be a condition of our obligation to patients, in this case it was the absence of personal engagement that I found difficult. It is possible that had I said something along the lines of 'all this seems very cut and dried, I wonder how frightened you are really feeling about becoming ill in this way?' I might have been able to make contact with him as a person. However, in any case, I could not fairly diagnose him as personality disordered. After all, patients not infrequently complain that the boot is on the other foot.

Success—and failure

Of all the other myriad forms of emotional or psychological distress that emerge in the consulting room most, on the whole, do not present too difficult a task in their management. Desperate and vulnerable people can, indeed, be persistent in their demands and become, through interactive processes, very dependent. However, although arduous at times, the mutual re-framing of symptom-laden narratives, whether or not leading to a diagnosis of mental illness, is nonetheless often straightforward and satisfying. People seem to get better, at least temporarily, and witnessing the change from distress to well being can be both poignant and uplifting. Having listened to and facilitated the telling of the patient's distressed story, we are then privileged to bear witness to its disentanglement, however temporary a resolution that might prove to be. Above all, we owe a duty of respect to the patient-as-other, a relationship that entails being *for* our patients, rather than simply being *with* them.

Things do not always work out well enough, however, and there are tragedies to be sure. In fact extreme actions such as suicide (see Chapter 14) are fortunately rare by comparison even though their impact is devastating. In my own experience, the suicide of a patient, almost without exception, comes as a shocking surprise. Because such extreme actions are very hard to predict, the management of risk can come to monopolize the attention of mental health professionals, especially when targets are set for reducing suicide rates. I am uncertain whether or not it is possible to discern reliably from the accounts of patients or carers the circumstances that will provoke so final a resolution. Some years ago, a psychiatrist wrote to tell me that a chronically depressed patient of ours was likely to commit suicide within the foreseeable future. The patient survives, albeit often in considerable distress, helped greatly these days by an e-mail group of similar sufferers.

Conclusion

What we commonly call mental illness is both banal and bewildering. Banal because so common and so much part of everyone's experience. Bewildering because attempts to capture it within a model, whether medical, constructionist, or psychodynamic, seem only to offer partial comprehension. Perhaps most of the time it does not matter greatly. To show respect and share our human understanding of a patient's predicament is often sufficient. Some clinical research would suggest that, certainly for depressed or anxious patients, whether or not we refer to a therapist or treat with anti-depressants makes little difference in the longer run (Churchill *et al.* 1999; see Chapters 14 and 19). It may, of course, matter greatly to the individual and for those with more severe illness the task can be crucial when so much in terms of personal dignity and autonomy may be at stake.

Finally, although physical illness is by no means immune from these processes, mental illness particularly falls prey to the vicissitudes of the discursive rivalries of different interest groups: lay, political, and professional. The physicist Werner Heisenberg, asserted that 'what we observe is not nature itself, but nature revealed to our method of questioning' (Broom 1997, p. 168). Different methods of questioning, whether those of empirical science or of discourse analysis, coalesce into alternative models of understanding. In the footsteps of Francis Bacon, empirical science discounts the 'bookish disputations' of poets and philosophers, and puts nature on the rack to force her secrets from her. However, some critics of scientific rationality and of the medical gaze, as Michel Foucault called it, go so far as to deny science's claim to a privileged access to truth, asserting that the much-vaunted objectivity of science is a sham. Its terms and practices, like those of any other discourse, are socially constructed, and hence inevitably culture-bound and value-laden (Nettleton 1995; Parker *et al.* 1995; Smith 1998, 1999). The medical model of mental illness, developed with scientific methods and aspirations, nonetheless retains a powerful influence on mental health policy (Rogers and Pilgrim, 1996):

> ...although the manuals would like us to believe that each category (of mental illness) is a pure form of pathology, the experience of practitioners is often of someone who seems both anxious and depressed, of people whose problems seem ambiguous and messy, not at all scientific. Indeed, it is unclear how often diagnoses are actually used in everyday clinical practice—often their only purpose seems to be administrative.
> *(Parker et al. 1995)*

As doctors, we cannot ethically ignore the evidence medical science provides and which informs current concepts of best practice. How successful and appropriate this model is for defining the human suffering we call mental illness and guiding our therapeutic responses, however, is open to debate. Whether lay or professional, our efforts to theorize nature, encompassing the rich complexity of human thought and emotion, only succeed through processes of abstraction and simplification—rational instruments of observation. There will always remain something beyond the field of view awaiting fresh understanding.

2 Body and mind

Richard Westcott

This chapter looks at the interaction of body and mind, mind and body as experienced in primary care. I start with a particular patient, who appears with what might be called a classic psychosomatic disorder. I show her presentation and the GP's reaction: the diagnostic process and approach to management. Recourse to an authoritative resource reveals illuminating differences between the worlds of secondary and primary care. I consider the nature of paradigms, their role in science generally, and how these (too often) implicit structures can be both helpful, yet obstructive in a consideration of the interaction between body and mind. It becomes clear that primary care discarded the biomedical model some time ago and has subsequently (albeit perhaps unwittingly) moved on from positivism, through social construction into a quasi post-modern world. Secondary care, however, has progressed less evenly, with some specialties in the teaching hospital apparently still firmly rooted in the earlier paradigm. These differences leave the primary care clinician with residual, often unidentified tensions, if he or she tries to struggle with traditional concepts of organic and functional illness, and phrases such as *somatization* and *psychosomatic illness*. I review some of the major transitions of life as opportunities to look at the subjective experience of illness and development of individuals within a context. All these provide the chance to develop a continuing relationship, as time passes, with the doctor, a shared language, self-knowledge (for all parties), and the realization that mental and physical health, the psyche, and the soma, are naturally inseparable.

To start with, a patient...

May is a slim, neat school cook in her early fifties. Over time I've got to know her quite well—she's had varicose veins (operated on), several episodes of (what would be called 'minor') depression, problems with a neighbour, and is the mother of two daughters, one of whom has Turner's syndrome. But what I'm most aware of at present is that she's been looking after her husband, who has disseminated cancer of the prostate. Now she has come to tell me about her abdominal pain and swelling. She's had it, on and off, 'a long time' but it's recently got worse; this is the first time she's told me about it. Having listened to her, I now ask some questions. Yes, the pain and swelling are relieved by passing wind or opening her bowels; her motions vary from sheep droppings to quite loose stools, and back again; the pain is worse when these changes are happening. No, she hasn't had any bleeding, her weight hasn't changed but she feels full quite quickly when she eats.

It must be difficult at home, one way and another, I suggest. May starts talking—about Don, his illness and their daughters (one cannot bear even to come to see him). She continues while I examine her. Everything is normal. Conscious of running over time, I need to wind things up. I wonder what to tell her at this stage. It seems almost certain that she has irritable bowel syndrome (IBS). I am aware that, even though she's told me a lot today and we've known each other for some time, there is much more to learn about her—her ideas, concerns and expectations, particularly about how she sees the future. I arrange blood tests, and ask her to make an appointment in a week's time, although we both know we'll be meeting tomorrow when I go to see her husband at home. The tests should all be normal, I predict to myself. In conclusion I say that it looks like IBS, and explain a bit about it, giving her a leaflet.

Afterwards, I think about May and her IBS. I know that IBS is the most common disorder encountered by gastroenterologists in the industrialized world, said to affect 20 per cent of all adults, and the most common functional bowel disorder seen in primary care. However, a chain of questions follows. Why has she got it now—how much is it to do with her husband's illness? Is IBS 'psychosomatic' (whatever that is)? A selection of symptoms—how do they become an illness, a syndrome, or even a disease (whatever *that* is)?

Trying to learn more about my patient's 'psychosomatic' disorder...

Certainly a good starting point for thinking about the interaction of body and mind is to study how the medical profession (particularly the different worlds of secondary and primary care) sees 'psychosomatic' disorder, and what paradigms and theories govern present thinking.

So, I set about learning about IBS.

My authority (Farthing 1995) starts his search for the cause and development of IBS in the gut, but evidence to prove that this is solely a matter of gut malfunction is incomplete. For disordered large bowel motility, 'few clear cut differences have emerged between healthy subjects and patients'. 'Clustered contractions' in the small bowel may be seen more often in IBS patients, but they occur in controls asymptomatically. A shorter transit time offered a possible explanation, but 'it is difficult to invoke a hypothesis that suggests that the irritable bowel syndrome is due to a primary motor disorder of the gut.' As for IBS patients having increased visceral sensation, 'this is probably not the primary defect'. He concludes that despite extensive research, there is little agreement on an understanding of its pathophysiological processes.

So, casting his net wider, and having noted that 'extra abdominal associations exist' the gastroenterologist wonders—'instead of merely (sic) an irritable bowel, there might also be an irritable oesophagus, an irritable stomach, an irritable bladder, and irritable vagina, and possibly irritable bronchi—or simply (sic) an irritable body.'

However, admitting that 'little doubt exists that emotional factors can alter the function of the gut', he concedes that it may result from an 'irritable brain'. Finally, after more discussion, 'a psychosomatic model for the irritable bowel syndrome' is invoked.

The traditional paradigm

Thus is demonstrated the traditional biomedical model, summarized by Neighbour (1987) as follows: it starts from the assumption that a state of normal health (as exemplified by the teaching hospital's disciplines of anatomy, physiology, and biochemistry) exists. Disease processes, defined in terms of departures from normal structure and function, can be studied via the science of pathology. A patient's symptoms represent illness (but if unacceptable, illegitimate, or unrecognized, do not), which can be investigated rationally, so that the malfunction can be identified as a diagnosis. The diagnosis allows selection of appropriate corrective measures from the repertoire of skills and resources available to the doctor—pharmacological, surgical, or some other technology. It is the role of medicine to fight disease and to restore the state of health, or at least to try to.

My example shows the approach in action: hierarchical, if not frankly Cartesian, it sees body and mind as distinct. From end organ to single system, then to multi-organ and whole body, later to brain and mind. Each stage is permitted by passage through the previous, so that were there convincing evidence at any earlier level, the process could have rested quite reasonably there. In this progress the physical retains primacy: the doctor strives to exclude the organic, before looking to the brain or the mind, let alone the 'psyche'.

Supporting the biomedical model is the theory of positivism, which confidently sees a patient suffering from a disease, able to be categorized as any other natural phenomenon. It allows a disease to be viewed independently from the person suffering from it and her social context. Mental and physical diseases can be considered separately, with provision for a group of psychosomatic diseases in which the mind appears to act on the body. Each disease has a specific discoverable cause, but individual susceptibility accounts for varying responses. The doctor, detached and scientific, diagnoses, and treats. This classic image of the scientist studying an object under the microscope represents the distance and difference between the observer and the observed, the ability to separate the cause from the result and the use of reliable 'hard' data. 'The emphasis on specific body parts, conditions and treatments assumes that these are universally constant, replicable facts' (Alderson 1998).

Born from the security of rationalism and nineteenth-century belief in progress, positivism catered particularly well for the classic infectious diseases and deficiencies. Either an organ, system or tissue shows evidence of infection, depletion, deterioration, or damage of some sort—or it does not. 'Organic' diseases are, therefore, definable. Thus, the biomedical model, based upon positivism, served its purpose well, seeming to satisfy everyone.

It gave a clear role to the doctor. The inchoate could be identified and uncertainty categorized, captured by a name—a diagnosis, no less. A logical process then determined the response, with *diagnosis* leading to *treatment*, two linked, but discrete activities—as we were taught in medical school:

> The doctor may insist on focusing on certain aspects of the patient's problem because they are the easiest for him to handle. He will then refuse to allow the patient to tell him anything else, or refuse to hear. To obtain his greatest satisfaction the doctor usually wants to find a patient with a serious, acute illness that has interesting features—elicited and recognized by him with great acumen—and one who responds rapidly, completely and gratefully to proper therapy.
> *(Royal College of General Practitioners 1972)*

For the patient, the scientific certainty of the organic diagnostic process is critically important. As soon as we are ill we fear that our illness is unique. Despite attempts at invoking sensible thinking, we are frightened that the illness, as an undefined force, is a potential threat to our very being and we are bound to be highly conscious of the uniqueness of that being. The illness, in other words, shares in our own uniqueness. By fearing its threat, we embrace it and make it specially our own. That is why patients are inordinately relieved when doctors give their complaint a name. 'The name may mean very little to them; they may understand nothing of what it signifies; but because it has a name, it has an independent existence from them.' (Berger and Mohr 1976). Armed with an organic diagnosis, the patient can feel equipped to fight that disease. The positivist process of organic diagnosis is to confer scientific recognition upon a complaint, recognizing it, and in its definition to limit and depersonalize it, and thus strengthen the patient.

However, the apparent certainties of this approach came at a cost. For positivism, to a greater or lesser extent, abandoned a variety of conditions that were not 'organic'. These were either totally ignored, causing predictable difficulties for both doctor and patient, or deposited in a less satisfactory, but essential category of 'functional' conditions, conventionally seen as representing a variety of behavioural abnormalities:

Patients come to their doctors with a great variety of different kinds of distress. Frequently the emotional and physical aspects of illness occur together and intimately reflect each other. Doctors have been trained in medical school to 'do something' and often play this role on occasions when 'being someone' for their patients may be more helpful.
(Elder and Samuel 1987)

Paradigm change and scientific revolution

McWhinney (1997) has summarized the Kuhnian theory of paradigm change. Rather than developing by gradual accumulation of individual discoveries and inventions, science progresses by integrating existing knowledge into a set of shared assumptions, which tend to become crystallized into a framework of received beliefs. This resulting paradigm dominates further research, exerting all the deeper a hold for not being made explicit. Kuhn (1967) describes scientific research as 'a strenuous and devoted attempt to force nature into the conceptual boxes supplied by professional education.' The formation of a scientific discipline begins with the promotion of the most convincing theory into its first paradigm. This paradigm then rules: the individual scientist not only accepts it, but can take it for granted. He or she can proceed comfortably, needing no longer to 'attempt to build his field anew, starting from first principles and justifying the use of each concept introduced'. Indeed, the acceptance of the paradigm provides a satisfactorily challenging and apparently appropriate research agenda for the scientist, and a secure arena for the professional worker to serve in confidently.

However, sooner or later paradigms run up against anomalies. At first, these may be ignored, or Procrustean attempts may be more or less successfully deployed to accommodate the discrepant or the inexplicable. However, the stage arises when 'normal science' can no longer solve the problem caused by the anomaly. If the paradigm cannot adapt, a new theory has to be developed. Since this process is concerned with implicit assumptions previously unquestioned, the ensuing dialectic can be expressed not just as conflict, but even as bitter and irrational struggle. Travelling widely over the history of science, Kuhn cites a fascinating range of examples of the structure of scientific revolutions. Along with recognition of unreasonable resentment, there are two characteristics that are relevant. First, he remarks on the difficulty the adherents of the old paradigm find in understanding, coming to terms with and using its replacement. Secondly, he points out that the new paradigm's advocates often come from a peripheral or indeed external group.

The Kuhnian hypothesis is helpful in trying to understand the difficulties primary care workers find themselves running into, as they struggle to work within the paradigm handed down to them from the centres of excellence, sources of their learning:

Medical students are taught by hospital specialists in a hospital environment. They are taught about diseases with signs and symptoms and are expected,

when faced with patients with signs and symptoms, to identify the diseases causing the patients suffering. The fallacious syllogism that because all cases of a certain disease have certain symptoms, therefore that set of symptoms always represents that particular disease, is perpetuated. The study of disease is made all-important, and the study of the patient as a human being and of the process of his (sic) communication with the doctor is neglected.
(Browne and Freeling 1967)

I try to learn more about May's IBS so that through understanding her condition—be it 'organic', 'functional' or 'psychosomatic'—I can help her better. However, what I read seems of limited relevance to me, her, or to her illness. I find myself becoming exasperated. Yet, this knowledge and advice comes from those to whom primary care turns (still) for the same, the supposed source of its enlightenment and to whom it pays fealty—the teaching hospital.

My irritated and perhaps unreasonable reaction is clarified by the realization that a similar response might be predicted from the other side: we are encountering a clash of paradigms no less. Different professional groups use words defined by themselves, which makes it hard for others.

Take 'somatization', for example. This has been defined as 'a pattern of clinical behaviour in which patients go to doctors believing that they have physical disease, but who do not, and do have emotional problems—commonly depression' (Gray 1994). Perhaps, but many would argue not only that patients like May have more insight than we credit them with, readily appreciating (as she did) that their symptoms are primarily related to their context and circumstances, but also that the stark categorizing of *either having disease, or not* implicit in the above sits uneasily with the Leeuwenhorst description (see below) and modern family practice.

As for 'psychosomatic', Bridges and Goldberg (1985) require that four conditions be satisfied:

♦ The patient must be seeking help for somatic symptoms.

♦ The patient must attribute these symptoms to some physical disorder.

♦ A specific mental disorder must be present.

♦ The somatic symptoms are due not to physical disease, but can be thought of as part of the mental disorder.

The requirement that a 'mental disorder' (whatever that may mean) has to be present is enough to stop any GP using the word, even if they felt so inclined. As I have already suggested, the knowledge that some seek to help their understanding can be more or less irrelevant to others:

This ever-recurring situation shows why it is so often futile for the specialist to adopt the role of a mentor and for the (family) doctor to persevere in his (sic) old status pupillaris. In these cases the specialist has nothing to teach, because the general practitioner knows far more—if only he dared to use his

knowledge. In fact he could teach the specialist a great deal, but that is a far cry.
(Balint 1964)

McWhinney (1997) rehearses some of the abundant evidence that a large proportion of people seen in family practice cannot be assigned to a disease category based on a physiological or anatomical abnormality. Only half of a group of patients presenting with chest pain in a general practice received an organic diagnosis. Although 265 patients with a headache were followed up for a year, only 27 per cent were specifically diagnosed; for adult males with abdominal pain, the comparable figure was 30 per cent. He concludes: 'The old paradigm has never had a very good fit with family practice where it has never been fully accepted.'

Of course, the causes of illness are far more complicated than the search for specific aetiologies suggests. Primary care recognizes that disease cannot be separated conceptually from the person or the person from their environment. The Leeuwenhorst Working Party of European general practitioners declared as long ago as 1974 that the GP 'will include *and integrate* (my italics) physical, psychological, and social factors in his considerations about health and illness.' Thus, the biopsychosocial model replaces the biomedical model.

I cannot even begin to understand May's IBS without reference to her past and present experiences, and to her relationships—with myself, her family, her work, and the wider community.

The exacerbation, if not the actual development of her symptoms—possibly even the entire syndrome—can be interpreted as being directly related to her circumstances. It does not demean May or diminish her suffering at all to recognize it as a reflection of her husband's illness. Her flare up of IBS represents the inadequacy of her own resources to maintain her present equilibrium: a state of health is temporarily lost and illness breaks in. This dynamic, but delicate balance naturally incorporates her (and my) knowledge of past experiences (many of which remain directly relevant, such as, for example, the small, but constant expenditure of emotional support called forth by a dependent daughter), the response of others (such as her other daughter's emotional inability to see her father in his present debilitation) and—I risk putting it crudely—*her need* for an illness now, to provide for time-off and acknowledgement of this at work, and perhaps to secure an additional means of communication with me, her doctor, at this time.

The new paradigm

The social construction approach represents a more accommodating paradigm for primary care. In contrast to positivism, this theory accepts that no single view can capture the full story, 'the truth'.

'We were forced to draw the conclusion, most important for the daily practice of family doctors...that one has to be very cautious indeed in assuming that information about the family given by one member agrees with the real truth' (Huygen 1978). The same thing can appear to be quite different from various places and conflicting stories need to be heard. Evidence varies, and even the act of observation alters that which is being assessed. With no neutral objective perspective, the personal experience of all participants (which must now include the doctor and those close to, as well as, the patient) assumes far greater importance. 'The mind's organization of perceptions, and emotions of fear or hope, affect physical pain in ways that positivism's separation of body from mind cannot address' (Alderson 1998).

Subsequently, much of primary care has moved further from positivism, into a variant of post-modernism. Here edges, identities, and behaviours have become blurred. Old bearings and certainties are lost as the particular, not to mention the universal, becomes ever more complex. The doctor wonders who is the patient anyway, patients comfort their physician, no one is sure what a disability is, let alone health...who knows what constitutes knowledge, and who can determine the validity or worth of any enterprise? Post-modernism's recognition of 'the boiling cauldron of life, infinite stratification of reality and the unravellable knot of knowledge' (Calvino 2000) better represents reality in the world of primary care. Certainly, GPs can feel more comfortable with such questionings and dissolutions, than with trying to work with a model, which fails to explain, embrace, or help resolve many of the problems our patients bring to us.

So at last in the developing world of social construction and post-modernism, GPs can admit with some confidence that their interest is in people—creatures made up of body and mind—first, and disease second (Davies 2000). They can be concerned with subjective experience of illness, its expression and development, with relationships and how the passing of time influences all. Working within this paradigm, all kinds of dualities including distinctions between body and mind, psyche and soma, organic and functional, even the pathological and physiological melt into a series of continua that correspond much closer to the reality of looking after people. 'GPs are interested in personality, family patterns, and the effect of these on the presentation of symptoms as much as in diseases themselves...(they are) trying to understand the relations between symptoms, health and illness, and specific diseases within communities' (Davies 2000). 'General practice is the only discipline to define itself in terms of relationships, especially the doctor-patient relationship' (McWhinney 1996).

Transcending the difference between body and mind

Moving easily from the physical to the psychological, and back again, via (if needs be) the social, GPs are strategically placed to override these boundaries. Of course, it is only by virtue of this unique privilege that they can work within the biopsychosocial paradigm. Arguably, it is only in general practice that the dualistic division, which runs through medicine 'like a geological fault', can be bridged. (No doubt this explains why it is that GPs have embraced this paradigm.) Most clinical disciplines are separated by this chasm: medicine and surgery to one side, the family of psychiatric specialties on the other (see Part IV of this volume). Physical doctors do not normally explore the emotions, while the psychological doctors avoid physical examination. However, in general practice, 'without this artificial barrier, the relationship between patient and doctor can develop through many encounters...in examining and attending to the body, we are also attending to the mind' (McWhinney 1996). Each aspect of the old dualism has naturally much to offer the GP working in this way. A physical examination can be a great help in confirming the diagnosis of a mental state, for example, depression or anxiety. Of course, listening, enquiring about feelings, sharing, interpreting, and summarizing enormously strengthens the management of physical conditions. 'It is as though when he talks or listens to a patient, he is also touching them with his hands so as to be less likely to misunderstand: and it is as though, when he is physically examining a patient, they were also conversing' (Berger and Mohr 1967).

In summary, May's consultation is far too complicated to be processed by the somewhat simplistic, reductionist biomedical approach. The 'extraordinarily complex convergence of philosophical traditions, feelings, half-realized ideas, atavistic instincts, imaginative intimations which lie behind the simplest hope or disappointment of the simplest person' (Berger and Mohr 1967) call for a real attempt at integrating the mind with the body, the biological with the social, the individual with the family, and illness behaviour with perceptions of health.

The biopsychosocial model at work

The classic demonstration of the biopsychosocial model at work is Huygen's book *Family Medicine* (Huygen 1978). Over some 30 years, individuals' illness episodes, presented to the doctor as consultations, were mapped on charts that included the same for other members of that family. During this time he learnt to look beyond the individual, as he tried to understand that person's illness: the doctor needs to focus on the relationship between the patient and others in the family, as well as the presenting patient. There is such a definite relationship between episodes of illness in different family members that the GP needs to see the family and its experience over time as the unit. Here, we see the interaction between body and mind in play not only on an individual level, but also between different family members.

For the most part Huygen is not concerned with whether the diagnosis was physical or psychological—his interest lies in how a family event such as birth, death, marriage, arrival, or departure precipitates imbalance expressing itself as a perceived need to see the doctor in one or more members. Some charts are devoted to showing how 'nervous disorders' can result from family events, but his main interest is in demonstrating the phenomenon of *inter-relatedness* and the role of psychosocial transitions as a cause of disequilibrium, manifesting itself, like May's IBS, as symptoms (be they physical or psychological) in an individual. Thus, one of Huygen's achievements was to demonstrate the way in which transitions in the life cycle can stimulate medical events in members of that family unit. External, but shared experiences can be seen to create symptoms, illness—even disease and disability. Such a process, in which body and mind, mind and body interact in a complicated network to produce these events at such significant moments is an experience well known in primary care. It is worth looking at in more detail.

The major transitions of the life cycle

Continuity alongside change, predictability with surprise—the circle of life can be seen as an ongoing process of change and development in which nothing ever stands still. It can be argued that all development involves disruption and disequilibrium following a period of stability. Various stages can be described as distinct phases, but whatever divisions are chosen, each brings different and specific problems. It is the transition from one to the next that requires adaptation and change. These specific turning points in the life cycle when imbalance is more likely may be identified.

Major transitions are critical times when biopsychosocial rearrangements have to be made, increasing the likelihood of insecurity, undermining confidence, and thereby encouraging the development of 'illness' (Markus *et al.* 1989), which can be expressed through the body or mind, as Huygen showed. Often disturbances arise because old solutions are tried for new situations.

At such times various different members of the primary care team may become involved. If GPs have something to teach their hospital colleagues, then they have much to learn from their own team members. In any event, primary care workers are well used to deploying the biopsychosocial model, recognizing that physical changes or problems may be expressed psychologically, and that physical symptoms may represent psychological, family, or social stresses.

Pregnancy and birth

There can be no greater time of personal physical change for an individual than pregnancy—inconceivable (literally) for those who have not undergone those extraordinary 9 months, during which the body changes astonishingly and the

mind adapts, or tries to. Even when completely normal – 'physiologically'—
this experience distorts not just reality, but perceptions too. The passing of time
itself changes, as surely as all changes with the passing of time:

> I am slow as the world.
> I am very patient, turning through my time...

Sylvia Plath's rumination on pregnancy in 'Three Women' explores this
intriguing territory where changes in the body alter the mind, and quaint old
medical distinctions between psychological and physical health become quite
meaningless. Along with other major transitions in the life cycle, this is a time
of both gain and loss. The gain in weight, the gain of a new person, the gain of
pride, pleasure, and love are all obvious. However, there can also be loss of
personal attractiveness, sexual activity, sleep, independence and liberty, money,
and (especially afterwards) attention. There is an increased risk of depression
(see Chapter 11), and a variety of physical symptoms and problems ranging
from stretch marks and breast changes, to piles, varicose veins, and perineal
damage.

The pregnancy and birth experience then represents a unique (though
paradoxically universal) personal life-altering event, both for the woman herself
and for her family, calling for an integrated body-and-mind-and-social
supporting approach from the primary care team.

Infancy

Huygen's charts confirm the experience of every primary care worker—that the
first few years of life see the greatest number of contacts with primary care. This
is certainly a time of major transition. It is interesting to note that distinctions
between mind and body never seem to have bedevilled the care of infants. All
would accept that an unhappy baby expresses itself physically and that a
distressed baby from whatever cause will respond to physical comforting.

However, this is also a turning point in the family life cycle. From its first
appearance, the newborn baby is not only a new member with its own definite
and specific requirements, but at least temporarily the most important person in
the family. Other members—particularly the parents—must adapt to this, for
babies are born with a powerful repertoire of tricks, which ensure that, in most
cases, their needs will be met. Vicious circles can appear quite readily. Thus, an
anxious or unsupported mother can transmit her worry to her baby (who will
have his own characteristics) and then there may be feeding problems, failure to
thrive, excessive crying, restless nights, clinging behaviour, hyperactivity, and
irritability (Markus *et al.* 1989). Any of these can be presented as physical
problems by the mother to the Health Visitor or GP. Moreover, the demands of
caring for a restless infant can, in turn, generate irritability in the mother, or she
may become over-protective—either way, compounding the problem. In

addition, she may well then develop her own symptoms: insomnia, loss of confidence, increasingly poor self-esteem, eating problems—or even an apparent full-blown depression (see Chapter 11). At any point along this pathway, the parents (and therefore the infant) can be helped by well-directed listening and attention to their difficulties from members of the primary care team. There may be a cluster of increased consultations for a variety of illnesses by different family members at this often-difficult time of accommodation to new demands. Huygen shows that these can be classified under different diagnostic headings, but as before only by bearing in mind the wider perspective derived from the biopsychosocial model can the GP understand and deal with them effectively.

Early childhood

An extensive and authoritative literature on the interaction of body and mind in children's illness attests to the general acceptance that in this age group above all, psychological problems can be expressed physically and vice versa. Apley's classic work studying abdominal pain in children laid the foundations (Apley 1974), so that paediatricians all now approach diagnosis using the biopsycho-social model, integrating the physical with the psychological, the child within its family and social context.

Unlike the paediatrician, however, the family doctor is often responsible for other family members' health care as well. This position enables the experience of helping one to benefit the care of another. Thus, tensions in one parent (or both) or between them may be picked up as a presented problem in the child or vice versa. This familiar cycle, which may be entered at various points, needs early identification. The GP earns her title of family doctor as she moves freely between the mind and body, and between the patient who presents and the family member whose needs have precipitated the problem (see Chapter 9).

Later childhood

Of course, childhood in its entirety may be seen as representing transition, but there are some major points of change even in a stable childhood, such as going to school and the first separations from parents. These occasions, along with other moments of challenge can produce symptoms, bodily or psychological, in both child and parents. In addition, the more major traumas of childhood may occur; frequent moves, divorce, the death of a parent, or being the victim of abuse. Anxiety in either party may generate overtly psychological problems or—as ever—these may be translated into physical symptoms. Equally, there might be relatively simple physical difficulties at this stage, such as tiredness from unaccustomed activities or poor eating from new meal patterns, which can manifest either in an obviously physical, or a more psychological way.

The GP needs to retain an understanding acceptance of the multiplicity of forms of expression of distress, generally avoiding the terms 'psychological' and 'physical'. Interestingly, families often seem happy to accept this holistic and practical approach, with parents having less need for body-mind distinctions than their doctors.

Adolescence

Whether or not the concept of 'adolescence' with its stereotype of storm, stress, and rebellion, is a twentieth-century Western invention or not, it is a time of rapid physical, intellectual, and emotional change, which brings symptoms and signs demonstrating the complicated inter-relationship of body and mind. Bodily and sexual developments leading to new powers, and changes of shape and size (see Chapter 12 on eating disorders), call for radical readjustments in the individual's sense of self. Moving from the protected, but dependent state of childhood towards more autonomy, adolescents experience a variety of anxieties in which physical and emotional turmoil, personal identity, and changing social relationships all inter-mingle confusingly, not only for themselves, but also for their peers and other family members (see the discussion in Chapter 1 of a teenage boy who presented distress about his body odour and later developed a psychotic illness):

> K. a fifteen year old boy consults complaining of bad breath. He is permitted, indeed encouraged, to talk of the problems he feels this causes for him in rela- tionships with people of his own age; a simple mouthwash is prescribed. At the next visit he says he feels his breath is cleaner and asks if he could be a homosexual; he finds he is very anxious in the presence of girls of his own age...
> *(Royal College of General Practitioners 1972)*

K. is testing his doctor, only progressing when and if he feels safe. Crucially, neither he nor his doctor makes any distinction between the physical, psychological, emotional, or social—although all are relevant. Instead, they work together, developing a 'fragmented yet continuous' consultation (Royal College of General Practitioners 1972) to discover about each other, learn what is acceptable and build trust. As these tasks assume greater priority than the biomedical demands of 'diagnosis and management', attention centres on the centrality and importance of the doctor–patient relationship. When the doctor attends to the patient's beliefs and emotions, she seeks a common ground of understanding and creates a basis for a 'mutual investment company' (Balint 1957) between patient and doctor. In this way, the patient-centred clinical method is evident. Adolescents consult doctors infrequently and are often acutely concerned about confidentiality. The GP has to have the imagination to establish contact swiftly and, if she succeeds, significant depths of depression or involve- ment with drugs and alcohol (see Chapter 15) may suddenly be revealed.

Parenting, families, and mid-life

Curiously, the literature on adult developmental processes is scant compared with those devoted to childhood, adolescence, and old age. It is impossible to do justice to the developmental tasks and transitions of adult life in the space available: forming relationships, achieving and sustaining parenthood for men and women, the vicissitudes of work in a technological age, ambition, success, failure, job loss and redundancy, infirmity and death of parents, relationship difficulties and breakdown, remarriage and reconstituted families, loneliness, and retirement.

The transition from the newly won independence of the young adult to a new inter-dependence and indeed dependence that parenting brings is one crucial turning point. This process places its own special demands on all concerned that, as before, blurs body and mind boundaries. Although modern society offers a wide variety of models for living together, having children, and supporting them in their turn through to achieving their own independence, the interaction between physical and psychological change and development for all parties in this process remains standard and universal. As I have argued throughout this chapter, Huygen argues that it is only by using an integrated biopsychosocial approach that GPs can understand and care for families.

Old age

All those caring for the elderly will have learnt that trying to draw clear distinctions between mind and body, body and mind is as unhelpful as finding differences between the 'physiological' and the 'pathological' in this age group. The physical changes of old age naturally produce restrictions: less activity and mobility, leading to and associated with a degree of social retrenchment. This predictable process of detachment is complex indeed. A slowing body—affected by stiffer joints, weaker muscles, a slower metabolism, and less acute senses—both engenders and is accompanied by, mental changes. Whilst ageing does not bring inevitable intellectual decline, mental agility does tend to lessen—which may in turn contribute to diminishing calls upon the physical resources of that individual. The circularity of these phenomena is obvious but perhaps it is helpful to restate it here, for at no other stage of life is the total interaction of body and mind more evident.

If these developments—be they 'physical' or 'psychological'—are severe, they tend to generate diagnostic labels. A GP may assess a hip joint (clinically and radiologically) and not be sure at what point the predictable attritional processes are ready for the conventional diagnosis of osteoarthritis—when does inevitable and natural wear and tear become 'pathological'? Similarly, there are times when a GP can make a relatively confident diagnosis of depression in a particular patient. However, it can sometimes be very hard when working with the elderly to be sure: is this state of loss of interest, withdrawal, awareness of loss and general state of sadness (perhaps realistic, perhaps exaggerated, but who am I to judge?) an entirely appropriate response, and therefore 'physiological'?

Such questions are unanswerable, but they illustrate how, with the elderly above all, there is such a substantial overlap between mind and body, that the GP on some occasions finds the best way is to move beyond the biopsychosocial model. A more modern, if not a post-modern paradigm, offering an awareness of the discomfort, difficulties, and ultimate impossibility of the diagnostic process gives the doctor permission to attend to what persists as an unclassifiable complexity. The GP can then concentrate on both the symbol and the reality, the language and the relationship. GPs know that patients can work comfortably with metaphors. Thus (as IBS was my way in), to feel something 'in my guts', 'to have a gut feeling', 'to hate someone's guts', or even Cromwell's famous 'I beseech you, in the bowels of Christ, think it possible you may be mistaken', all show that 'guts' can represent the body's core of unsophisticated honesty or be the seat of strong feelings. In this more 'metaphor-aware' stance, whilst continuing to attend to the ailments that the elderly bring, and to the relationship between his patients and himself, the GP is better able to listen to the whole individual, as the life cycle turns, and old age brings decline and death. The hospice movement has reminded primary care and taught the wider profession, that a holistic approach, which acknowledges not just the variety of needs every individual has, but their inter-relatedness, is essential in caring for those who face death. The process of adjustment to deterioration and loss (whether physical or mental), disability, loss of personal function, or grief for another person is a developmental task, along with all other transitions.

Conclusion

In an attempt to comprehend the complexity of the primary care experience I have taken two approaches. An individual journey with a particular patient and a more general, universal examination, which reviews the spectrum of work that family practice encompasses. Both confirm that 'all kinds of interaction exist between the somatic, psychological and social fields. A disorder in one of the fields can manifest in another and be treated in still another field', as Huygen put it succinctly in the 1970s, quoting earlier work from the 1950s. This phenomenon underlines the importance of adopting an approach to 'mental health' that starts within the bedrock of primary care.

As the GP begins to work with the more complex models outlined in this chapter, 'health' itself becomes harder to define. The definition of health by the World Health Organization as a state of complete physical, mental, and social well being has been seen to be a misleading and unrealistic fiction. When Huygen investigated a number of volunteer families who regarded themselves as healthy and happy he found problems—sometimes serious—in the majority. Most 'healthy' people usually have several complaints, either bodily or mental. 'Illness, death, mishaps and unhappiness are with us at all times and a family doctor witnesses this, although he (sic) sees only part of it' (Huygen 1978).

Balance can be achieved in the presence of such adversities—perhaps this is 'normal' life—through the growth and development of individual capacities. 'Health' then may be more usefully interpreted as a state of *dynamic equilibrium* or at least a measure of temporary harmony in that process of continuing change and integration of new experiences that life represents (Browne and Freeling 1967). The physiological is to be found alongside—confused with and hard to separate from—the 'pathological', all illnesses affect the patient at multiple levels, and the relationship between doctor and patient has a profound effect on the illness and its course. A 'body and mind' model must then be abandoned in favour of the integrated and synthesizing approach, which is arguably the defining characteristic of primary care—only GPs simultaneously treat physical and emotional problems (Gray 1994; McWhinney 1996).

Of course, none would dispute that there are times for using conventional disease categories—to make the right therapeutic decisions and for communication within the health care system, to help both patient and doctor. To diagnose and treat angina, for example, a positivist model may be appropriate. However, to begin to understand how angina is presented, not to mention exacerbated, experienced, interpreted, managed, and in the longer term prevented, we have to look to more developed paradigms (Alderson 1998). For 'the idea of disease as an entity which is limited to one person, and can be transmitted from one individual to another, fades into the background, and disease becomes an integral part of the continuous process of living' (Huygen 1978). According to these later paradigms, disease is neither separated conceptually from the person, nor the person from his or her environment. Life and living brings change, and the need to adapt to that change—which may be seen as physiological or pathological, as health or illness, as physical or psychological. Such complexity is more usefully interpreted holistically in the context of that change, with awareness of relationships, not least of that between GP and 'patient'.

Back to my patient

I saw May the next day at home, when I visited her husband. It was a positive visit. The community nurse had set up a syringe driver, which was controlling his symptoms better. We sat together on his bed talking for a while. May came to see me a week later as planned. She felt better, she said. There was a pause. Could she tell me something personal? Of course, I replied automatically: that was what doctors are for—but then I felt slightly anxious. It was really personal, she reiterated. I told her that it was fine. I had no choice—I was now committed, but what was coming? I felt my heart beating faster, wondering what *really personal* meant. My mind raced through possibilities: what had I done or not done, what was it she wanted to say about me, was she going to tell me that I had something like halitosis? It came out suddenly: she needed to tell me about a time a couple of months ago, when they'd made love. It had been perfect—she would always treasure it, she remembered it now and, well, whatever happened, and she knew he was dying, that moment was special.

I felt a confused surge of relief and happiness. Their wonderful Liebestod may have been past and momentary, but in that orgasm—body and mind, mind and body, she and he, and now even a part of me too—all was fused. For one moment, we were both transfixed in a moment.

'How much then can a moment contain?' asks Berger. Perhaps enough of the particular to represent the universal.

He died soon after. May and I have met several times since, but there has been no reference to that memorable consultation. Her IBS seems to be better now, on no treatment. She has retired early and has bought herself a puppy.

3 Biological and narrative time in clinical practice

Brian Hurwitz

> ...the ticking of a clock. We ask what it *says*: and we agree that it says *tick-tock*. By this fiction we humanize it, make it talk our language...tick is our word for a physical beginning, tock our word for an end. What enables them to be different is a special kind of middle.
> *(Kermode 1968)*

> I can only answer the question 'Of what am I to do? If I can also answer the prior question 'Of what story or stories do I find myself a part?'
> *(MacIntyre 1981)*

Neither seen nor felt directly, not heard, nor tasted, nor smelt, time is dimensional to being and inherent, therefore, in medicine (Elias 1992; Heidegger 2000). Clinical encounters typically focus on discerning time sequences, on relationships of before and after, on discussion of beginnings and endings. Setting out and manipulating temporal relationships are processes as central to consulting as they are to storytelling; in both, time passing and changes happening are existentially entwined.

I recently registered one of my patients blind. The day was a sad occasion for both of us. I have been Doris Smith's GP for 16 years. During this period, I have developed some feel for her mental illness, which is episodic and severe, I am able to recognize its early manifestations, and have a reasonable understanding of what's likely to precipitate serious breakdown. We have a trusting relationship; I've written many a note to Doris about aspects of her care—concerning letters from hospital specialists, abnormally high blood glucose results and missed clinic appointments—to which she has always responded. However, I probably 'know' Mrs Smith in the sense of being acquainted with her personality and domestic circumstances better than I understand her.

During the period of our relationship, the suspected link between onset of diabetic complications and blood glucose control has been clearly established by a number of impressive trials. It is now known that the product of average blood glucose concentration and time predicts the onset of sight-threatening disease, the relationship probably being causal, since control of blood glucose delays (and may prevent) eye disease. An unfelt risk factor has been found to exert harmful effects over time (UK Prospective Diabetes Study Group 1998a,b,c). Findings such as these undercut Leriche's view, that 'health is life lived in the silence of the organs' (Canguilhem 1978) and underpin treatments aimed at modifying today's risks in order to prevent tomorrow's undesirable outcomes.

During over a hundred consultations in general practice I have endeavoured to influence Mrs Smith's *future* by intervening in her *present* lifestyle—advising changes to her diet, exercise habits, and medication, discussing with her daughter (with whom she occasionally resides) the overall aims of diabetes management, and referring her to specialists. Now, reluctantly, I prepare myself for sad scenes in her unfolding biography: an elderly, vulnerable woman, living alone in inner London coming to grips with being blind.

In general practice, the biographies of patients and doctors intersect and interact (Williams 1997; Heath 1998). Contact is inter-generational, episodic, and may extend over many years. Successes and failures unfold over variable time spans; events bringing happiness and loss are shared, feelings of affinity evolve towards closeness and fondness, those of repulsion towards dislike and even hostility. Such relationships evolve in the context of a wide stage-set provided by the NHS, with all its workings and facilities, and by the 'stage directions' operative at the time. In the case of someone like Doris the stage directions for a GP, the medical goals of professional activity, define my remit as one of 'social physician': over time, to monitor, treat to prevent future possible outcomes, and to coordinate health care, taking account of the latest evidence of effective treatment and national targets for morbidity prevention (Department of Health 1998, 1999; Porter 2000).

Time frames

Accounts of illness experiences are typically punctuated by time. Some diseases are associated with slow, unfolding awareness of difficult-to-pin-point sensations. Others cause instantaneous, 'thunderclap' symptoms, such as stabbing pains, flashing lights, and then blindness. These extremes encompass a spectrum of innumerable other sensations that may come and go, move about with unaccountable tempo, and vary in quality, intensity, and rhythmicity.

Time, which marks out continuous processes of growth, development, and ageing, allows different stages of the life cycle to be the focus of specialisms: embryology, foetal medicine, neonatology, paediatrics, gerontology—each attends to a particular segment of our temporal span (Armstrong 2000). Many disciplines inevitably make common use of time: in selection of screening and re-screening intervals, in defining medication regimens, response to treatment, periods of recovery, infectivity, incubation, and prognosis. Values are recorded over time, on growth charts, kick charts, or temperature charts; devices plot variables against time, such as forced expiratory volume, the electrical activity of heart muscle, and 'real time' ultrasound echoes.

Time, titrated in a multiplicity of ways, in the movements of the heavens and the motion of clocks, in schedules, timetables, appointments, and diaries finds pervasive and polymorphous expression in life. As a measurable duration spanning events and actions, Aristotle considered time the 'calculable measure of motion with respect to before and afterness' (Aristotle 2000). In the unending flow of occurrences, time marked out by before and after provides the framework in which different positions, sequences, values and functions can be compared and juxtaposed (Elias 1992).

By delineating occurrences along a time axis of before and after, relationships essential to clinical understanding are charted: 'For *how long* have you had these symptoms? Were they troublesome *before* (or *after*) your wife died?' are questions aimed not only at clarification, but at discerning the onset of a concomitant flux of events.

Lacking itself material qualities, time has been judged the necessary presupposition of experience and thought. Existent or not in the universe, anthropologists report no cultures lacking a concept of it. In shaping ideas and experiences of time, Edmund Leach believes repetition is the key: 'Drops of water falling from the roof are not all the same drop, but different'; and in order to recognize them as different we must first distinguish and define intervals of time: 'Time intervals and durations always begin and end with the same thing, a pulse beat, a clock strike...' Leach writes, an observation that applies to measuring and marking time metronomically, though not to how it is perceived and experienced (Leach 1971).

We term the second of the two related clock sounds 'tock' (not 'tick'), Frank Kermode suggests, precisely to defeat the tendency of the interval between tick-tick to empty itself of any meaning other than mere duration and chronicity: 'The clock's tick-tock I take to be a model of what we call a plot, an organization that humanizes time by giving it form...Tick is a humble genesis, tock a feeble apocalypse' (Kermode 1968).

Narrative and time

Kermode is referring here to the fictional devices of stories, in which duration and meaning are paradigmatically structured in a triadic form: beginning, middle, and end. His insight is helpful to clinicians who spend much of their lives listening to story fragments, and eliciting connections between experiences and processes in which precise temporal relations, the *order* in which events unfold, can be crucial signifiers of their meaning and significance (Box 3.1).

Galen conceived symptoms to be special experiences that disclose disease as reliably as a shadow follows the body on a bright day (King 1992). Though our bodies cannot directly speak, changes in internal environment variably coded,

Box 3.1   **A GP consultation and the temporal order of things**

Johnny, a crane driver, had always assured me he was HIV negative. An intravenous heroin user for whom I prescribed methadone, Johnny insisted further HIV tests were not necessary: he'd had three while in prison and these had shown him to be negative.

When I realised he had a girlfriend—also a patient of mine—I quizzed him again about his HIV status and whether he'd discussed the risks with her. He hadn't, because he thought himself negative. I persuaded him to let me write to the Prison Medical Service for details of his test results.

Three HIV tests had, indeed, been performed, over a period of twelve months, the last of which was positive. Johnny had been informed, and offered monitoring. That was four years ago.

I asked him again about the tests. Johnny knew the third one was positive, but seemed unconcerned about it. To him two out of three tests—a clear majority—were negative. The *order* in which test results were declared was not of crucial significance; Johnny appeared to deny that two negative tests followed by a positive result were more likely to indicate he had been infected than a positive result from a first test followed by two negative results.

perceived, and encapsulated in language thereby give rise to symptoms. In encoding, recalling, and communicating such experiences, processes of narrative selection and classification take place.

Discerning the temporal relationships of such symptoms is one of the main tasks of consultations. In general practice, patienthood arises because people feel a need to share with health advisers snippets of experience and life story that concern them, and about which they invite interpretation. Not self-consciously framed as stories with a beginning, middle, or an end, these fragments typically display variable threads of story-like structure, as simple chronological sequence, as dramas of gradually unfolding awareness, or as more or less complex meandering observations reported by patients themselves, relatives, or friends.

Narration involves recounting, shaping, and the ordering of events (their 'emplottment'). Though fragmentary and episodic in clinical settings, it is through the constant telling of stories that we manage to make sense of the internal and external world:

It is through hearing stories about wicked stepmothers, lost children, good but misguided kings, wolves that suckle twin boys, youngest sons who receive no inheritance, live riotously and go into exile and live with the swine, that children learn or mislearn both what a child and what a parent is, what the cast of characters may be in the drama into which they have been born and what the ways of the world are.
(MacIntyre 1981).

A fundamental part of discourse and culture, some investigators view the story-telling impulse to be a part of an evolutionary survival kit. The experimental neurologist, Antonio Damasio, for example, believes tripartite narrative structures to have biological parallels in the excitatory processes of perception and memory. According to Damasio, the way organisms interact with objects—in perception and in memory—is best understood 'as a simple narrative without words. It does have characters (the organism, the object). It unfolds in time. And it has a beginning, a middle and an end. The beginning corresponds to the initial state of the organism. The middle is the arrival of the object. The end is made up of reactions that result in a modified state of the organism' (Damasio 2000).

The structure of beginnings

Conceiving or perceiving a beginning places a phenomenon apart, while simultaneously signifying linkage to certain other processes or developments. A beginning generally designates a point in time, place, action, or intention at which a process or idea first comes into existence. Edward Said explains: 'beginning is designated to indicate, clarify, or define a later time, place or action' above all, to signify precedence in relationship, the first step of something relating to what follows. But how does it relate to what follows? To speak of a beginning signifies the initial manifestation of something that has both duration and coherence of meaning—whatever belongs to the beginning endures, at least for a while, being connected in some way to subsequent events or consequences (Said 1985).

Beginning usually invokes a classification made *after* the event (Said 1985). However, once a beginning has been identified its recognition allows classification of a course of events and paves the way for intervention. Take the pain of shingles: not itself causative of the rash by which it is more usually diagnosed, the pain heralds the beginning of a condition that unfolds predictably. Prior connections—temporal, clinical, and pathological—have linked pain of a particular distribution and sort with the subsequent onset of a distinctive rash. Diagnosing the condition on the basis of pain alone (its clinical beginning) can help to re-plot its course with effective treatment and prevent later complications.

Nevertheless, with no necessary connection between beginnings and causes, beginnings are infused with causal significance. Implied relationships of casuality—between what is begun and its origination—contribute to satisfying the desire for events and occurrences one day to 'manifest a deeper kind of belonging of one thing with another than the mere juxtaposition which now phenomenally appears' (James 1956).

Experiences manifesting narrative kinds of belonging put feelings, sensations or events into an order of sorts, frequently a successive, chronological one.

However, although time is almost always constitutive of narrative, temporal succession alone does not turn description into narrative; rather, it is by establishing *how* occurrences and episodes are *linked together* in a particular way (how they fit logically, biologically, historically, or genetically) that narrative coherence in medicine is manifest (Rimmon-Kenan 1983).

Hearing stories

To listen, remember, and interpret the many fragments of experience patients bring to consultations requires sympathy, patience, and an interest in the temporal patterning of events. These are aspects of sensibilities not dissimilar to those involved in appreciating stories (Hunter 1991). A meticulous concern for relations of succession, association, and causation, an attentive interest in the unusual, in deciphering and piecing together the meaning of words, gestures, and expressions are qualities required of good clinicians.

However, the narrative nature of medical consultations is very different from that crafted by literature. In literature, stories need not be constrained by chronology (Box 3.1); positions in time may jump about (Box 3.2), even reverse (Amis 1991), and the usual assumptions concerning external reference—correspondence between what takes place in fiction and what can occur in everyday life—can be relaxed.

Box 3.2   **Extract from the beginning of *The bridge of San Luis Rey* by Thornton Wilder**

It was very hot noon, that fatal noon, and coming round the shoulder of a hill Brother Juniper stopped to wipe his forehead and to gaze upon the scene of snowy peaks in the distance, then to the gorge below him filled with the dark plumage of green trees and green birds. He had opened several little abandoned churches, and the Indians were crawling in to early Mass. Perhaps it was the pure air from the snows before him; perhaps it was the memory that brushed him for a moment of the poem that bade him raise his eyes to the helpful hills. At all events he was at peace. Then his glance fell upon the bridge, and at that moment a twanging noise filled the air, as when a string of some musical instrument snaps in a disused room, and he saw the bridge divide and fling five ants into the valley below.

Thus it was that the determination rose within him at the moment of the accident. It prompted him to busy himself for six years, knocking at all the doors in Lima, asking thousands of questions, filling scores of notebooks, in his effort at establishing the fact that each of the five lost lives was a perfect whole. Everyone knew that he was working on some sort of memorial of the accident, and everyone was very helpful and misleading. (Wilder 1972)

In a preface to his last book, *To the Hermitage*, Malcolm Bradbury (2000) sketches out the fictive stance he has adopted (Lamarque 1994). By alluding to transformations in time, place, and landscape, he awakens our interest in the story's formal features, including its period and perspective, and stakes a claim for the authorial omnipotence of the novelist (Box 3.3; Bradbury 2000). Though clinical narratives are clearly constrained in ways that fiction isn't, they too may jump about in time, place, and temporal sequence. Alteration of perspective can achieve significant changes in interpretation, the proverbial wisdom of medical hindsight stemming, at least in part, from the angle it offers on a narrative viewed from a vantage point further forward in time. In medicine the fictive stance is also not unknown: because clinical stories are assembled from imperfect processes of perception, memory, and censorship, and are subject to influence from various motives and emotions— embarrassment, shame, guilt—concealment and distortion of information can engender fictive components in them.

Whereas all the elements in a novel possess some meaning stemming from deliberate inclusion within the story, those in life may not (Bell 1994). GPs in the UK undertake 8000–10,000 consultations annually, in many of which the search for a diagnosis may not be a major concern, and does not provide the key to the fragments of experience that thereby come to be discussed. On the contrary, many experiences considered reflect 'lived temporality,' a status quo of symptoms and sensations not necessarily related to underlying medical or psychological conditions.

Box 3.3   **Preface from *To the Hermitage* by Malcolm Bradbury**

This is (I suppose) a story. I have altered the places where facts, data and info, seem dull or inaccurate. I have quietly corrected errors in the calendar, adjusted flaws in world geography, now and then budged the border of a country, or changed the constitution of a nation. A wee postmodern Haussman, I have elegantly replanned some of the world's greatest cities, moving buildings to better sites, redesigning architecture, opening fresh views and fine urban prospects, redirecting the traffic. I've put statues in more splendid locations, usefully reorganized art galleries, cleaned trans- ferred or rehung famous paintings, staged entire new plays and operas. I have revised or edited some of our great books, and republished them. I have altered monuments, defaced icons, changed the street signs, occupied the railway station. I have also taken the chance to introduce people who never met in life, but certainly should have. I have changed their lives and careers...(Bradbury 2000)

Personal time

The experience of duration is bound up with an awareness of change and with the relative span of feelings, bodily sensations, and events (Fraise 1963; Goody 1968). A sense of inner time connects ideas and memories of past experience with the present, linking knowledge of who we once were with whom we have become. 'Making sense of one's life as a story is…not an optional extra', writes the philosopher, Charles Taylor, 'for in order to have a sense of who we are, we have to have a notion of who we have become, and where we are going' (Taylor

---

Box 3.4   *So many different lengths of time* by Brian Patten (1996)

How long is a man's life, finally?
Is it a thousand days, or only one?
One week, or a few centuries?
How long does a man's death last?
And what do we mean when we say, 'gone forever'?
Adrift in such preoccupations, we seek clarification.
We can go to the philosophers,
But they will grow tired of our questions.
We can go to the priests and the rabbis
But they might be too busy with administrations.
                    *   *   *
So how long does a man live, finally?
And how much does he live while he lives?
We fret, and ask so many questions –
Then it comes to us
The answer is simple.
A man lives for as long as we carry him inside us,
For as long as we carry the harvest of his dreams,
For as long as we ourselves live,
Holding memories in common, a man lives.
His lover will carry this man's scent, his touch;
His children will carry the weight of his love.
One friend will carry his arguments,
Another will still share his terrors.
And the days will pass with baffled faces,
Then the weeks, then the months,
Then there will be a day when no question is asked,
And the knots of grief will loosen in the stomach,
And the puffed faces will calm.
And on that day he will not have ceased,
But will have ceased to be separated by death.
How long does a many live, finally?
A man lives so many different lengths of time.

Box 3.5   **Time's Chariot. 'Rethinking Anthropology' by Edmund Leach**

'The feeling that most of us have that the first ten years of childhood "lasted much longer" than the hectic decade of 40–50 is no illusion' writes Edmund Leach, for 'biological processes, such as wound healing, operate much faster (in terms of stellar time) during childhood than in old age. But since our sensations are geared to our biological processes rather than to the stars, time's chariot appears to proceed at ever increasing speed. This irregular flow of biological time is not merely a phenomenon of personal intuition; it is observable in the organic world all around us. Plant growth is much faster at the beginning than at the end of the life cycle; the ripening of the grain and the sprouting of the sown grain proceed at quite different rates of development' (Leach 1971).

1989). A sense of self and personal identity depend in part, therefore, on the intactness of an inner story (the story of one's life) extending through time (Orona 1990).

The poet, Brian Patten, asks how long a life is and surmises a person lives many different lengths of time (Box 3.4; Patten 1996). As individuals, we age at a pace that is slowing down in relation to the sequence of stellar time (Box 3.5), with awareness of time's passing affected by ill health and by mood. Whereas severe pain blots out all sense of a past and a future, uncertainty and grief can so empty the present of meaning that the flow of time becomes suspended (Box 3.6; Scarry 1985).

Box 3.6   **Waiting with time**

Recently, or was it years ago, my wife found a breast lump which turned out to be malignant. She's 36. Since then, time has become distorted, the objective measures of calendars and clocks becoming meaningless as appointments, results, operations, and treatments have approached and passed. Minutes, hours, and days have become prolonged and compressed... Six months have sped by... what about the waiting? What to say to each other at the start and end of each day when there is only one date, and time, and result on your minds?... as the end of active treatment looms, there is the hardest wait of all. Life is no longer measured in terms of 'expectancy' but rather as 'survival'. (McLeary 2000)

Conclusion

Phenomena, concepts, and experience of time are intimately bound up with existence. Paul Ricoeur (following the tracks of a long line of philosophical investigation) evokes the mystery of the relationship when he writes: '…time has no being since the future is not yet, the past no longer, and the present does not remain. And yet we do speak of time as having being. We say that things to come *will be*, that things past *were*, and that things present *are passing away*' (Ricoeur 1984).

Time's immaterial flow is revealed by the processes of ageing, measured out by the ticks of technology and titrated by medical instrumentation. Biologically and narratively time flows in the direction of causality, along an axis from before to afterwards. Experientially, time offers us a 'platform' from which we live our lives and through which—in hopes, plans, and projects—we exercise some control over its course. Ill health can disrupt this 'assumed futurity', and distort or slow down time's subjective flow (Davies 1997).

Clinical medicine articulates together measures of time, subjective experience, and objective biological processes. *Taking* a medical history (as the process of interpreting what patients tell doctors continues to be termed) remains the central approach to clinical investigation, and is predominantly a process of decipherment, for which narrative and interpretative skills are required (Greenhalgh and Hurwitz 1998). In the varied descriptions patients bring to doctors, time signifies change, and duration and sequence mark relations essential to emplotting experience of ill health (Good and Good 2000).

Clinical narratives co-exist and co-evolve alongside other possible stories— some displaying similar beginnings and different endings, or different middles and the same endings—featuring identical actors performing different actions. Did Doris Smith's blindness result from her schizophrenia, which compromised her ability to adopt the right diet; or was her poor diet really all due to poverty? Intensive insulin treatment could have led to a better outcome in terms of Doris's vision; were my fears that insulin treatment would cause serious iatrogenic complications sufficient to justify not offering it her? Such cognate stories are not the hypothetical fictions of mere 'thought experiments', but reflect the central purpose of clinical medicine—to shape for the better the temporal, biological, and narrative course of human lives.

Acknowledgements

Thanks to Ruth Richardson, Andrew Elder, John Launer, Helen Watson, and James Willis for helpful comments on earlier drafts of this chapter.

4 Mental illness, general practice and society

Iona Heath

My work as a general practitioner is based on an attempted articulation of clear distinctions between concepts of illness, disease and health (Heath 1995). Illness describes the patient's subjective experience. It is the first vague feelings of something being not quite right and it is, and was always, the starting point of the whole endeavour of medicine. In illness, the body makes its presence felt in a way that does not happen in health. No one notices his or her throat until it is sore. Illness is necessarily lonely because no one can share the direct experience of a symptom, and almost all illness carries implicit fear of a diminished life or untimely death.

Disease is quite different and is the stuff of biomedical science. It is a theoretical construct and the means by which humanity has tried to control and make sense of the experience of illness. Each disease is a reified abstraction developed by a process of describing patterns of both symptoms and physical signs, which different patients appear to have in common. As these patterns are refined, the patients come to be described as suffering from the same disease. Thus, biomedical science is based on a series of relatively crude generalizations, which we recognize as diseases. If we group people together according to these disease categories, we can extend our knowledge about the phenomenon that they have in common—be it diabetes or epilepsy. As a direct result, there has been enormous progress in clinical medicine and public health. The great danger is that the spectacular success of biomedical science has lead directly to the common and dangerous delusion that the 'objective' facts of disease are true in a way that the subjective experience of illness is not. The experience of disease is often lonely, but not necessarily so, because once a disease is diagnosed there are, by definition, fellow-sufferers with whom experience can be shared. The diagnosis of disease brings with it the possibility of treatment and some estimate of prognosis that makes explicit the hidden fears of illness.

Put at its simplest, illness is what people have on their way to see the doctor and disease is what they have on the way home. They come with a sore throat;

they go home with tonsillitis. They come with a tummy pain that comes and goes; they go home with irritable bowel syndrome. Almost all disease involves illness, but illness is not necessarily a sign of disease, and exactly similar symptoms can be caused by both disease and unhappiness. Scientific medicine has transformed the human experience of many diseases for the better, but it is not an entirely benign endeavour. One of the crucial tasks of general practice is to strive to distinguish illness caused by disease from that caused by unhappiness, because, if symptoms caused by unhappiness lead to investigations or treatment within the framework of disease, the patient will be exposed to all the dangers, but none of the benefits of biomedical science. The task is to resist the medicalization of ordinary human distress.

Health is quite different again. It is positive, all embracing, and closely related to a sense of being at ease in the world and with oneself. Health has much to do with how society is organized in terms of cohesion, equity, and shared culture. Illness belongs to the individual patient; disease belongs to scientific medicine; health is the gift of an inclusive society.

All the considerable problems of definition in physical illness are heightened in mental illness. The borderline between symptoms caused by unhappiness and disease is even more blurred, and is often scarcely distinguishable. This blurring is manifested in the research finding that more than half of unselected patients in a general practice waiting room have symptoms that fulfil a definition of clinical depression (Kessler *et al.* 1999). Such a finding must raise fundamental questions about definitions of normality and disease, and whether there is any constructive purpose to be served by a definition of disease that includes such a large proportion of the population. If a core task of general practice is to resist the medicalization of illness, this seems to apply with even greater force to mental illness where symptoms are a universal response to existential distress. As general practitioners, we must constantly ask ourselves at what point does it become helpful to the patient to concretize their mental distress as mental illness (Heath 1999).

The shifting sands of definition

In 1917 the American Psychiatric Association recognized 59 psychiatric disorders. With the introduction of the Diagnostic and Statistical Manual, the DSM, in 1952 this rose to 128. The second edition in 1968 had 159, the third in 1980 227, and the revision of the third (DSM-III-R) in 1987 had 253. Now we have DSM-IV, which has 347 categories (Wesseley 1998). What does this mean? Does it represent the progress of science or, somewhat less honourably, an epidemic of medicalization that threatens to engulf an ever-greater proportion of the population (Manning 1999)? Is this degree of definition helpful to the sufferers or does it merely provide intellectual exercise for researchers and specialist clinicians? Patients and general practitioners can perhaps be forgiven some scepticism about the nature of psychiatric diagnosis (Wallace 1988). Anyone reading through the medical records of a patient with a chronic and enduring mental illness will notice the tendency for the diagnosis to shift over time (Blum 1978). Most general practitioners will recognize my experience of patients whose diagnosis has varied along an apparent continuum, which includes schizo-affective disorder, psychotic depression, borderline personality disorder, and schizophrenia. The remarkable thing is how consistent the suggested treatments have been in the face of the changing diagnosis. The cynical view is that the diagnosis seems to matter little as the treatment options are few and are nearly always permutated until a relatively stable, more or less satisfactory outcome is achieved.

The journey to being a patient

Many general practitioners have the extraordinary privilege of knowing patients and families over many years and several generations. We can see mental illness and disease being generated slowly and inexorably and encroaching on the patient's life over a long period of time. We watch as individuals are progressively damaged by the actions and attitudes of families, strangers, the wider society, and themselves (Beitchman *et al.* 1992). Not all of this is malevolent, but the gradual undermining of coherent meaning and self-esteem within the story of a life can be profoundly pernicious. The resources that constitute mental health are systematically eroded, and the process is disturbing and distressing to witness.

The mental health consequences of domestic violence provide one example of this process. Domestic violence is the cause of a shocking amount of private pain and sorrow (Hallett 1995), and as many as 25% of women are estimated to have been exposed to domestic violence at some point in their lives (Mooney 1994; McWilliams and McKiernan 1993). Being a repeated victim of violence is intensely demeaning and demoralizing, and as a result, victims tend to lose their self-esteem and begin to accept the counter-accusation that they themselves are somehow to blame:

> I said Make your own fuckin' tea. That was what happened. Exactly what happened. I provoked him. I always provoked him. I was always to blame. I should have kept my mouth shut. But that didn't work either. I could provoke him that way as well. Not talking. Talking. Looking at him. Not looking at him. Looking at him that way. Not looking at him that way. Looking and talking. Sitting, standing. Being in the room. Being.
> What happened?
> I don't know.
> *(Doyle 1996)*

There is a profound toll on the psychological well being of those who are subjected to repeated abuse, as there also is for their children. Women who have experienced domestic violence suffer a high incidence of psychiatric disorders, particularly depression, and various self-damaging behaviours, including drug and alcohol abuse, suicide, and parasuicide (Jacobson and Richardson 1987; see Chapter 17).

Mad or bad

The murky hinterland between madness and badness pervades the conceptualization of mental illness. The effective practice of medicine depends on the doctor's ability to imaginatively understand the patient's predicament. Only in this way can patients' crucial subjective experience of their symptoms be properly scrutinized. Effective imaginative identification depends on positive regard—an actively fostered willingness to think well of the patient's aspirations and intentions. This is perhaps even more important and more difficult in general practice, where relationships with patients must be sustained over long periods of time. Positive regard implies the rejection of judgmental attitudes, and underpins an attempt to make sense of the patient's attitudes and actions in terms of the reality of their life situation. The increasingly blurred boundary between madness and badness, combined with an enduring moral disjunction between the two, challenges this, and perhaps explains the ever-increasing medicalization of non-conforming or deviant social behaviour. Historically, the criminal and the insane have been treated equally badly by society and often within the same institutions. The development of psychiatry has been a great force for good in improving the life opportunities and experience of those suffering from psychiatric illness. However, today we seem to have arrived at a point where psychiatric discourse has been extended to become the only acceptable means of humanizing society's attitudes to the bad. The result is the conundrum of the personality disorder (Eastman 1999; Mullen 1999; see Chapter 5).

The cynical view from the front-line of general practice is that personality disorder is a convenient diagnostic label, which enables the psychiatrist to evade responsibility for some of the most difficult and challenging patients. The counter argument might be that general practice is even more prone than psychiatry to use 'medical model' reasoning to explain behaviour, which would otherwise be unacceptable. It is probable that this process does a disservice to those whose need for psychiatric care is beyond doubt and it certainly sets GPs an impossible task.

Moral luck

The notion of moral luck, first discussed by Bernard Williams in 1976 (Williams 1981) and further explored by Thomas Nagel (1979), is deeply entangled in the distinction between madness and badness. Nagel described moral luck as follows:

> Where a significant aspect of what someone does depends on factors beyond his control, yet we continue to treat him in that respect as an object of moral judgment, it can be called moral luck.

We all try to make sense of our lives by finding explanations for the events that befall us. We search out explanations for the behaviour of others and, crucially, we hold each other responsible for attitudes and actions. In so doing, we make moral judgements about them. A plea of illness is one of the few grounds that society sanctions for being excused this responsibility, and thereby the moral judgements of others. Those who become criminal and those who suffer serious psychiatric illness tend to share similar life stories and have often been subject to violence, abuse, and loss. Do those of us who have had the moral luck of life stories free of such deep scars, have the right to condemn? When does an explanation of violence condone it and when does it not? Such questions arise whenever a general practitioner, often favoured with moral good luck, meets a patient, burdened by an excess of moral bad luck.

The abuse of psychiatry

The lack of a clear demarcation between madness and badness also goes some way to explaining psychiatry's peculiar susceptibility to political abuse. Fugelli (1999) maintains that:

$$\text{Medicine} = \text{biology} \times \text{individuality} \times \text{culture} \times \text{politics squared}$$

and the preponderance of political influence is underlined by our increasing understanding of the power of the socio-economic determinants of health. Poorer people live shorter and sicker lives. There is a socio-economic gradient for the prevalence of almost every major disease and these gradients are often at their steepest for psychiatric diseases (Thornicroft 1991). The four-fold difference in the rates of male suicide between social classes I and V provides just one example (Gunnell et al. 1995; see Chapter 14). However, at what point does psychiatry become an agent of social control and, beyond that, a tool of political repression? The history of psychiatry demonstrates that it is peculiarly susceptible to being used in the medicalization of political, socio-economic, racial, and homophobic oppression—the medicalization of 'otherness'.

The discontent of the socio-economically deprived will always have the capacity to drive social unrest. However, if the discontented can be described as depressed or found to be suffering from psychological distress, they can be treated with pharmaceuticals or offered counselling. Social unrest is averted, the discontent is subverted and the injustices of society remain untouched. Nothing then disturbs the comfort and complacency of those on the gaining side of injustice. Many general practitioners feel implicated in this process (Berger and Mohr 1967) and implicated more deeply with each prescription for an SSRI written to help someone put up with unacceptable housing conditions.

Those struggling to retain their dignity and to cope at the bottom of a steep socio-economic gradient are marginalized, and excluded from many of the conventional rewards of life. This exclusion may well be reflected in a rejection of 'normal' mainstream attitudes, priorities, and behaviour, and at the extreme of this process, behaviour comes to be regarded as either mad or bad by the rest of society. There is a constant need to guard against the tendency towards normalization that exists within psychiatry. These difficulties are further compounded by issues of cultural diversity and the differing understanding of different behaviour patterns in different cultural contexts. The continuing excess rate of compulsory hospital admission for Afro-Caribbean men remains a major cause of concern:

> It [dysthymic disorder in DSM-III or neurotic depression in ICD-9] may hold coherence in the more affluent West, but it represents the medicalization of social problems in much of the rest of the world (and perhaps the West as well), where severe economic, political and health constraints create endemic feelings of hopelessness and helplessness, where demoralisation and despair are responses to real conditions of chronic deprivation and persistent loss, where powerlessness is not a cognitive distortion but an accurate mapping of one's place in an oppressive social system, and where moral, religious and political configurations of such problems have coherence for the local population, but psychiatric categories do not.
> *(Kleinman 1987)*

Subject/object

The grounding reality of medicine is the patient's subjective story. Everything that comes after is an abstraction from and an approximation to that reality. Illness belongs to individual patients; disease belongs to science. The former is subjective; the latter 'objective'. The patient tells us the story of their illness; we must then summon our knowledge of biomedical science, which by its very nature turns the patient into a standardized human object, and make a judgement as to whether the patient's illness fits into a useful model of disease. The expectation is that such a model will offer effective treatment or even cure.

Medicine is a science whose object is also a subject and there is great danger in thinking about a human being as an object. The dangers are already great with physical illness where the patient can readily feel that the particularity of their experience has been lost and that the doctor can no longer see the person behind the mask of the disease. However, at least in physical illness, the objectification of the body is a process that is already familiar to the patient. The sick body obtrudes into consciousness in a way that the healthy body does not. The body becomes an object that impedes the person's planned or desired activities (Toombs 1993). There can be no exact parallel in mental illness—no one can perceive their own mind as an object. The mind is essentially and inevitably subjective. We experience our own minds as subjects and we also experience the minds of others not as objects or as third persons but as a second person—a 'you'—as another and autonomous subject. This essential subjectivity seems to me to undermine the application of the biomedical model of science in psychiatry in a very fundamental way. The steps of objectifying and generalizing are inevitably partial in the face of the unique individual subjectivity of each human mind.

The discipline of general practice is characterized by the longevity of the relationship between patient and doctor. A doctor and a patient can accompany each other through more than thirty years of shared life history, and a crucial part of their joint task is to try to share some understanding of the patient's experience of illness and disease. Within the rich context of an individual life, the crude simplifications of diagnostic labels can come to seem increasingly irrelevant. Individuals suffering from diabetes can be so different and their experience of illness so various that the doctor begins to wonder whether this is really a unitary phenomenon. However, at least in diabetes, the diagnostic label provides a framework for treatment that is of proven benefit to the patient. The case in psychiatry can seem much less certain:

> we find that labelling is always a dangerous process...because it connotes problems as fixed or invariant.
> *(Anderson and Goolishian 1988)*

Does the too ready use of a label impede the necessary understanding of the individual's particular experience and distress, and the place of that distress within their life story? Marshall Marinker has argued that throughout medicine the diagnosis does not usually precede and rationally dictate the treatment (Marinker 1973). Instead, the diagnosis is used retrospectively to justify a treatment that the doctor has already chosen. Perhaps there are good reasons for this to be the case. The diagnosis of schizophrenia encompasses a great range of abnormal experience, and individual biography and often the treatment is dictated more by the detail of the patient's symptomatology, and the doctor's reactions to it, than by the label itself. This seems to reinforce a tacit recognition of the pre-eminence of the subjective in psychiatry. If the focus on the importance of the subjective was made more explicit, the services for patients with mental illness might become more responsive and sensitive to the particularities of individual need.

There is a large research literature that criticizes general practitioners for their failure to diagnose depression (Goldberg and Huxley 1992), but a crucial part of that failure is the general practitioner's commitment to resist the medicalization of unhappiness (Kendrick 2000). Many patients share their doctor's unease about the diagnosis of depression and seek to make sense of stressful life experience in a way that internalizes it into a coherent life narrative, and sustains the dignity and self-esteem of the sufferer. This process of internalization prevents the progression of illness to disease and is impeded by too ready a diagnosis of disease. Again, a focus on the detail of patients' experience, and their understanding of it, can seem much more constructive than the identification of a diagnostic label and a consequent protocol of treatment. Perhaps psychiatrists, like general practitioners, should be content more often, to confine their efforts to accompanying the patient and witnessing the suffering brought by illness without reaching too quickly for a disease and a treatment (Heath 1995):

> He never separates an illness from the total personality of the patient—in this sense, he is the opposite of a specialist. He does not believe in maintaining his imaginative distance: he must come close enough to recognise the patient fully...He very seldom sends a patient to mental hospital for he considers it a kind of abandonment.
> *(Berger and Mohr 1967)*

Clearly, if effective treatment is available, it should be offered, but it is far more likely to be accepted by the patient in the context of a relationship in which the patient feels heard and understood (Britten 1998).

Stigma

Despite much effort, mental illness still carries a significant stigma (Porter 1998). Part of this seems connected to the fact that being ill relieves individuals of some of their responsibilities to the rest of society. In this respect, the subjectivity of mental illness can become a liability. Physical illness provides apparently objective proof of the existence of illness beyond the control of the sufferer. In contrast, the subjectivity of mental illness makes it much more elusive and less open to any form of objective verification. Sufferers are excused their responsibilities, but also excluded in a way that, whilst no longer as cruel as it once was, often remains judgmental and condemnatory. The pervasive, atavistic fear of mental disintegration means that the apparently 'normal' can be keen to draw a clear demarcation between themselves and those others who suffer mental illness. This barrier nurtures the stigma that many sufferers feel. The public perception that severe mental illness lies at the root of much violent crime further stigmatizes sufferers and this impression is easily exacerbated by sensationalist media reporting (Ferriman 2000).

Discrimination

Stigma is compounded by discrimination and, regrettably, discrimination against those suffering from mental illness remains endemic within the organization of National Health Service. Increasingly rigid geographical catchment areas for mental health services mean that patients are given no choice of specialist mental health care. This is in stark contrast with most physical illness for which the general practitioner will have a range of referral possibilities to offer the patient.

The elderly mentally ill face even worse discrimination, to the extent that those suffering from Alzheimer's disease and similar conditions have seen their health care needs systematically excluded from the universal provision of the NHS. The vast bulk of these health care needs are for intimate personal care, and for stimulation and encouragement. These are all low-technology skills and this has allowed them to be redefined as social care that can be charged for on the basis of a means test (Heath 2000).

Sensibility and insight

Despite the very widespread stigmatization and fear of mental illness, there are tantalizing connections between madness and creativity. Many major creative artists have had serious mental illnesses and many more ordinary patients with mental illness seem to have an exceptional sensibility. Many of the patients I have known seem to have had an emotional susceptibility which gives them great insight into human nature and its predicaments. However, this insight also leaves them vulnerable to the loss of balance that seems to lie at the root of so much mental illness. Many patients seem to be aware of both the rewards and the risks of their sensibility and have a very accurate appreciation of how much it is blunted by 'tranquillizing' psychiatric medication:

> Whenever their lives were set aflame, through desire or suffering, or even reflection, the Homeric heroes knew that a god was at work. They endured the god, and observed him, but what actually happened as a result was a surprise most of all for themselves.
>
> No psychology since has ever gone beyond this; all we have done is invent, for those powers that act upon us, longer, more numerous, more awkward names, which are less effective, less closely aligned to the gain of our experience, whether that be pleasure or terror... What we consider infirmity they saw as 'divine infatuation' (*áte*). They knew that this invisible incursion often brought ruin: so much that the word *áte* would gradually come to mean 'ruin'. But they also knew, and it was Sophocles who said it, that 'mortal life can never have anything grandiose about it except through *áte*'.
> (*Calasso 1994*)

Part of the stereotypical description of patients suffering mental illness is that they lack insight into their own condition. Gadamer (1996) points out what an odd notion this is. Denial has always been part of the human response to illness and the more serious the illness the more likely is the patient to deny something of its reality. Paradoxically, such denial is often regarded as courageous in the face of physical illness, but reprehensible in the mentally ill.

Physical health and mental illness

All bodily illness has consequences for the mind and all mental illness affects the body:

> As living things we are wholly taken up by anger, completely shaken by fear. We are not angry or fearful in just one part of the soul.
> *(Gadamer 1996)*

The chronically mentally ill often have very poor physical health (see Chapter 13) and a significantly reduced expectation of life. The increasing separation of mental health services within NHS, exacerbated by the creation of Mental Health Trusts, illustrates and institutionalizes the enduring fiction of the mind–body split. The physical consequences of poor mental health are more and more widely recognized, and yet the re-organization of the health service will locate the specialist care of physical illnesses and mental illnesses at geographically separate sites. This will run the risk of systematically distancing those with the most serious mental illness from the physical care that they need. The increasing numbers of patients who suffer both a serious mental illness and a serious physical illness, such as diabetes, epilepsy, or asthma, have a very poor prognosis. Yet, there is very little research on the best and most effective ways of managing such patients, particularly when the situation is further compounded by significant abuse of alcohol or drugs. Care based on guidelines formulated for people suffering a single disease is very unlikely to be effective.

Listening and hearing

General practitioners strive to approach their patients closely, to understand the detail of the experience of illness and distress, and not only to listen to stories, but to hear them. The challenge is always to approach closely enough: not to delude ourselves about the nature of what we see and hear, and not to seek the shelter of the familiar structures of biomedicine before we have recognized and acknowledged the experience that the patient brings. The inevitable yet essential reductionism of biomedical discourse is always an impediment to understanding, and needs always to be balanced by a valuing of experience that does not fit:

> I am also convinced
> That you only hold a fragment of the explanation.
> It is only because of what you do not understand
> That you feel the need to declare what you do.
> There is more to understand: hold fast to that
> As the way to freedom.
> *(Eliot 1939)*

The whole enterprise of medicine is predicated on the patient being able to communicate the nature of their distress to the doctor. The patient can trust the doctor's intervention and treatment only if he or she feels that their experience of illness has been understood. A too rapid process of diagnostic labelling can undermine this understanding. The meanings of illness, the threat, the fear, the suffering, and the endurance can only be interpreted, ordered, and contained if both doctors and patients can find and agree on the right words. In this, the task of the consultation parallels that of poetry:

> Poetic form is both the ship and the anchor. It is at once a buoyancy and a holding, allowing for the simultaneous gratification of whatever is centrifugal and centripetal in mind and body. It is by such means that Yeats's work does what the necessary poetry always does, which is to touch the base of our sympathetic nature while taking in at the same time the unsympathetic reality of the world to which that nature is constantly exposed. The form of the poem, in other words, is crucial to poetry's power to do the thing which always is and always will be to poetry's credit: the power to persuade that vulnerable part of our consciousness of its rightness in spite of the evidence of wrongness all around it, the power to remind us that we are hunters and gatherers of values, that our very solitudes and distresses are creditable, in so far as they, too, are an earnest of our veritable being.
> *(Heaney 1995)*

Language enables us to mirror human experience and to find meaning in it that can be shared with others to make us feel less alone. Poets and novelists make use of the whole resource of language, and 'that sedimented reason which resides in all use of language' (Gadamer 1996), and doctors need a similar aspiration. Any restriction of language to a particular discourse closes off the possibility of understanding. At its best, the consultation allows both the 'buoyancy' of a detailed exploration of individual suffering and the 'holding' of a careful setting of that suffering within the context of our shared human experience of a frequently hostile world.

Understanding the distorted and tumultuous experience of the psychotic mind poses particular challenges:

> O that awful privacy
> Of the insane mind!
> *(Eliot 1939)*

> The final difficulty of reading madness... is that in the act of doing so, one dissociates oneself from it or associates oneself with it, and in either case becomes disqualified as an interpreter. To read madness sanely is to miss the point; to read madness madly is to have one's point be missed.
> *(Neely 1991)*

Yet, the universality and inclusiveness of language will always have the potential to make the connections necessary to at least begin a dialogue (Roberts 1999):

> What takes place here between doctor and patient is a form of attentiveness, namely the ability to sense the demands of an individual person at a particular moment and to respond to those demands in an appropriate manner... It is an attempt to set in motion once again the communicative flow of the patient's life

> experience and to re-establish that contact with others from which the person
> is so tragically excluded.
> *(Gadamer 1996)*

The changing focus of mental health services

Over the last 25 years, there have been huge changes in the configuration of mental health services. The key change was the closure of the large long-stay mental hospitals during the 1980s. Since then there have been many more people with serious and enduring mental illness living within communities and registered on general practitioners' practice lists. Many patients cope extraordinary well, but others have great difficulty managing the necessities of daily living, and quickly lapse into degrees of self-neglect and even squalor. The extraordinary prevalence of severe mental illness among the street homeless remains an indictment of current systems of care (Bhugra 1996). Mental health professionals have been forced to re-orientate their services to focus on the needs of the severely mentally ill, and to attempt to minimize the risks that such patients pose to themselves and those who might come into contact with them. Somehow this seems to have led to an emphasis on processing and labelling at the expense of the depth of engagement, which could perhaps hold out greater hope of making a real difference to the quality of people's lives. Less seriously 'ill' patients (however disabled) have been increasingly excluded from specialist services and the possibility of preventing deterioration seems to have been reduced accordingly.

How could things be better?

We need a mental health service which:

- is grounded in the notion of positive regard;
- is built on listening and 'enabling' (Howie *et al.* 1999);
- provides a response to all degrees of seriousness of mental ill-health and tries to prevent less serious problems becoming much more serious over time;
- provides an accessible service to all subgroups within the population—particularly the most vulnerable—adolescents, the homeless, some members of ethnic minority communities, refugees and asylum seekers, the old, single unemployed men, etc.;
- is aware of the genesis of much mental ill-health within damaged and damaging families and attempts to provide intensive therapeutic support to such families;
- provides an adequate response to the very steep socio-economic gradient in mental ill-health;

- is properly integrated with services for those who misuse drugs and alcohol;
- is aware that many of those suffering chronic mental illness also suffer physical ill-health;
- is multi-disciplinary, involves all members of the primary health care team and extends beyond that team to make uses of resources within local communities, local authorities, and patients themselves;
- uses medication frugally, sceptically, and in an appropriately evidence-based manner, and reassesses the continuing need for medication at regular intervals;
- enables equity of access to the psychological and psychotherapeutic treatment modalities;
- is aware of the dangerous potential for abuse within psychiatry.

The main barriers to achieving such a service are the lack of time, trust and resources, and the background of an unjust society that distributes opportunity and hope in a profoundly inequitable manner. Primary care professionals and mental health professionals need to work together to maximize the former and to advocate at every opportunity for the alleviation of the latter.

Conclusion

Current sources of information for establishing 'population needs' for mental health care are largely confined to hospital admission rates and the prescribing rates for various forms of psychotropic medication. In some areas, disease registers (see Chapter 13) have been created for patients with severe and enduring mental illness, but these have usually been constructed from repeat prescribing records and may miss those who have stopped their medication. Registers of such potentially stigmatizing conditions also raise serious questions of patient confidentiality and whether appropriate consent has been obtained for the inclusion of names on the register. There is an urgent need for Primary Care Trusts and similar organizations in the other home nations, to find more subtle and sensitive ways of describing and measuring the burden of mental ill health within communities. Those who plan services need to work much more closely with those working in the front-line of primary care who witness the generation and life course of almost the whole extent of mental illness and disease. If this could be achieved, we would have a firm foundation on which to build improved mental health services and, perhaps in this way, society could be made a better place for the mentally ill and for those who try to care for them.

Part II
Reflective practice

5 The difficult patient

Eia Asen

Anyone working in primary care will have had their fair share of difficult patients—and probably a paucity of 'easy' patients. In this chapter we look at patients who are not just difficult, but who are a considerable problem to their doctors or other primary care workers. The first step is to examine the term 'difficult patient'. It is vague and ill defined, and likely to evoke a whole range of associations. For example, aggressive and challenging patients will come to mind for some workers, or those 'heart sink' patients who turn up seemingly endless times for consultations and who do not respond to any of their doctors' best efforts (Wamoscher 1966). Most annoyingly to their doctors, these patients tend to present with somatic symptoms that wander from one part of the body to another (Van Eijk 1983). Then there are those patients who some doctors find difficult simply because they want to have long explanations for whatever is wrong with them and who repeatedly question the wisdom of their doctors' remedies and prescriptions. It can be seen that what is a difficult patient for one practitioner may be an ordinary one for another. Calling a patient difficult is probably as much a reflection of the doctor's prejudices or tolerance level as having to do with the patient's specific characteristics.

The patient in context

When patient and doctor meet, each brings a whole set of individual characteristics—beliefs, wishes, hopes, and fears—into this encounter. Together they create a context—the consultation—that can be experienced in many different ways by each participant (Neighbour 1987). One possible outcome of a consultation is that the doctor experiences the patient as difficult. This means that the doctor locates the difficulty as being only inside the patient. Yet, an outside observer, perhaps a registrar, may well have a different perception of the patient—and the doctor. The observer may focus on the interaction between doctor and patient, and perceive the interaction as being difficult, rather than just blaming one party. The patient, on the other hand, may find his doctor difficult. Who then is right? The answer is simple: nobody and everybody!

The difficult patient needs to be viewed in context—that of the doctor–patient relationship. The interactions are between doctor and patient, with one person requesting a consultation and treatment from the other, on the basis of special qualifications and experience. The outcome is primarily determined by:

- the nature and context of the consultation;
- the characteristics of the patient;
- the characteristics of the doctor.

Examining each of these three dimensions may help to de-construct the notion of the 'difficult' patient.

The nature of the request: buying and selling health?

Balint (1957) and many practitioners after him (Bourne 1976; Temperley 1978; Elder 1987; Wiener and Sher 1998) have examined the different conscious and unconscious requests patients make when they present with symptoms to their doctor. Influenced by psychoanalytic thinking, this work has looked not only at the patient's mind, but also focused on the interactions between doctor and patient. In this chapter a different metaphor for describing aspects of the doctor–patient relationship will be introduced—in line with the current political obsession with 'purchasing' health care. Patients—more fashionably now known as 'users', having survived a previous incarnation as 'customers'—can be seen to be going to their general practitioners to 'buy' some health. The market metaphor of buyer, vendor, and goods may be useful in clarifying how the concept of the difficult patient—and, indeed, the difficult doctor—emerges interactionally. Using the market metaphor permits the construction of a range of possible scenarios.

A common scenario is that of the patient who wants to buy the goods that the doctor has to sell. For example, the patient who is depressed may wish to purchase examination, diagnosis, and relevant medication from the doctor. If these 'goods' are on sale, and patient and doctor agree on the purchase, then both patient and doctor are likely to be satisfied. Here, we have the scenario of a 'good' doctor and a 'good' patient. The doctor is likely to think of the patient as normal if not 'easy' (as opposed to 'difficult')—and the patient may have very similar thoughts about the doctor.

However, what if the doctor really wants to sell a psychotherapeutic intervention, counselling, for example, but the patient simply wants medication? Most doctors tend to believe in user choice and will eventually allow the patient to decide. Even if doctors are disappointed at the outcome of the consultation, they will hardly think of the patient as 'difficult'—at least not the first time round. However, if this situation keeps happening, then it is likely that the doctor will feel increasingly misused by a patient who does not want to buy the recommended products. Patients who want to buy what the doctor does not really want to sell run the risk of becoming—sooner or later—defined as 'difficult'. It is equally likely that doctors who repeatedly do not want to give their patients what they want, will also be defined by their patients as 'difficult'. In this scenario, the patient's complaint fits with what the doctor has on offer, but the doctor's preferred remedy is not purchased by the patient.

The scenario of the patients' symptoms not fitting the doctor's remedies is very different. There are patients who are preoccupied with their bodies, consulting their doctor endlessly for what appear to be minor physical complaints, from fatigue to unspecific joint pains, from dizziness to vague abdominal pain (Markus *et al.* 1989). None of the investigations reveal any evidence of pathology, none of the remedies offered seem to work. Frequent attenders—also known as 'the fat file syndrome'—are a time-consuming group of 'heart sink' patients and doctors tend to become increasingly impatient, if not anti-patient, with them. These patients seem to want to purchase further expensive and time-consuming investigations, and have a tendency of asking for referrals to specialist services, much against the doctor's inner convictions or judgment. There comes a point when all the resources—and the doctor's patience—are exhausted. When the doctor states to the patient that there is 'nothing physically wrong with you' and therefore not much more that can be done, the patient usually feels misunderstood, misdiagnosed, or neglected. This is the point when patients can become 'difficult', as they are unlikely to be satisfied with the explanation that there is 'nothing wrong' with them: why would they see their doctor if they felt all right? To these patients their symptoms are real and the obvious response is to ask for more rather than less. They may become more demanding and difficult, making a formal complaint or expressing the wish to see another doctor in the same surgery. Despite all the hard work going into explorations and investigations, the doctor no longer has any goods to sell—in fact, doctors often feel at this point that they have 'sold out'. The doctor's self-image of being a competent professional is not nurtured by a continuation of such interactions, and sooner or later the patient gets blamed. Doctors, like any other human beings, tend to defend themselves by projecting their own hopelessness into others. Another difficult patient is born.

Here is another familiar scenario: the patient seemingly buys what the doctor has to sell, but then does not use the product, putting it on the shelf or flushing it down the toilet. The so-called non-compliant patient is familiar to all general practitioners, saying that he tried the prescribed remedy just once, but that the side effects were just too strong. No efforts on the doctor's part is sufficient to convince the patient to give it another try and allow the remedy to work. The patient asks for a new tablet and the doctor knows only too well that there is no chance whatsoever that the patient will make appropriate use of it. The more the doctor tries the less the patient complies. It is not difficult to see how such an interaction will result in the doctor seeing the patient as being rather 'difficult'.

The scenario of the patient apparently complying with the remedy provided, but this making no difference to the symptoms, is not an uncommon one. The symptoms may shift from one part of the body to another despite all good efforts. The patient is dissatisfied and the doctor does not know what to do next. Increasingly, the doctor will feel blamed for selling the wrong product, and a whole range of similar or different interventions will be tried, as well as increasing or decreasing the dose or frequency of medication or psychological treatment. The doctor starts doubting the diagnosis and wonders whether it is he or the patient who is 'wrong'. When the doctor decides that all that can be done has been done, it is the patient who will eventually end up being classified as 'difficult'. Here, it would seem that all the known goods the doctor can sell are useless, with the patient sampling half-heartedly what is on offer.

Some patients insist on their doctor selling more goods than he or she would really like to. Demanding patients, with ever increasing new requests, seemingly insatiable, can be experienced as very difficult. Requests for more and more investigations or medications escalate. Amongst this group, drug addicts for whom doctors prescribe methadone are particularly difficult to satisfy, with their frequent requests for urgent appointments and even more frequent non-attendances. These patients tend to be demanding and difficult to contain in general practice. Doctors can find this group of patients difficult because of their ability to be dishonest and to play one doctor off against another, particularly when targeting registrar GPs or locums in the hope that they might trick them into prescribing extra amounts of drugs.

When the patient repeatedly insists on *buying a product that is simply not on sale*, we have another scenario that can result in the patient being called 'difficult'. Patients at times appear to have come to the wrong address. It appears that they want help with financial issues, housing or legal advice. The patient who attributes all his problems to his appalling living conditions and asks the doctor to get him re-housed is a common example. The doctor can re-direct the patient to the appropriate agency or professional, but at times this may be fruitless as long as the patient persists that it *is* the doctor's job.

These are some of the scenarios that are common in general practice. The metaphor of buying and selling health, limited though it may seem at one level, not only helps to understand some of the interactions between doctor and patient, but also enables the formulation of survival strategies. Doctors can reflect on what it is that the allegedly 'difficult' patient wishes to purchase and whether the desired product is 'in stock'. They can then consider whether they wish to sell this item or recommend another one, and speculate about the consequences of either action. Furthermore, doctors can ask themselves whether they should stock up some new goods in their 'shop' or whether they should help the patient to choose one of the goods already available—or, indeed, no goods at all.

Typology of difficult patients

Describing the phenomenon of the difficult patient simply in interactional and contextual terms would be a one-dimensional approach. Clearly, personal characteristics play a big role and can affect the doctor–patient relationship very much. Some individuals seem to be intrinsically difficult, and almost anybody interacting with them might end up with very similar impressions. Traditional psychiatry has invented a typology for difficult or 'impossible' patients, once referred to as 'psychopaths' and nowadays called 'personality disorders'.

The term 'personality disorder' is often invoked when patients appear to defy the doctor (see previous chapter). When appropriately used it refers to an 'enduring pattern of inner experience and behaviour that... is pervasive and inflexible, has an onset in adolescence or early adulthood, is stable over time, and leads to distress or impairment' (DSM-IV 1994). Ten different specific personality disorders are identified in diagnostic manuals of mental disorders and they can be grouped in three clusters, based on descriptive similarities:

- Cluster A includes the paranoid, schizoid and schizotypal personality disorders, with patients often appearing peculiar or eccentric.

- Cluster B contains antisocial, borderline, histrionic and narcissistic personality disorders, with patients presenting in demanding, dramatic and challenging ways.

- Cluster C consists of patients in whom anxious and fearful behaviour patterns dominate; the personality disorders in this group are categorized as avoidant, dependent and obsessive-compulsive.

It is obvious that human beings are infinitely more complex than any system of classification can hope to encompass, and there is often a problem in making a person fit all or most of the required features of a specific disorder. The actual psychiatric diagnosis of 'personality disorder' is dependent on the presence of quite a number of specific criteria. Very few of the patients experienced by their doctors as being 'difficult' are likely to meet these criteria and thus warrant the diagnosis of personality disorder. However, quite a few patients may well have personality traits some of which fit the descriptions. Having such traits does not qualify someone to be described as having a personality disorder—otherwise many of us would walk around with that label. Moreover, there is also an important clinical issue in that it is often (wrongly) stated that there are no effective treatments for personality disorder: if this label is too readily applied to a difficult patient, then this patient may be effectively written off by the doctor. If the patient feels his doctor is giving up on him, he will become more 'awkward' and demanding, with the result that this, in turn, will only confirm the doctor's 'diagnosis'. Here, the diagnosis of personality disorder is at risk of becoming a self-fulfilling prophecy. However, this does not invalidate the concept of personality *traits* and in the following section those traits that tend to be associated with causing difficulties in primary care are described.

Patients with *paranoid personality traits* present themselves finding it very difficult to trust their doctor, refusing to answer personal questions, and reading hidden negative meanings into benign remarks. Such patients tend to misinterpret compliments or view a simple mistake by the receptionist as a deliberate attempt to slight them. It is not unusual for patients with paranoid personality traits to bear grudges against members of the helping professions, exhibiting a marked unwillingness to forgive 'insults' or 'bad treatment' they feel they have received. Minor conflicts arouse major hostility that can last for a long time. It is interesting that patients with other related personality traits, such as schizoid features, cause less discomfort to primary care workers, probably because the affected individuals often have flat emotions and are odd and shy, with a seeming indifference to the approval or criticism of others.

Antisocial traits manifest themselves in a variety of ways that make these patients difficult at times: aggressiveness, disregard for safety of self and others, impulsivity, and deceitfulness. Impulsivity is also an important feature of borderline traits, expressing itself in recurrent suicidal threats and gestures, as well as self-mutilating behaviour. Patients displaying borderline traits often involve potential helpers in complex rescuing missions, eliciting simultaneously hope and despair in the professionals working with them.

Histrionic personality traits can be on occasion difficult for doctors, with affected individuals interacting in inappropriate sexually seductive or provocative ways. These patients' sense of self-dramatization, their theatricality and exaggerated expressions of emotion are often perceived as entertaining by their doctors, and this tends to reinforce the display of these traits.

Patients presenting with *narcissistic personality traits* may be irritating, but they are rarely seen as 'difficult'. Their often grandiose sense of self-importance and of being 'special' is perceived by outsiders as arrogance, and their inability or unwillingness to recognize and identify with the feelings and needs of others may lead doctors to show less and less interest in them over time. *Avoidant personality traits* are rarely a cause for experiencing a patient as difficult or troublesome. Individuals with these traits view themselves as inept socially and inferior to others, and thus show restraint about getting involved in intimate relationships and avoid activities that involve significant interpersonal contact.

This is quite a different matter with *dependent personality traits*. These include a difficulty with making everyday decisions without an excessive amount of advice and reassurance from others. Primary care workers often get drawn into endless discussions on seemingly trivial matters, giving advice where much identical advice has already been given. Ironically, with each new helper becoming involved, the patient's dependence grows, with others assuming more responsibility for major areas of his or her life. The lack of self-confidence, inadvertently reinforced by the increased presence of helpers, contributes to the patient's inability to initiate projects or make plans. After initial periods of irritation, doctors gradually become more impatient, and attempt to challenge the patient. The patient usually finds it impossible to express disagreement for fear of losing professional support, increasing her efforts and going through excessive lengths to obtain nurturance from others. When it seems impossible to break this cycle, the patient will be called 'difficult'.

Patients with anxious and *obsessive-compulsive personality traits* tend not to be seen as 'difficult' by their doctors—even though their families often feel irritated if not terrorized by these traits.

In summary, it is generally more useful to think of personality *traits*, rather than be too quick to diagnose a personality disorder—because of the closure and finality that such a label usually implies. It is very rare that a whole personality is disordered and it is a more positive approach to think of personality or character traits that may be present but can be complemented by or balanced with other good traits and personal strengths.

Hateful patients

Another way of looking at difficult patients has been suggested by Groves (1978), with grouping patients who evoke strong feelings in their doctors into four stereotypes. *Dependent clingers* escalate from appropriate requests for reassurance to endless cries for all forms of attention imaginable. Their self-perception of bottomless need is matched by their belief in the doctor as inexhaustible. Flattery may initially 'seduce' the doctor though the patients' developing intense dependency eventually creates a sense of aversion in primary care workers. *Entitled demanders* use somewhat different tactics—intimidation, guilt induction, and disqualification. The effects on doctors can be devastating—from feeling useless, to becoming fearful about reputation, to getting angry that the patient is not co-operative. Fear often leads doctors to counter-attack, setting up a cycle that corners the patient who then feels even more entitled to make more and more unrealistic demands. *Manipulative help-rejecters* are another category of patients described by Groves (1978), only too familiar to most practitioners. They behave as if they believed that no treatment could possibly help, returning again and again to the surgery, reporting that the regimen did not work. Sooner or later these behaviours elicit in the doctor anxiety that a treatable illness has been overlooked, and eventually lead clinicians to experience feelings of guilt and inadequacy. *Self-destructive deniers* present with chronic forms of seemingly unconscious self-harming behaviour, such as serious drinking when liver failure is present. Caregivers, getting increasingly impatient, eventually secretly wish that the patient would die and 'get it over and done with'.

What most of these 'hateful' patients have in common are strong dependency needs that stimulate a series of negative feelings in most doctors. Practitioners who feel aversion or even hatred towards one of their patients need to set limits on dependency. Naming these needs and becoming curious about why it is that the patient requires the doctor to fulfil requests and demands that cannot be met, is a first step to addressing these.

Typology of difficult doctors

Difficulties may also result from the doctor's personality and his reaction to the patient. Doctors, for example, who are excessively independent may be rather impatient with patients who are prone to self-pity, dismissing them as undeserving of their care. By contrast, doctors who tend to feel sorry for themselves may give in to any requests patients make for advice, treatment, and domiciliary visits, indirectly encouraging their patients to become dependent on them. Livesey (1996) lists a few medical personality types, which include the controlling doctor, the excessively sympathetic practitioner, the excessively conscientious doctor, the busy, and the jolly doctor (see next chapter). Each of these personality features may be brought out by some specific patients and the resulting interaction will make the doctor seem 'difficult' in the patient's eyes—and the patient 'difficult' in the doctor's eyes.

As already outlined, the context of the consultation and the personal characteristics of the patient are two of the three main factors that determine whether a patient receives the label 'difficult'. The third dimension concerns doctors' own individual features and histories. These often enter the consultation in overt or covert ways. Doctors and other primary care workers, like any professional group, have their own experiences and beliefs, all of which inform their view of the patient. For example, a doctor whose husband is tired and low all the time, is likely to be affected by this daily reality. It is quite possible that she may be particularly sympathetic to a male patient presenting with non-specific complaints of being low and tired all the time (TAT). However, it is also possible for the reverse to happen in that she could find this patient increasingly 'difficult'—particularly if he fails to respond to her good advice and bio-psychological interventions.

Other doctors may be informed by different experiences, present or past:

Dr Clot, for example, felt seriously affected by a patient some years ago that he had diagnosed as suffering from mild tension headaches. Despite the patient's continuing complaints over a period of a whole year, Dr Clot continued to believe that the symptoms were essentially evidence of psychological distress. This proved wrong when an underlying, by then inoperable brain tumour was discovered. This experience sensitized Dr Clot and made him very anxious about any somatic presentation, however vague. His practice partners accused him of being over-investigative and he replied that he had to do this 'to be on the safe side'. To Dr Clot no patient ever seemed to be too 'difficult'—however much they were demanding his attention.

Another category of doctors is those who do not believe in the importance of emotions or psychological problems. They tend to have what is euphemistically known as a 'matter of fact approach' and find difficulty with any display of emotion. They try to talk their patients out of 'fussing too much' and ask them 'to pull yourself together'. Those patients who are reluctant to oblige get some direct or indirect encouragement not to return for further consultations—if they have not voted with their feet already. It is not uncommon that when seeing another doctor in the practice, that same patient gets redefined as being 'sensitive'.

Doctors can often be unaware of the difference between their perceived medical functions, and their personal attitudes and feelings towards the patient (Courtenay and Hare 1978). Certain patients will provoke a reaction rather than an understanding from certain doctors. This can have different reasons: an explosive 'fit' between the patient's and the doctor's deeper personal issues; a growing desire to control the patient rather than to remain responsible for aspects of the patients' health; a genuine inability to contain some patients' worries and anxieties. It is usually in the patient's interest that the doctor retains some measure of control, but only enough to discharge his responsibility (Courtenay and Hare 1978). If doctors are not secure in their own self-knowledge and aware of their strengths, as well as limitations, they can become 'difficult doctors' with certain patients. They become defensive, and their patients experience them as awkward or remote. Doctors, like other professionals, employ conscious and unconscious defences to protect themselves from an emotional engagement with some patients. Yet, some of these defences can be out of proportion and prevent doctors from being able to share the patient's feelings in helpful and therapeutic ways (Main 1978). Certain predisposing factors, such as tiredness, illness, preoccupation with personal problems, anger with practice team members, stress caused by shortage of time, all make it more likely that doctors avoid subjective encounters with their patients' feelings (Salinsky and Sackin 2000). Gaining some insight into the reasons for their defensive reactions enables doctor to slow these down and to modify them—for the benefit of their patients.

Reflective doctors

Another type of practitioner is what we shall term the reflective doctor. When experiencing a patient as difficult, this doctor starts an *inner conversation*, reflecting on the nature and context of the consultation, the patient's individual characteristics and traits—as well as engaging in some self-reflective practice. In doing so, the doctor needs to become curious about his or her own position: what is it that might be going on in his own life that could resonate with the patient's predicament? How might the doctor's own personal characteristics, traits and issues 'fit' with those of the patient? This self-reflective curiosity (Cecchin 1987) aims to generate questions that beg for hypotheses that can lead to some speculative answers.

When thinking of a patient as 'difficult', reflective doctors are aware of both their own and the patient's personal characteristics and histories, as well as the specific context that is created through the interactions in the consulting room. Whilst this may be a desirable state, in practice, time constraints and other limitations make it unlikely that this can be practiced with each and every patient. In fact, too much reflection might well result in paralysis and inaction. However, when feeling at a total loss with a difficult patient it may save time and energy to become reflective.

Strategies for survival

It seems that the type of doctor described as 'reflective' above, has the best chance of surviving difficult patients. How then can doctors and other primary health care workers learn to engage in reflective practice? In this section a step-by-step guide is presented to assist professionals deal with what seem to be difficult patients.

The first step is to take time to reflect on the nature and context of the consultation, possibly using the purchasing and selling health metaphor. The doctor can ask herself: what sort of scenario is this? What does the patient want to 'buy'? What can I—what do I want—to sell? An example may help to illustrate this point:

Mrs Diff is a frequent attender at Dr Law's surgery. She usually presents with minor ailments. Fixing an appointment with the receptionist proves a major task as no time or day ever seems ever right and negotiations can take up considerable time. She telephones a lot, expecting to speak to Dr Law in person then and there because of some urgent 'problem'. The receptionists have found many different strategies for protecting the doctor from these unwanted telephone calls. Mrs Diff seems only too aware of her limited access to her doctor and never stops complaining about 'not being allowed to speak to my doctor'. Once in the consulting room Mrs Diff talks solidly for the first five minutes of the consultation, listing a whole range of new and old symptoms. She also makes frequent references to not being liked, everyone ganging up against her and having nobody to talk to. Through-out this very repetitive and familiar stream of words Dr Law is mostly preoccupied with how to get Mrs Diff out of the consulting room. Mrs Diff leaves the surgery thirty minutes later, armed with the next appointment for a few days later. Dr Law generally feels totally helpless and useless in relation to this patient and has given up hope of finding a better strategy—other than just to be there.

In considering how to work with this difficult patient the practitioner might first feel tempted to look at Mrs Diff's personality issues. On the face of it, there seem to be some paranoid and dependent traits present. One could leave it at that or think about the effects of these traits on anyone interacting with Mrs Diff. Making massive demands on reception and professional staff often provokes the opposite of what may be consciously intended: after initial attempts to be helpful, avoidance manoeuvres on part of the staff will set in. Of course, such responses reinforce the feelings of dependence, rejection and of not being liked. Most paranoid ideas have some basis in (external) reality and people with these traits tend to act in such ways as to confirm their view that the world is against them. Thinking about this might lead the practitioner to examine the context of the consultation. The patient wants to buy something that is in short supply. At one level she wants to be examined and prescribed a remedy for her physical complaints. At another level she might want to buy affection, perhaps some physical contact in the course of an examination, perhaps some psychological or social contact through the conversation with the doctor. Dr Law might just want to sell what he is best at selling: a thorough physical examination and some placebo medication. Here there is a discrepancy between what buyer and vendor want. Dr Law may well have to consider offering something quite different from what is usually on offer—otherwise the patient will continue the stuck relationship pattern with the practice. Before changing tack, Dr Law may also wish to reflect on his own disposition in relation to Mrs Diff: what does she trigger in him? Who in his life may have similar ways of relating to people? What are the personal issues preoccupying him at this point in his life?

It is not suggested that general practitioners should always reflect in such detail on every patient—there is simply not enough time. However, when it comes to dealing with difficult patients, this may be quite an economic way of taking stock. These patients tend to absorb much energy—and time. Patients perceived as being 'difficult' can evoke extreme emotional responses in their doctors: high anxiety or boredom. Doctors need a survival kit to combat these emotions. Perhaps the most important weapon to avoid burnout is that of curiosity (see next chapter). As long as the doctor remains curious about the patient, and his or her predicament, the difficult patient is not at risk of becoming impossible. It is therefore the doctor's task to find ways of becoming and remaining curious (Cecchin 1987). One way of doing this is continuously to create new perspectives on the patient's symptoms and predicament, thus widening and changing the field of observation. The curious doctor—curious about wanting to find out why a particular patient is seen as difficult—will try to make the connections between otherwise unseen aspects of the patient's life and relationships, past or present, examining how the mind speaks for the body at one moment and the body speaks for the mind at another (Elder 1996). This can be done in a number of different ways.

Family orientated questions

One way of opening up new perspectives is to introduce the family dimension through gentle probing. Dr Law may ask Mrs Diff a series of questions, aimed at getting the patient to contextualize her symptoms:

Who in your family knows about your tummy aches? How are your aches affecting members of your family? What sort of responses do you get? Who is most sympathetic? Who least? Who or what tends to make the aches better? Is there anything you yourself can do (or not do) to make them get better? If your tummy ache could speak, what might it say?

These and other questions aim to examine the context in which the aches occur. This not only reawakens the doctor's interest in his patient by focusing on another dimension of her life, but it also raises questions for Mrs Diff. She is invited to become curious about the various aches, their fluctuations, the effects on others, and the effects of those near and dear on the aches. In this way the symptoms become connected with the outside world, rather than just being located in her body. Such a consultation need not last more than 10 minutes, and can be followed up by asking the patient to keep a diary about the aches or pains, day by day, when they occur, how long they last for, and what makes them better or worse. Another appointment can be made a fortnight later to look at the findings and further consultations can follow with doctor and patient, like a pair of detectives, jointly hunting for the patterns surrounding the symptoms, united in their quest to identify the guilty part(ies). It is this joint quest that may be a new experience for the patient who has hitherto felt isolated and marginalized. The task challenges her alleged paranoid and dependent ways of behaving—a new context is created. The patient is turned into the investigator of her own aches and pains, and thus becomes a collaborator in the diagnostic and treatment process. The process of self-observation and the recording of onset, duration, and circumstances of the symptoms often helps patients to make some important connections (Asen and Tomson 1992).

The process of questioning can be powerful in that it helps patients look at their symptoms and themselves in a new light. Patients are encouraged to view other people in relation to themselves, as well as speculating how, in their view, others see *them*. In this way the patient perceives himself and his relationships through the eyes of another person, and compares this with his own perceptions. It is a way of interviewing that releases 'latent' information and enables individuals to make their own sense of their living situation. The process of asking questions that make patients reflect about themselves and others gets them involved in writing or re-writing their stories: disjointed and random events become connected, fixed scripts start crumbling with new connections being weaved. Some of these questions are known as circular questions (Selvini Palazzoli *et al.* 1980), as each question is based on the feedback the patient provides. In this way, a kind of circle is formed, whereby the patient is involved in his own feedback from which further questions are constructed by the doctor. Box 5.1 lists possible questions that may be relevant in some consultations in general practice (see also in chapter 9).

This list may seem somewhat overwhelming and it is certainly impossible to ask all of these questions within one consultation. There is no need to hurry, questions can be asked—and answered—in different consultations and over a period of time. The questions stimulate both the doctor's and the patient's curiosity, and help them to put the pieces of the puzzle together.

Other family methods

Drawing *a family tree* or *genogram* (see Chapter 9) is another way of widening the perspective for both doctor and patient. The initial focus is on illnesses, pains, and aches, and then shifts to the exploration of family relationships in current and previous generations. A good-sized piece of paper is needed and it is best if the doctor draws up the genogram, with the help of the patient. The developing chart becomes the centre of interest as both doctor and patient look at it. This is a non-threatening way of proceeding, as eye contact can be avoided if necessary: difficult matters do not have to be discussed face-to-face, but can be put down on paper. This can help patients to gain a different perspective (Asen and Tomson 1992).

The Family Circles Method (Geddes and Medway 1977) is another technique that can be used within the context of a consultation. The doctor introduces this task by explaining to the patient that he, the doctor, feels a bit stuck as to how best to help. He suggests that a new approach is tried to look at things from a different perspective. The doctor then proceeds to draw a large circle on a piece of paper, stating that this circle stands for the patient's life. He then asks the patient to draw inside the large circle some smaller circles to represent all the important persons, passions, hobbies, illness, and other issues. The circles can be touching, overlapping, or far apart, large or small. Once the patient has completed this picture, in no more than 3 minutes or so, she explains to her doctor how she sees her life, relationships, and the place of illness within it. A conversation can then develop exploring connections that have become visible through this exercise. The Family Circles Method is

Box 5.1   **Examples of reflexive and circular questions**

1. **Problem/symptom questions**
   Purpose: to get a definition of the problem and contextual responses to it
   - Who noticed your problem/symptom first? Who second? Who last?
   - What is your explanation for the symptom/problem? What is your spouse's/father's/mother's explanation?
   - Who does what in response to the symptom?
   - When you're have pains, who responds to it first...What does s/he say or do? What happens next? How do you respond to that? What happens then? What's your response to that?
   - How does the problem affect your spouse/father/mother/child?
   - How does s/he form the opinion that you could act differently?
   - How do you know this? What else might they think or feel that they don't let you know about? How might they talk about your problems in your absence? What would you have to do to find out?
   - If you did, what sort of responses might you get?

2. **Help questions**
   Purpose: to determine who wants help for what, as well as discovering the implications of seeking help
   - Who in your family thinks that you need help—who wants it most/least?
   - What is your explanation for these differences?
   - Who is most/least distressed about your problem?
   - How did you discuss this and with whom? What were the sort of responses?
   - Supposing you weren't coming here for help, how would you deal with this problem? Does coming here for help make it easier or more difficult to discuss these things with him/her?
   - Who would be most/least in favour of you coping on your own, rather than coming to the surgery a lot?
   - What will happen in the future if nothing is found that will help the problem?
   - What will happen in the future if there is no longer a problem?

3. **Change questions**
   Purpose: to explore the implications and consequences of change
   - What sort of observations would you make that would convince you that things were getting better?
   - How would your father/partner notice that you were getting better?
   - How would your relationship with mother/partner/child be affected if you got better?
   - Who would be most/least affected by you recovering?
   - Supposing you were able to consciously produce your symptoms— what would you have to do? How would you go about doing this?

4. **Relationship questions**
   Purpose: to get patients to look at relationships, communication, and interaction patterns in the family

- How do you see the relationship between X and Y (e.g. your son and his father?)
- How do you think X sees her relationship with Y?
- How would Z (e.g. your mother) see the relationship between X and Y?
- How do you explain the differences?
- If X was sitting here and heard you say this, what might s/he say? How would you then respond?
- Who is the closest/most distant to father/mother? Who second/third most?
- Who agrees with you that X is closest to Y?
- What happens/would have to happen for this to be different?
- Was there ever any time when this was different?
- What were things like before and after such and such happened?
- Who suffered most/least from X's illness/death/birth?
- Who can cheer up/depress X or Y most?
- When do you feel most like a daughter, when like a mother, when like a wife? What happens? Who else makes you feel like that?
- Who is most/least upset when A or B happens?

5. **Hypothetical questions**

   Purpose: to get patients to examine the implications of different scenarios and hypothetical situations
   - If you weren't around...how would your family get along without you?
   - If you had not been born, what would your parents' marriage be like?
   - If you got suddenly better, who would next be in line for having health problems?
   - You have already got some experience with doctors and other helpers. What would I have to do to make this treatment/therapy a failure too?
   - Supposing your partner had been a fly on the wall throughout all our meetings...what would s/he think about it all? Would you agree?
   - Supposing you asked your son to leave and insisted that your husband spends more time with you...how would that affect your headaches?

a quick and graphic way of gathering, assessing, and working with personal and family information.

There are other techniques and tools to generate new information, some of which are described elsewhere (Asen and Tomson 1992). What they all have in common is to engage both doctor and patient in a joint quest for a new and different understanding. Patients who feel that their doctor is interested in them tend to be less 'difficult' than those that have a 'difficult' doctor who dreads having to see them and who communicates this indirectly.

Psychodynamic approaches

Of course, it is not always possible for doctors to muster sufficient interest or curiosity, particularly if there is a long history of difficulties. Some patients do not respond, whatever the approach, and their doctors then feel totally drained of energy. Here, the concept of projection might be usefully employed. The practitioner can ask herself: 'what is it that the patient is doing to me that I feel so drained? What is it that the patient wants to get rid of?' Some patients have remarkable abilities for getting rid of their unwanted feelings or problems by off-loading these onto their doctor. Characteristically, the patient enters the consulting room visibly distressed, then unburdens himself, and exits some 10 or 20 minutes later, clearly relieved, leaving behind a doctor who feels bad and burdened. There is no need for doctors to accept unquestioningly the projections of patients. Self-reflective doctors can ask themselves:

> why do I always feel like this at the end of every consultation? What is it that I do that permits (or invites) this patient to continue loading me with all their bad feelings and problems? What would happen if I no longer made myself available in that way? What can I do that will lead to a different outcome in the next consultation?

It is possible to start talking to some—not all—patients about these issues, letting the patient know about the effect she or he has: 'every time you leave the surgery I feel really bad—bad about your life, bad about not being able to help you at all. I would like to help you—so, how can you help me not feel so burdened or paralysed by what you say? How can you make me feel less bad?' Some doctors might think that such an intervention could make the patient feel guilty. It depends on the tone with which these words are delivered: if it is reproachful, then the patient might feel guilty. However, if it portrays how lost the doctor feels in such circumstances then this can result in some responsibility being put back to the patient. If patients want to have useful doctors, they need to look after them—at least a little bit. Some patients will respond to this intervention, others will not. In that case the doctor may have to be even more blunt:

> I feel I am totally useless in helping you, but I would like to be useful. Doctors need to feel that they are useful. How can you help me to be useful because if I continue to feel useless, I cannot think of how to help you. What would I have to do to be helpful? Give me some advice.

Living with failure

Doctors generally like providing the appropriate remedies for their patients to get better. These remedies range from physical to psychological interventions, from straightforward advice to sophisticated therapy. There are times when the presenting problems and distress seem resistant to any kind of intervention, and doctors may need to accept that there is no help that can be given. This acceptance can itself be beneficial for the doctor-patient relationship as it acknowledges the limitations of medical knowledge and psychological intervention. To return to the market metaphor: if there are no goods to sell, but the patient insists on shopping for the sort of health that cannot be bought, then it may be useful to state simply:

> Sadly medicine is so limited at present that I can think of nothing that would help. This makes the situation very difficult, but I do not want to give up on you. Perhaps I can help you to face the fact that there is no remedy for your problem(s) at present. All I feel I can do is to help you to live with it—it is like learning to live with a disability.

This type of framing puts both doctor and patient at the same level—they join forces to live with the problem, rather than spending further energy fighting it. By describing the situation as 'difficult'—rather than seeing the patient as 'difficult'—there is potential for a new opening, and therefore a different future relationship between doctor and patient.

At times it may be useful to introduce a face-saver. Identifying some kind of physical 'cause' that might be responsible for the symptoms can be the beginning of building a bridge. One example is persistent treatment-resistant back pain. Instead of attributing the symptoms to stress, it may be more helpful to consider providing a physical explanation, say a 'bony' abnormality that might be demonstrated on an X-ray, but which cannot be corrected by physical means. This 'explanation' validates the patient's subjective symptoms and allows talking about how to live with this problem. It pays sufficient respect to the symptom, whilst at the same time identifying strategies for living with it.

Second pairs of eyes

Difficult patients often tend to be 'chronic' and, given the nature of general practice, they may be around for decades. Some simply cannot change. When totally overwhelmed by a patient perceived as very difficult, doctors may well consider asking for one of their colleagues in the practice to give a second opinion. Part of the survival kit for dealing with difficult patients is the possibility of inviting someone else in, with a new pair of eyes (and ears). This can provide a new perspective—or, at worst, transfer a difficult patient to a practice partner—who, to everyone's surprise, may not find that very same patient difficult at all. However, there are situations when there seems nothing left other than to refer such a patient to a specialist, be that the practice counsellor or a psychiatrist. Sadly, difficult patients do not always respond well to the suggestion of being sent to other professionals and they tend to question their doctors as to the rationale for such a decision. Honesty in these situations is the best policy.

Conclusion

The notion of the 'difficult patient' is a construction, usually arrived at by the doctor after a number of complex interactions with a patient. It is usually an unhelpful notion in that, once labelled in this way, the patient–doctor relationship becomes stuck. In attempting to deconstruct the notion of the difficult patient, doctors and other primary care workers can examine three different dimensions: the patient's and doctor's individual characteristics, as well as the nature of the request and its context. This can contribute to a better relationship between patient and doctor. A starting point is for the doctor to ask a series of self-reflexive questions:

Why do I allow myself to see this patient as difficult? What is it that the patient does to me that makes me think he is difficult? How would I have to change the context and nature of this consultation so that I no longer need to experience this patient as difficult?

These and other questions are an excellent starting point to make this often difficult work a bit easier.

6 Stress, strain and burnout: support and supervision

Jane Milton

This chapter will address the strains and stresses the general practitioner faces, besides the satisfactions of the job. It will look at how these arise, and then how the doctor can be helped and supported. Relevant questions include: why do people become doctors? What do they expect from their patients? What does society expect from its doctors and how does it regard them? What transactions, conscious and unconscious, happen between doctor and patient, and what can go wrong? Doctors' stress goes beyond the everyday strains of unsocial hours and annoying paperwork, and we need a complex and multilayered way of understanding their tasks and relationships. I use a psychoanalytic frame of reference to inform the discussion about conscious and unconscious aspects of human concerns and relationships, trying to think about them in developmental terms.

People are endlessly preoccupied with doctors, watching TV dramas about them, praising their skill and devotion, or swapping horror stories of callousness and neglect. It hardly needs saying that the role of doctor is a highly significant and powerful one in our lives. Historically, the awe doctors attracted long predated their effectiveness; the sanitary engineers who in truth saved more lives in previous centuries lacked the same cachet. Although the distant hospital specialist may be more idealized, the GP, who is the first port of call, who enters our homes, and has the licence to probe every orifice, retains a special power. Those who attempt to denigrate the GP's role into that of a simple gatekeeper only reveal their unease by the vehemence of their contemptuous dismissal.

The power of the GP-patient relationship

The role of doctor is an extremely powerful one in the eyes of society, of individual patients, and not least of doctors themselves. The effect on the doctor varies. In some cases pride in identity as a doctor changes to smugness or omnipotence, nicely summed up in the joke: 'What's the difference between

God and a doctor? God doesn't think He's a doctor'. This entails a sense of moral superiority over patients and impatience or pity for frailty. The often-impossible workload and hours on duty for the junior hospital doctor probably contribute to this by breeding a 'macho' culture—a manic attitude helps to keep the exhausted young doctor awake to 'save lives' and then to swap horror stories in the mess with bravado. Other doctors react differently, becoming anxiously awed and ground down by the responsibility they have taken on, and become hyper-conscientious in a miserable and driven way. Patients' needs are then experienced as endless, reproachful, persecuting. The hoped-for outcome of a doctor with enjoyed competence and confidence touched with humility may be hard-won over years.

Social attitudes

Society's attitude to doctors' power varies with the mood of the times. Currently, the awe and veneration of earlier decades is giving way to challenge, and out-rage at failure and imperfection—idols have further to fall than ordinary human beings. Hierarchies are breaking down, and individual autonomy and choice is at a premium. Now it is recognized that doctors, too, have feet of clay, there is disappointment and righteous indignation at this loss of an ideal. Resentment of those with special skills and knowledge was earlier controlled by the process of idealization. This put doctors safely beyond both reproach and envy. Now that doctors are seen as more human, the envy has become more active and virulent, leading to witch-hunts and public humiliations. There is a push towards dethroning the professional institutions that have become seen as shielding doctors from accountability.

In the midst of this revolution in social attitudes, doctors are often on a knife-edge. They are needed more than ever, but may have to be humiliated, even destroyed, with the rest of the previous elite. In post-communist Russia, most doctors in the public service still occupy a relatively degraded position; their already very low pay is frequently docked for small omissions in form filling. Doctors as members of society and as patients may see the good aspects of our own current bloodless revolution; the need for them to have realistic challenge and proper accountability. As professionals though they are likely to feel besieged, even scapegoated and demoralized by what is happening.

When doctors are forced to give up the old privileges—from the doctor's exclusive dining room to the unquestioning acceptance of their diagnoses—they have something to mourn as individuals and as a profession, however much the loss may have been inevitable, even ultimately welcome. To mourn a loss is dis-ruptive and emotionally demanding, although it can lead in time to greater internal strength. When mourning fails, we are left with anxiety, depression, or grievance, and this contributes to burnout, as I will discuss later.

Helplessness

In spite of the current challenge and debunking, what still gives the doctor's role its peculiar power and intensity? Few fail to be a patient at some point in their lives. Those who are doctors as well may partially and temporarily avoid true patienthood by belonging to the 'club'. They need only think back though to their pre-medical days, or to times of serious illness and helplessness, or to the illnesses of friends and relatives. To be ill and not to know what is going on inside is to be fearful and vulnerable. The reassuring predictability of the world and of mind and body is suddenly lost. In the presence of the doctor we are all to an extent anxious, appealing, deferent, or dependent (or pugnaciously defiant as a counter-reaction). This can be seen as inevitable and even a necessary regression in the service of getting help. We lose some of our thinking and reasoning ability, needing the thinking to be done for us. We want confusing and indecipherable disease to be rendered meaningful and coherent, and effective action prescribed. The doctor is allowed, indeed, must be able to touch and to invade the most intimate spaces of body and mind.

The doctor is also often called upon to give judgement and can feel (and act) like a moral judge (see earlier discussion in chapter 4), not simply a professional giving an opinion. Is the patient allowed to take time off work, to drive a car, fit to take a particular job; is he or she 'really' ill or just malingering? In extreme cases, the doctor can even take the patient's liberty by forcing psychiatric admission. Finally, the diagnosis of incurability may seem like a death sentence pronounced by the doctor.

Re-living early patterns

Where else in life does such an intimate sort of relationship occur, so deeply involving the body, so asymmetrical in terms of power, knowledge and skill? Only in infancy and early childhood, where the power of the parents is at first absolute. The reality of early helplessness and parental power is so common-place that it ceases to shock as much as it might. This early situation shapes our lives in many ways, having echoes in the many later relationships we encounter where there is asymmetry in power and knowledge. Although the hospital specialist may attract more immediate awe than the general practitioner, the depth and continuity of the relationship with the GP, and their 24-hour responsibility, means that they are put in a more thorough-going 'parental' position. This is heightened by the natural (and probably useful) regression triggered by the discomfort, helplessness, and confusion intrinsic in being ill and seeking help.

Relationship patterns that the patient has internalized in childhood act as unconscious scripts or templates, which come to imbue the GP patient relationship; the way the GP is perceived and misperceived, the way he or she is reacted to and related to. This happens particularly in patients who are chronically ill, physically or psychologically fragile, and hence frequent attenders at the GP surgery, though even a one-off consultation in a usually-fit individual may have powerful resonances, with the patient finding him or herself unaccountably tongue-tied, emotional, or defensive. GPs also will unconsciously bring their own internalized parent–child templates to bear on the relationship.

Both the patient and the GP thus unknowingly bring to their interaction a complex of perceptions and identifications about parents and children. These deeply-embedded relationship templates in the idiosyncratic, subjective inner world of each of us influence the way we both treat and experience all significant others throughout life. With time, if all goes well, we move towards a more realistic picture of the world and others, but this process may get very stuck. This can lead to repetitive patterns that are either benign or imprisoning.

A child who has learnt the need to be sensitively tuned-in to the fluctuating moods of a chronically unhappy mother or father may become an adult with antennae alert to the unhappiness of others. He or she may unconsciously seek out a partner who needs the same sort of careful handling as mother or father did, as such people have become the main objects of interest and attachment. This search is driven by a longing to 'make the ill parent better'. Such a person might be drawn towards entering a caring profession like medicine because of this. This child's and later this adult's ordinary aggression may have been inhibited through fear of what it might do or, in phantasy, has done in the past. Conversely, a child with tolerant robust parents will tend to establish inside— internalize—much stronger figures who evoke far less worry, and who allow the freedom to get attached to stronger sorts of people in adult life.

Temperamental factors may be accentuated or mitigated by early experiences. Thus, an innately careful, wary baby may be reassured by a mostly happy and confident mother, or made more suspicious and withdrawn by a disturbed, unpredictable mother ambivalent about her child. The internal parents, who provide such important templates for later relationships, will be formed from a complex amalgam of actual experience and expectation based on phantasy. Small children show through play their lurid phantasy models of what people do to each other, and of what they would like to do to their loved (and hated) ones. These are often based on primitive body functions (rival siblings getting killed and eaten; frighteningly violent, excretory ideas about parental sexuality; fears of important bits getting chopped off for misdemeanors). Neglectful or cruel parenting will exacerbate this, whereas benign experience will tend to mitigate it. Such primitive phantasies mostly become unconscious, though they may emerge in dreams. They tend to be activated again, in some form, at times of great stress in intimate relationships, in psychosis, or when the body itself frighteningly malfunctions during illness. When we are sick we often become a bit 'paranoid', and our fears become less realistic and more nightmarish.

Inner lens

Depending on the state of relationships and the emotional tone in the 'internal world', acting as a filter or distorting lens, no two patients will see one GP in quite the same way. Dr A may be seen by Ms B as kindly and very confident, but by Mrs C as overbearing and paternalistic. A third patient, Mr D, may have a dominant view of Dr A as someone who needs gratitude and appeasement. Then finally a psychotic patient Mr E may have a quite different, more disturbing view of Dr A as someone who is cruelly experimenting on him. Some, or all of these perceptions may reflect aspects of the true Dr A, of his actual conscious and unconscious ways of relating to his patients. Alternatively, one or more of these views may be quite distorted versions based on projections, which indicate more about the patient than about Dr A himself. However, to further complicate matters, Dr A will almost certainly be drawn into relating a bit differently to each of the four patients; they will unconsciously provoke certain responses, tap into certain of his latent predispositions, this in turn tending to confirm each patient's preconceptions.

Like it or not, the GP is drawn inexorably into a web of relationships which are intense and complex. The internal forces which nudge both doctors and patients into adopting their reciprocal roles of parent and child cannot be abolished, only perhaps noticed a bit more and taken into consideration. Early in the consultation there is often a rapid, automatic exchange between patient and doctor, where the patient gives up some of his or her adult self-control and reasoning capacity. This is, instead, invested in the doctor, who automatically takes on this 'projection' by becoming exaggeratedly the only one of the two capable of thinking and acting. The pressure on the GP to respond by taking action, fulfilling wishes and expectations, (e.g. to issue prescriptions, over-investigate and over-refer) can be enormous, especially in the inexperienced doctor. Doctors who are always taking action like this may be criticized as poor listeners. They can be experienced as though they are 'fathers', impatient about feelings, solving problems through action. On the other hand, a doctor who is too swamped by what he or she hears and feels in the surgery may become a helpless, ever-available 'mother' swamped with distress, popular, but always running late, getting more and more ragged.

This unashamedly caricatured reference to mothers and fathers leads on to a point about general practice as compared to hospital medicine. The stereotypical, but often-useful division of labour between nursing and medicine in hospitals is less available for GPs, who are often called upon to provide both traditional paternal and maternal roles for their patients. Practice nurses mostly do not fulfil the same intensely maternal roles as hospital nurses, the latter so intimately involved with feeding, changing and dealing with excreta in a way that complements the doctor's more paternal function. The GP will by temperament probably be better at one gender role than the other (and this will not necessarily reflect their actual gender), but he or she will more often have to do things alone. In a hospital, as in a family, there is likely always to be a couple or team involved in thinking about patient care. This is analogous to the way a mother often has the child's father or her own mother, or another available adult, to think with, to reflect and process her own responses to her small child.

The internal observer

Intensely private though the GP-patient relationship may appear, in a sense there is always an invisible 'observer' present in the consultation, in the form of the doctor's own judgement of herself and her work, fed into by her sense of society's judgement of the doctor. The most harmonious scenario involves a confidently competent doctor, feeling appropriately respected, supported, and rewarded within his institutional setting, society, and profession. This internal observer stands benignly behind this doctor, however fraught and difficult the individual consultation may feel. In another scenario, however, the doctor may feel watched at work in a critical and undermining way, by a figure that is waiting to pounce on the smallest mistake. She feels under-valued and swamped by the need to fill in forms for a faceless, suspicious bureaucracy that seems to question her honesty and diligence. Sometimes the patient seems to the GP to gang up with this outer authority by approaching the consultation in a suspicious, denigrating way, treating their doctor as an unskilled referral-machine and automatically mistrusting what is on offer in the surgery. Both the individual GP and the wider society contribute to this internal observer. In the worst case a GP's own habitually harsh self-doubt is only too horribly confirmed by society's mistrust and readiness to blame.

A culture of blame

General practice, like many aspects of our culture, is in a turmoil of change at the moment, with disruption of the old accustomed roles, leading to mixed messages and confusion for both doctor and patient. There is a current push towards breaking down 'paternalism' within all professional relationships, not just medicine. Some would seek to do away with any inequality, advocating that patients should and could be empowered to take charge of their own bodies and minds, in equal partnership with their doctors. Although the justice and good sense in this seems self-evident, such an utopian aim fails to take account of the psychological dynamics outlined above. In the case of medicine, we come up against the bedrock of naturally-occurring and inevitable asymmetry between doctor and patient that I have described. This is not to say that there may not be scope for improvement in mutual understanding and respect.

Paradoxically, alongside the yearning for 'equality' between patients and doctors, there are spiralling demands for perfection and omniscience on the part of the doctor. The old too-uncritical acceptance of failure gives way to a demand for flawless, super-human practice. Human failing in the doctor is increasingly pounced upon with outrage and complaint, ultimately through the courts. This is linked to a generally increasing expectation of the right to freedom from pain and disease. Where ill health and failures of treatment used more to be mourned as bad fortune, they are now increasingly seen as due to failure and incompetence on the part of doctors—someone must be to blame. Indeed, blame and seeking vengeance spares one the pain of mourning, and one's own guilty and helpless feelings. The average GP may feel beleaguered by this. This will be particularly stressful and demoralizing for a practitioner who is already burdened by images of sick, reproachful figures from childhood. It will be particularly undermining for the GP whose basic self-esteem depends on constant reassurance about effectiveness and popularity. In many GPs, the impact of a complaint by a patient or a relative is deeply traumatic, attacking as it does an already-conscientious and self-critical individual to the very core.

Who becomes a doctor?

What sort of person wants to take on these awesome responsibilities? Most teenagers don't see it this clearly when they enter medicine. The average applicant to medical school is bright, interested in science and wants to be helpful and effective. They may have been inspired by a relative or by fictional doctors. They probably like the idea of being important and admired; they like the idea of a guaranteed job with reasonable pay and, to an adolescent looking at it from the outside, the heroism of long, hard, unsocial hours can seem rather romantic.

Less consciously, other factors may play a part. In an important subgroup of doctors, the wish or need to help may stem from having a chronically ill parent or sibling. They may have grown up feeling subtly guilty and responsible about a disabled younger brother, or a chronically depressed mother. Something more hidden or unspoken in the family may have had an influence too: a series of mis carriages mother had in the distant past or a terrible history of persecuted refugees, or perhaps a suicide in the grandparental generation. Depending on temperament, the aspiring doctor may be led internally to deal with such frail inner figures via the vigorous and decisive action of being a surgeon, or by choosing the competent detachment of the laboratory scientist; or perhaps, via the GP surgery, by the apparent opportunity to sort the whole internal family out!

'Reparative' needs in people are universal, often nothing to do with pathology or problematic childhood relationships. It is a human need to be effective and useful, or creative in some way and work sometimes provides it satisfactorily; sometimes it has to be found in other ways. Many jobs can satisfy a need to repair, rebuild, and heal, though not usually in such an appealingly concrete way as medicine and surgery. The degree of desperation and omnipotence with which such needs are held, though, will have important consequences. Some individuals hate the feeling of helplessness and 'not-knowing' so much that they are driven to rushed, even manic action; the tolerance of waiting and uncertainty is unbearable. The loose ends, muddle, and general unsatisfactoriness (in terms of instant healing opportunities) of much of what patients present to their GPs will be anathema to such doctors. Such people, if they stay in general practice, could become intolerant, perhaps even cruel, to their more recidivist patients, although they may be very good at organizing new initiatives and treating clear-cut physical illness.

Another influential unconscious factor may be an intense curiosity about what goes on inside people. Psychoanalytic ideas suggest that at a primitive, unconscious level, this might be related to the frustrated curiosity of the small child in his or her early researches about sex and babies. Again, this can be seen in the play of small children, eager in imagination to get inside the mother's or father's body, find out what is going on within and between them; what are they being left out of; and what are their hidden, often sexual, secrets. One finds a lovingly-tinged version of this curiosity associated with reparative wishes to investigate and cure. However a more aggressive version of this, associated with aggrieved feelings of exclusion, may become linked with something more unconsciously aggressive and meddlesome in the doctor later on. This manifests itself vividly in two stereotypical extremes; the one, sensitive, patient, restrained, and reparative; the other verging on meddlesome, even cruel, with the patient's needs taking second place to the chance to cut open and fiddle around inside. Compared with surgeons, GPs have less of a chance to get inside the body and act things out so obviously, but the same dynamic can take more subtle forms in the way they treat their patients' minds and bodies.

Needing the patient to 'cure' the GP

No doctor is free from these unconscious primitive reparative and curiosity needs—indeed, they often help. Also doctors, like everyone else, need a certain level of satisfaction in their work or they feel depleted, as if they were feeding other people, but not being fed themselves. Problems can occur when there is over-dependence on patients with a need for them to get better, be grateful, perhaps even suitably dependent and respectful. Where unconscious, unfulfilled childhood needs are paramount and predominantly driving the choice of medical career, problems will occur. The doctor will over-invest in the work, needing to be 'cured' by the patient getting better. Ordinary stresses will become more pronounced, as so much emotional significance is hanging on the work. It will be hard to keep an ordinary reflective and professional distance from patients, particularly patients who resonate with unconscious needs:

Thus, one middle-aged male GP gets bogged down in consultations with several elderly women on his list who are lonely and depressed. He is unable to set boundaries to consultations or deny home visits; the latter become too social—he is unable to say no to food and presents—he feels more and more under a special obligation to them. He feels preoccupied outside work in a hopeless way with their misery and discontent, guilty that he cannot improve their lives. He remains unaware of the link with unresolved feelings about his mother, a chronically depressed woman who never seemed to get much better in spite of all his efforts. His irritation with her made him feel so guilty he has squashed all conscious awareness of it. Another, younger GP, dislikes consultations with certain middle-aged brash professional men on her list. She finds herself alternately bullied into making unnecessary referrals or stubbornly resisting referral when they demand it. She finds it hard to keep a thoughtful professional stance and rely on her clinical judgement in such cases, being too caught up internally (and, again, the link is unconscious to her) in unresolved issues in relation to her bullying and demanding childhood father.

On a more ordinarily optimistic note, most doctors, the majority of whom are not seriously driven or impeded by their unconscious needs, will tend to find their niche in a practice as time goes by. A self-selection process is operated automatically by both doctors and patients within a practice. The particular skills, preferences, and vulnerabilities of the GPs determine which patients tend to end up with which doctors. Thus a sufficient fit develops over time between the patient's need to be known and to be helped, and the doctor's need to know and to help. The knowledge soon gets around the practice that Dr R is really understanding and helpful if you're depressed. Dr S doesn't give you so long to talk, but you can rely more on his surgeries running on time, and he's excellent at sorting out joints and backs. Then although you know that part-timer Dr T won't have an appointment free for 2 weeks she's not sceptical about alternative medicine like the others; she may even recommend a homeopathic remedy.

The 'containment' process: gaining perspective and internal support

A patient comes to her GP a few months after her husband's death. She talks of her loneliness and misery. The GP feels helpless, deeply affected by her patient's loss, worried there is nothing she can do for her. She can't think of much to say, but manages to convey that she can see how awful it is, how empty her patient's life feels at the moment, so soon after the bereavement. She encourages the patient to come to see her again soon.

Another GP sees a patient he referred with a breast lump six months ago. The patient has now been told by the hospital of widespread secondary disease. As he listens to her rather listless flat story, he finds himself feeling furious on her behalf about the unfairness of it, and wishing there was something he could do. He says something about how terribly unfair it must seem, and she comes more alive, and cries furiously for a while. Then she starts to discuss with more energy how best to talk to her children about what is happening to her. After a ten minute consultation she leaves with a more determined air and a repeat appointment.

As they sat feeling painfully helpless, listening to their patients, these two GPs considered an action—in both cases the action would have been prescribing an anti-depressant without very clear clinical indications—but both refrained, for the moment at least. They were instinctively aware, without spelling it out to themselves, that they were already performing an important function for their patient. What they were doing could certainly not be dismissed as 'just listening'. Importantly, they were allowing themselves to feel and experience painful emotions on behalf of the patient, without acting precipitately to rid themselves of these. Both GPs were working hard in these consultations; often this sort of thing is not recognized as work at all. What is more, it is vital work. Human beings actually require, in order to function properly, that at times of severe distress they are known and understood in this way—something needs actively to be 'taken in', felt and thought about by the other.

The psychoanalyst Wilfred Bion (1967) termed this commonplace, but vital process 'containment', and suggested that it has a prototype in the ordinary way a mother helps to make things bearable and meaningful for her infant. She becomes the recipient of inchoate, as yet un-named and unthought disturbance, for example, related to hunger, wind pain, cold, fear of falling. The mother has to be able to experience some of the awfulness on behalf of the baby, but to process and think about it, too. This gives the infant the message, through her response and action, that she can bear it a bit more than the baby can, and make some sense of it. For Bion this process sets the scene for the child to be able to name feelings and to develop the capacity to think itself. However, it is something the mother can only properly do if *she* has developed the ability to experience enough of a reflective space inside herself, related to *her* own sense of another's inner containing presence.

This process remains important throughout life and is part of the way we communicate with each other without words. To be the containing person is hard work and can be draining; part of why it is exhausting to be the parent of an infant or to be a GP. The ill patient, somewhat regressed, and presenting often-inchoate distress to a figure automatically perceived and related to as parental, is often going to need to evoke just this 'containing' sort of response. As with infancy, bodily and mental disorder is often confused or indistinguishable when the patient first presents to the GP, and the GP may be bombarded with mental or bodily distress, or both at once, and have to do a lot of sorting out.

A given GP can only be expected to perform this function for some patients some of the time without partially shutting herself off or, alternatively, taking some premature action to put a stop to the painful feelings the patient is 'projecting'. The GP, like most professionals who are used to making decisions and taking positive action, may find it particularly hard not to know the answer to things, not to be able to resolve uncertainty. Even if he or she does it well for some patients in some surgeries, it will not be humanly possible to do it well all the time. Worthy of note here is Donald Winnicott's (1965) concept of the 'good-enough mother', a human being, rather than an unrealistic paragon of motherhood. A clear extrapolation can be made to the 'good-enough GP' or a 'good-enough' consultation or series of consultations. In general practice, patients usually have the chance to come back and have another go at getting through.

All doctors, from their vulnerable late adolescent years onwards, face the extremes and variety of human life and suffering—birth, death, disease, disfigurement, madness, sexual problems. Above all they encounter fellow human beings in states, sometimes extreme, of fear, pain, and distress. It is hardly surprising that the task of containment is found to be so hard by junior hospital doctors. Again, this is somewhere where nursing and other members of the team can help out. GPs are not protected and supported in quite the same way. They are also not protected by the relative predictability of a specialty; anyone, with any problem, may walk in next.

All GPs know it is important to listen to distressed patients. However, they tend to under-value this activity in comparison with functions that are more visibly active and doctor-ish. They also tend to assume (again perhaps a hangover from the macho junior hospital doctor culture) that they do not need to be listened to much themselves. The reverse is certainly true. Later I will discuss in some detail how the GP himself might be contained personally and within the practice in order to go on performing this vital function for patients.

What is 'burnout'?

The most frequently cited definition of burnout is that of a syndrome consisting of three components: emotional exhaustion, depersonalization of others, and a feeling of lack of personal accomplishment. There is increasing concern about this syndrome in GPs. Kirwan and Armstrong (1995) among others have investigated the prevalence of burnout among GPs, and a number of other good studies have been published on psychological distress in GPs (Sutherland and Cooper 1993; Chambers and Campbell 1996).

The burnout syndrome makes psychological sense as both the over-strained and exhausted GP's response to, and last-ditch defence against, the huge emotional demands of the job. This is in the context not just of inadequate emotional support, but of the increasingly persecuting culture in which the GP works. A 'burnt-out' GP is depleted emotionally, has little sense of job satisfaction, and is forced to depersonalize his or her patients in order not to experience any more of their unbearable emotional demands. A distinctive feature of burnout as it has been described is that it grows insidiously, and is linked to years in clinical practice and age. It might be compared to a long-standing unhappy couple that have forgotten why they were drawn together in the first place; love is lost; they feel flat and disillusioned, bring out the worst in each other and grow to feel bad about themselves. For both, 'the other' becomes a de-humanized source of grievance, rather than a suffering fellow human being.

Factors found empirically to be associated with depression, anxiety, and burnout are: working long hours, which include heavy on-call duty and being single-handed; working in non-training practices; living alone; and having poor social support networks. Interestingly, Sutherland and Cooper (1993) found female doctors to be significantly less distressed than their male colleagues, and wondered whether this was associated with their better use of social support networks. Part-timers also seemed to fare better. Important stressors were fear of complaint and assault, high patient expectations, and adverse media publicity. They noted that GPs were also adversely affected by new organizational structures over which they experienced little control and felt ground-down by mundane administrative tasks in the face of inadequate resources. They felt increasingly more visible and open to criticism, but less supported. Sutherland and Cooper (1993) found job satisfaction levels significantly lower than when surveyed in 1987.

Some of these findings pose interesting questions. Might it have been more tenable at one time to work long hours, say as a single-handed GP, when one could be confident in a relatively benign sense of the outside observer, confident in one's own power and prestige, and in the deference of society? What is the significance of the finding that women are faring better? Is this something to do with the breakdown of a 'macho' culture in medicine, with increasing patient demand for sharing and listening? Or is it simply related to the fact that more women GPs work part-time? The findings overall indicate that in a culture that is more suspicious and less deferential, GPs are being shown empirically, as well as through commonsense, that they need to work together more, to be realistic about workload, and to support each other. Attempts to maintain omnipotence are increasingly going to fail, perhaps particularly in the mid-life of the GP, often a time in one's working and personal life, where unrealistic goals have to be modified and limitations faced; also a time of potential flowering of creativity (Jaques 1965).

Supporting structures for the GP—internal and external

The final common pathway for all forms of support is through their effect on the GP internally. To survive emotionally and to do good, fulfilling work, the GP needs competence, appropriate confidence, energy, curiosity, enthusiasm, patience—the list goes on. Thus, the supporting structure comes from within, but can only be created through interaction with others, past and present. Self-knowledge is always helpful, together with curiosity about and tolerance of one's own emotional reactions. Some GPs are interested enough or aware of particular need to seek this in a formal way through personal psychotherapy, but most would try to develop it in the ordinary way, through their lifelong experience in personal relationships.

An important quality for the GP to be able to develop, for his or her own survival as much as for the patient's sake, is a curiosity about and a tolerance, hopefully even an affectionate tolerance, for human foibles (see Chapter 5). Honesty about one's own shortcomings will help one to tolerate weakness and failure in others, and to be interested in and respect the multiplicity of odd ways in which people choose to live their lives. The moral high ground is an ultimately pointless place to inhabit and trying too hard to change people will usually have the opposite effect, besides being exhausting and demoralizing. Such a tolerant attitude will help the GP not to feel too irritated and got-at by the patients who appear to regard the surgery as their home, who won't do what they're told or who have apparently taken up ill-health as a way of life.

Although it takes time, effort and an element of personal exploration, finding a frame of reference for thinking about relationships can help the GP become more understanding and tolerant. This might for example be psychoanalytic theory, systems theory, or attachment theory. Such a framework might help the GP make sense of why human beings can become, for example, clingingly dependent, chronically angry, help-rejecting and self-defeating in so many ways (see Chapter 5).

It is important for a GP to be able to recognize, and accept his or her emotional and physical limits. Going back to the containment model above, even if the doctor allows only a fraction of his or her patients to 'get inside' emotionally each day, every occasion on which this occurs will be significant. As already said, processing other peoples' distress is not always sufficiently recognized as work (analogously, parenthood is a vital, but denigrated activity), but work it certainly is. It can be rewarding, but one has only a finite capacity for it on a day-to-day basis. It can be tempting for certain doctors to collude with the omnipotence assigned to them and act as if they were invulnerable; a strategy that is unlikely to work indefinitely.

Holland (1995) pays particular attention to the GP's need to set respectful limits on patients' more unreasonable demands—for instant service, unnecessary visits and so on. This is another important component of the containment process. To use the parent–child analogy again (without intending to be patronizing), parents have ultimately to help the anxious child to cope with waiting, and develop his or her own resources. This is where the structure and 'rules' of the practice can be of great help to the GP. The opposite risk is then one of a defensive and rigidly unresponsive setting, with too much division between the caring GP and the 'dragon' receptionist.

How may the GP find support and protection from the catastrophic or gradual attrition of her ideals, expectations, and internal resources that lead to burnout? First, there is a need to develop an internal space for reflection, somewhere from which a perspective can be achieved on both the patient and the self. As long as this space exists or can be reclaimed, creativity is possible, and professional curiosity and enthusiasm can be kept alive. Such internal space is achieved and maintained ultimately through the support of personal and professional relationships. This is where the academic side of general practice, formal and informal, can be very helpful.

Paying attention to this academic side, to one's medical home base, is the constructive side of continuing professional development or CPD, which must be set against its more bureaucratic and persecuting aspects. General practice can be a lonely job and a group of other GPs on a course or at a conference all know what a difficult (even impossible) job it is without having to be told. One of the dangers of having to collect CPD 'points' is that the doctor regards this as a chore, rather than making it work for him or herself. More points tend to accrue from short technique-based courses, but a longer course with more chance to reflect with colleagues over time may actually prove more replenishing.

Reality of teams

The mutually supportive image conjured up by the phrase 'primary care team' can be something of a myth in actual practices, where the GP is often forced to work mostly alone, under great pressure. Some people choose general practice because they prefer to work autonomously. It is important, however, that the individual doctor resists the pressure to collude with a system that drives him or her into increasing isolation. The 'macho' tradition can see team meetings and case discussions as luxuries, taking time away from 'real work', but this is seriously misguided and falsely economical of time. Sometimes the fear of discord between partners leads practices to avoid meeting and talking. Certainly, a group of forceful and individualistic professionals may argue fiercely now and then in meetings, but this can be creative. The danger of not allowing this to happen is that conflicts go underground and are acted out in harmful ways within the practice.

Practices need to think seriously about setting time aside for such work (see Chapter 8). In a healthy practice, patients' needs can be thought about at depth and colleagues' needs can also be acknowledged. A practice that functions well in this way will have the space to be able to take responsibility collectively for partners who are overburdened or failing, and to take appropriate action before things deteriorate too far. Good care by colleagues is particularly necessary in the current climate. A practice that works together well and reflects on its workings will develop good self-esteem. This will help to counter the demoralizing effect of increasing criticism and bureaucracy imposed from outside, and protect against burnout in its partners.

Some practices tacitly make use of an in-house counsellor or psychotherapist to stimulate them informally into thinking more deeply and psychologically (see Chapters 9 and 10); a few practices even employ an outside facilitator to lead discussions about the psychological aspects of their work. In the Balint tradition (see next chapter), this function happens outside the practice itself. Formal groups like these where time is set aside for reflection on the doctor–patient relationship, with a group of GPs from different practices, are often available during training for general practice. However, for a variety of reasons, GPs only rarely allow themselves such a space subsequently, although Balint groups remain a thriving minority interest. GPs are more likely nowadays to pursue short courses in psychological techniques like interviewing skills or in the application of dynamic or systems theory to the consultation. These will in themselves provide some space, and renew professional pride and identity, besides teaching an actual skill. It is, however, important that the GP should not come to feel that he should *really* learn to do something else other than general practice itself, as if the role of counsellor or therapist *per se* were somehow superior.

Conclusion

I have reflected on general practice from the point of view of the complex relationships it involves—with patients, with colleagues and with society generally. Human relationships can be intensely rewarding, but they are also one of our greatest sources of pain and distress. The GP regularly witnesses some of the worst of human experience, in a context of both idealization and increasing suspicion, and cannot go on doing this for years without support. It is a challenge for individual GPs and to the profession itself to adapt to our new and evolving social conditions, keeping professional enthusiasm and compassionate curiosity about human beings alive.

7 Training for GPs

Paul Sackin

It must be apparent thus far that working on mental health in primary care is not just about understanding mental illness. Human relationships, in all their complexity, are absolutely central to the work of general practitioners. The training and continuing education of GPs need to take this into account. The curriculum needs to cover far more than preparing GPs to follow evidence-based guidelines or complete a list of consultation tasks, important as these might be. This chapter is about how GPs can become prepared to work in the emotional world of general practice. These emotions include not just those surrounding sick patients, but also members of the primary care team and, as Jane Milton (see the previous chapter) has so powerfully shown, the GP herself. These factors are important at all levels of GP training—undergraduate, vocational training, and continuing—though the emphasis may be different.

What has been happening up to now?

Undergraduate education

The traditional approach to medical education seems far away from the world depicted in the preceding chapters. Would-be GPs are expected to specialize in science from the age of about fourteen and to obtain at least three Grade 'A's at A-level in physical and biological sciences. Their pre-clinical phase centres on detailed learning of anatomy and physiology. Then their clinical work is based on the grand teaching hospital and powerful consultants. No wonder that, by the end of their undergraduate training, many students have become less in touch with their emotions and have lost much of their sense of vocation (Barbee and Feldman 1970; Preven *et al.* 1986).

Fortunately, there are signs that this is beginning to change. Most medical schools now base their curriculum around a problem-orientated and patient-centred approach. Such programmes were, to some extent, models for the General Medical Council (GMC), when it reviewed undergraduate education, and published its findings and recommendations in *Tomorrow's Doctors* (General Medical

Council 1993). The recommendations are based on the 'need for enhancement of attitudes to learning and for acceptance by students of greater responsibility for their own education: '...Above all, we have recommended changes in the style of the undergraduate course in the belief that they will bring about reduction of the curriculum overload...' Many of the principal recommendations are relevant to education in primary care and for dealing with mental health issues. The proposal for a core curriculum, which would presumably include these essential areas, is one example. Others are the emphasis on communication skills and the inculcating of appropriate attitudes of mind and behaviour.

The publication of *Tomorrow's Doctors* in 1993 obliged the more traditional medical schools to make radical changes to their curricula in order to comply with the GMC's policy. The focus has noticeably shifted from specialists ensuring that as much as possible of their particular speciality is 'covered', to a more generic education. There is much more opportunity to learn from health professionals other than doctors and, most important, from patients, their families, and their carers. These are welcome developments, but there is still some way to go.

Vocational training

When it comes to vocational training for general practice, arguably the education received by many GP registrars is less satisfactory today than it was in the 1970s and 1980s. In the early days of vocational training the vision of the early pioneers (Royal College of General Practitioners 1972) was translated into innovative training programmes. There was a great deal of excitement in the air as general practice, still the Cinderella branch of medicine, began leading the way with its educational innovation. The day release programme that I attended as a trainee in the mid-1970s, for example, was greatly influenced by John Stevens (1974). Stevens' approach was based on what he considered education to be:

> [It] concerns itself with the joy of discovery; the discovery of useful ideas, their use, testing and throwing them into fresh combination...Education is concerned with the central problem of preventing intellectual pollution by inert ideas, with training the imagination, and teaching a learner to teach himself, now and throughout his life...It will teach him how to ask the right questions and how best to attempt the answers.

In his James Mackenzie lecture, Stevens (1974) listed the main educational methods used on his courses. These included:

- symposia on major clinical problems at the end of each of which 'a consensus of good clinical practice will be printed out and fed back to the practices for audit';
- random case analysis to 'gain insight into our performance in the consultation';

- project teaching and learning—presenting a project to the peer group enabled GP trainees to 'integrate, reinforce and internalize' their new knowledge;

- sensitivity training so as to 'learn to handle and gain insight into feelings— feelings of dependency, anxiety, aggression, sexuality, and collusion—in ourselves and in our patients'.

While Stevens was successfully running release courses for GP trainees, Paul Freeling (Freeling and Barry 1982) had set up the influential Nuffield course, aimed to train GP course organizers to deliver the sort of training that Stevens envisaged. Even if some of the details may have changed, their approach looks as relevant, progressive, and exciting now as it did then. Some of the vision has been incorporated into contemporary GP training, but sadly, and in ways predicted by Stevens in his Mackenzie lecture, the 'golden age' of the 1970s and 1980s is long over.

One of the problems with this 'golden age' was that it was only 'golden' for a few people. Until about 1980, GP training was voluntary and the quality of training on offer was variable, both in the practices and on the day-release courses (Sackin 1986). There was a danger that the better schemes and the better trainees would get better, and the worse ones worse. In the 1980s and 1990s there was, therefore, a move towards setting minimum standards for training and increasing accountability for the trainers. Ideas that people like Stevens had pioneered began to be incorporated into new regulations for training and for summative assessment. In so doing, there was (and is) a danger that exciting approaches to learning would become stale.

When to learn what

So much for the background. What should today's students, registrars, and established GPs learn in order to be competent and confident in the emotional world of primary care? The rest of this chapter describes some of the areas that are of key importance. These include consultation skills training, Balint groups, learning how to listen effectively, the systemic approach, multi-professional learning, and learning to manage serious mental illness. I do not always indicate exactly at what stage one or other approach is most appropriate. This is because most of the approaches are suitable for all levels of education, whether undergraduate, vocational, or continuing, but different stages vary in their educational aims and, therefore, the methods that might be used.

I have outlined above some of the aims for undergraduate education and for vocational training. Underpinning these is a belief in the principles of adult learning (Brookfield 1986). Learners should be actively involved, the learning should be progressive, there should be no compulsion to participate in any particular exercise, and there should be support available. The content should be based on the learner's experience. This may not always be possible at undergraduate level or even in vocational training, as learning has to take place in a wide variety of areas that it might be difficult for a student or GP registrar to experience directly. For continuing professional development, however, reflection on experience is fundamental. It is through such reflection that the individual can discover his learning needs and so attempt to meet them.

Consultation skills training

Consultation skills are an area of obvious importance for training in primary care mental health. Traditionally, vocational training has been the main place for this teaching, but it is essential that undergraduates have some grounding in consultation skills, as these are obviously important for any clinical interaction.

The history of consultation skills teaching in many ways mirrors the history of vocational training in general. The starting point was the pioneering work of Byrne and Long (1976), who made audiotapes of large numbers of consultations. They proposed a model for the consultation and began to make judgements as to its quality. The implication was that specific skills were required to consult effectively and particular skills might be needed for different 'phases' of the consultation. Pendleton and colleagues (1984) developed and popularized the idea of a skills-based approach using feedback on video-recorded consultations. Once their methods had been refined and developed by others, the video recording became used for assessment, as well as for learning. While it is understandable that efforts should be made to ensure that those entering the profession should be seen to be consulting to a minimum standard, the introduction of videotaped consultations into summative assessment may prove to be counterproductive. Inevitably, examinations dictate the curriculum (Marinker 1984). GP registrars are liable to concentrate on achieving just the minimum standard needed for the examination. Much time and effort is used on overcoming the technical obstacles to producing reproducible recordings and, by the time they have passed, many registrars have such negative feelings about the method that they never want to engage in video consultation analysis again. The examination has sapped the registrars of the creativity to which they originally aspired (Hambling 1998).

Salinsky and Sackin (2000) have considered elsewhere the value and limitations of communication skills training for general practitioners. Such training can help to make doctors more secure in the traditional, but still important 'disease' model. Its main function, however, is to help doctors work in the 'illness' model (McWhinney 1997), albeit one in which patients' ideas and concerns are taken into account at all stages of the consultation. Communication skills training gives young doctors a useful structure in which to work, and so helps them to develop their skills in a secure and systematic way. Perhaps the most important limitation of this approach is that the doctor's feelings are not always considered enough. A doctor may know exactly *what* to do, but be unable to *do* it because his feelings have been disturbed by something in the patient and/or by external circumstances. Traditional teaching does not take into account the fact that all patients give rise to an emotional response in their doctors. How to deal with this response and to *use it therapeutically* is an essential part of training for general practice.

Some modern devotees of the behavioural approach to communication skills training are aware of this need. Draper and Weaver (1999), for example, have devised an ingenious series of exercises to help participants to understand the emotional blocks that might prevent them from listening properly to their patients. Further exercises help trainees to find ways of overcoming these blocks. Such an approach is extremely valuable, but arguably insufficient to deal with the sort of emotional issues highlighted in the previous chapter.

Emotional education

Perhaps it is not surprising that dealing with the emotions can still be little more than a postscript in medical education. Ian McWhinney (1999) has quoted Crookshank writing in 1926 about the handbooks of clinical diagnosis that appeared in the early 1900s. 'They give excellent schemes for the physical examination of the patient whilst strangely ignoring, almost completely, the psychical'. McWhinney argues that this approach reflects 'the distrust of the emotions in Western culture', which is still a legacy of the Enlightenment and is only now just beginning to change. Even psychiatry often avoids getting too involved in the emotions:

A woman in her mid forties was getting strange attacks of semi-consciousness. She saw a neurologist who felt that the attacks were not organic in origin. She was therefore referred for a psychiatric opinion. The senior registrar whom she saw in the clinic took an extremely detailed psychiatric history. Her past history, family history and mental state were recorded in several pages of clearly written notes. In the end the doctor decided she was depressed (though there was little evidence of this) and prescribed an anti-depressant.

At follow up there was no improvement so she was admitted to hospital. As the SHO I spent a long time talking to Mrs A whom I found remarkably 'normal' and not at all depressed. But I got no nearer to understanding her strange 'attacks'. In desperation I asked the consultant to see her. He asked her about her family and her circumstances and she often talked of going home. Suddenly the consultant asked her what came into her head when he said the word 'home'. 'Dog', she said immediately. It turned out that her dog had died and Mrs A's dilemma was that she realized subconsciously that she had been more attached to the dog than to her son who was in hospital care (this was in the 1970s) with severe learning difficulties caused by tuberose sclerosis. Mrs A had told me about the death of the dog and about her son but it never occurred to me either that anyone could be so attached to a dog or that the two events might be connected. I left this post while Mrs A was still a patient and her parting shot was that she would buy me a dog for Christmas!

The senior registrar's history was exactly analogous to the medical student's traditional clerking. All the facts were elicited, but none of the feelings. A successful outcome was achieved by the combination of the consultant's skill in encouraging the patient to free associate and by my 'doggedly' listening to my feelings in a way that I had become familiar with as a result of having attended seminars run by Michael Balint when I was a student.

Balint seminars

In the 1950s, general practice in the UK was at an extremely low ebb. GPs were often regarded (by themselves as well) as doctors who had 'failed' to climb up the consultant ladder. It was hard for doctors to become GP principals, and they were often exploited as assistants or junior partners with few prospects of promotion. Their feelings of frustration and insecurity were not helped by the realization of the more conscientious doctors that working with patients was difficult, demanding, and required skill and sensitivity. Specialists could help in the diagnosis and management of specific diseases, but even psychiatrists did not seem to help with those unhappy, often polysymptomatic patients whom their doctors found so draining.

There was, therefore, an enthusiastic response to the announcement of a 'research-cum-training' seminar to be led by the psychoanalyst Michael Balint at the Tavistock Clinic in London. The results of this seminar were published in the famous book, *The Doctor, His Patient And The Illness* (Balint 1957). Thus, Balint groups were born. Half a century later we perhaps forget how revolutionary they were. For one thing, GPs were mainly single-handed in those days and often regarded their colleagues with suspicion, worrying that they might poach their patients. It was therefore a considerable achievement that a small number of doctors agreed even to meet together in a group. It was quite remarkable that they were willing to disclose intimate details about their work with their patients and, indirectly, about themselves.

What were the essential features of these early Balint groups? Perhaps the key point was that they helped participants to listen to their patients. Balint's work was very much based on the psychoanalytic principle that people reveal aspects of their unconscious in all sorts of everyday ways. Thus, clues to what was going on for patients lay not so much in traditional history taking ('If you ask questions all you get is answers'), but in observing how they behaved, what they did not say, etc. Even more important was how they made their doctor *feel*. A key contribution of Balint's work was that these feelings could then be used therapeutically (the drug 'doctor'). This new way of working for GPs did, in Balint's view, 'inevitably entail a limited, though considerable, change in the doctor's personality'.

The group discussion and the relationship of the presenting doctor to the group would reflect the doctor–patient relationship. The presentation of the case had to be done without notes as omissions, hesitations, etc., were clues about the doctor–patient relationship, rather than signs of incompetence in the doctor. This basic principle characterizes Balint groups today. John Salinsky and I quote a dramatic example of it (Salinsky and Sackin 2000):

> Doctor B presented a case of a woman who had recently been discharged from hospital with the diagnosis of ?stroke. The group was puzzled by the doctor's distress in talking about the woman and her family and the doctor felt that the group did not understand him. It was only on a subsequent occasion that it came to light that the discharge note had actually said '?stroke ?suicide attempt'. The presenting doctor had 'forgotten' to mention the crucial '?suicide'. He later revealed that this case had stimulated him into thinking about the traumatic suicide of his grandmother when he was a newborn baby and its profound effect on his mother and, indirectly, on himself.

The group in which this case was discussed was doing research into doctors' defences. Revealing such personal details is not a feature of most Balint groups and such revelations were entirely voluntary even in this research group. Balint was always at pains to point out that his case discussion groups were not 'therapeutic' groups for the doctors. They were designed entirely to help the GPs work better with their patients and, if the doctors needed 'therapy', they should seek this elsewhere. Perhaps this view is somewhat paradoxical when taken in conjunction with the 'change in personality' referred to earlier. Yet the focus of the groups was, and still is (at least in the UK), on the doctor–patient relationship and the leaders ensure that members do not hijack the group to try to use it to solve their own problems.

An important characteristic of a well-run Balint group is that it encourages creativity. Group members should, in effect, freely associate with the clues that come up, whether they come from something spoken, the way the group is behaving or the way people are feeling. Fostering creativity is so crucial in picking up clues from patients with psychological difficulties and helping them. Balint groups provide a refreshing change from the predominant medical culture of asking questions and generating solutions. However, even in successful Balint groups this culture can be hard to change. Many leaders now ask the presenting doctor to sit a little apart from the group and not join in the discussion for a while, once a few initial questions of fact have been answered. This allows the other group members to do the work themselves, using the information and evidence that has already been revealed.

A useful side effect of the Balint approach is that, although the work can be challenging, the atmosphere is highly supportive. The culture is one of equality among group members. For example, the case quoted above was from a doctor with lots of experience of Balint work who has been a GP for 30 years. Yet he was seen to be 'learning' just as much, though probably in a different way, as an inexperienced doctor or student.

Do students and young doctors *have* to take part in a Balint group in order to gain the required sensitivity and emotional awareness? It is certainly the norm in Germany and Switzerland, and Balint groups feature strongly in American residency programmes for training GPs. It is a method that has undoubtedly stood the test of time. It would be good if it featured more prominently in GP education in the UK, the country in which it all started. Some, including a distinguished member of Balint's original group (Horder, J. P., personal communication), argue that, even if formal Balint groups are few, Balint's influence pervades vocational training courses anyway. It is certainly true that most of the early pioneers of these courses had attended Balint seminars and used the model for setting up small groups of GP trainees. We have already seen, for example, how important the Balint approach was for John Stevens. Yet when I visited over 30 case discussion groups on vocational training courses (Sackin 1986), I felt that only a few of them were effective in helping the participants to understand their work with patients. Perhaps the situation has improved since then. It would be good to think that small groups on the day-release course can help GP registrars adopt the basic principles of Balint's approach. Attendance at more intensive groups could then be voluntary.

Learning to listen

If Balint groups are to be voluntary, students and young doctors should certainly not escape from learning how to listen well. 'Listening is at the same time a skill, and a way of being a physician. When we are in this state of mind, we can listen to our patients with total attention'. Ian McWhinney (1999) goes on to point out how attentive listening not only allows physicians to behave with compassion, but it also heightens their awareness of patients' bodily symptoms. Doctors need to listen attentively in order to hear and understand their patients, whatever the presenting problem may be. An extremely successful way of learning listening skills has been described by some Australian authors (Greco *et al.* 1997). The basis of their approach with GP registrars is to use 'triads'. These consist of a speaker, a listener and an observer, with a medical educator to act as facilitator and to help with debriefing. The speaker is asked to present a current problem, which can be a difficult case, but could be from any aspect of his life. The listener reflects the content and feelings of the speaker. 'He must follow three rules: no judging, no solutions and no diverting'. The observer observes what is happening between speaker and listener.

The three essential objectives for the work in triads are:

♦ Each registrar has an opportunity to practise active listening, allowing the subject to explore the problem themselves, with the listener avoiding interjections and not steering the course of the subject's thoughts.

♦ Each registrar to experience being listened to well, thus gaining some insight as to how patients feel when their doctors are good listeners.

♦ The observers gain insight into what happens when active listening is practised.

The work in triads is part of an active listening module in which the registrars also have the opportunity to practise active listening with real patients and to take part in case discussions.

At about the same time as Greco and colleagues were developing their methods with GP registrars, my colleagues and I were launching co-tutoring for established GPs (Sackin *et al.* 1997). The principles are very similar. GPs meet regularly with a colleague and are given equal time to be speaker, with their partner being an active listener. Speakers choose their own agenda. They may wish to use the session to talk about a current problem in their practice or in their personal life. Other participants have used these sessions to understand their learning needs and to develop a personal learning plan. Co-tutoring was designed principally to help GPs to feel listened to and supported, and participants bear witness to its success in this respect. They also report that it has helped them in their work with patients and in their relationships with colleagues. Originally, co-tutors usually worked in pairs, but more recently we have found, like Greco and colleagues, that a third person in the group acting as observer adds a considerable dimension. Like in the 'triads', the three members of the trio have the opportunity each time they meet to be speaker, listener, and observer.

Co-tutoring requires outside facilitation. We expect co-tutors to attend a 2 day residential course before they start co-tutoring, so that they can hone their skills in listening, giving and receiving feedback, and emotional awareness. Like with Balint groups it is salutary to see how much even experienced GPs can learn in these areas. The group attending each course then meets for follow-up days to gain ideas, keep up the momentum, and give each other support.

Clearly, methods such as co-tutoring and triads are adaptable to students and doctors at any level. There is good evidence that peer support by students can enhance their learning (Goodlad 1995). Students in groups can engage in simple paired listening exercises as a start and might then be encouraged to move into a deeper relationship with colleagues. Given some basic skills in listening and support, students can work together on projects or other assignments to the benefit both of their relationship and of the better achievement of the task.

The systemic approach

In Chapter 9 Graham and Mayer describe systemic approaches specifically designed to respond to the needs of families in primary care. However, exercises designed to train students and doctors in systemic thinking can teach them far more than that. The principles involved have been well stated by Launer who, with Caroline Lindsey, has run successful courses in systemic family therapy for primary care workers at the Tavistock Clinic (Launer and Lindsey 1997; Launer 1998a,b, 1999a,b,c).

Launer explains that the exercises are designed in a way that helps participants to 'unlearn' conventional linear thinking. There is less emphasis on concepts such as simple cause and effect, the single diagnosis or medical objectivity. Launer argues that, while these traditional ways of thinking are appropriate at times, 'we see our role as being to introduce some significant difference into participants' understanding of how consultations might be conducted. Our exercises (see Chapter 5) are therefore governed by the following emphases:

- ◆ interaction, more than individuals;
- ◆ process, more than content;
- ◆ beliefs and values, more than objective truths;
- ◆ multiple perspectives, more than single ones;
- ◆ empowerment, more than paternalism;
- ◆ allowing evolution of solutions, rather than problem solving.

The exercises that Launer describes in his series of articles are designed for established professionals, be they GPs or other primary care workers, but there is no reason why such an approach should not be used for medical or nursing students. Indeed, it might work particularly well for these groups as less 'unlearning' should be necessary. The set of exercises covers all the principles that Launer sets out. They include:

- ◆ introductory exercises to help participants feel how relationships in families work and to construct a geneogram;
- ◆ interviewing skills which emphasize the need to generate multiple hypotheses so as to be open to all possibilities;
- ◆ using an observing team to give feedback and offer supervision;
- ◆ dealing with complex, but common, situations in general practice such as the patient's agenda being very different from the doctor's;
- ◆ how to deal with suspected child abuse.

These exercises reflect very much the principles of adult learning discussed earlier. The systemic method leads to the understanding of many important concepts, while being grounded in the participants' daily work.

One could argue at length as to which is 'better'—the Balint or the systemic approach. Such a debate is unlikely to be helpful as both methods offer a great deal. The value that participants find in them is likely to be related to the enthusiasm and skill of the facilitators, and to the learning styles of the learners. Perhaps the systemic approach offers some clearer ideas as to 'how to do it' or at least 'how to listen', so as to understand the patient's ideas. In constructing a geneogram, for example, clues may become quickly available as to the dynamics of the relationships within the family. A key strength of Balint groups is the depth of emotional understanding that participants can gain. They may become more confident in making interpretations and sharing these with their patients, which can help to improve insight and understanding. A possible weakness is that it can take a long time for the learners to be clear what they should actually do when faced with a 'difficult' patient.

Both the Balint and systemic approaches become increasingly hard to assimilate the longer that those new to them have been working within the traditional medical model. Launer and Lindsey (1997) describe how 'even highly motivated [participants] such as ours habitually use interviewing techniques that are severely constrained by ideas from the dominant professional culture'. These unhelpful approaches include inappropriate persuasion, paternalism, and perhaps above all, an over-emphasis on problem solving. Both the systemic and Balint approaches depend on listening and feedback in order to increase the patient's understanding. The earlier in their training that students adopt this approach, the better.

Multi-professional learning

Although it would be a mistake to deny the key importance of the therapeutic relationship between the patient and his GP, doctors no longer work in isolation. Much of the care for patients with mental health problems may be given by professionals other than doctors. Even if the doctor is the key worker, others are still almost inevitably involved, especially if such important team members as receptionists, secretaries, or pharmacists are included. It is only commonsense that GPs need to develop appropriate attitudes and skills during their training, so that they can understand the roles of their colleagues, know how to work most productively with them, and respect the philosophies that underpin their approaches. Here, again, the traditional medical view of the doctor being invariably the leader of the team often gets in the way.

How is this multi-disciplinary approach to be achieved? There certainly seems to be a considerable gap between a belief in the value of multi-professional learning and actually putting it into practice. Perhaps part of the difficulty is the confusion between doctors learning *about* or *from* other professionals, and learning *with* them. The latter concept has been promoted for many years and is sometimes known as inter-professional education (Whiteman 2000). There have been isolated examples of where it seems to work well and yet it has never really been adopted on a wide scale. This has not stopped the Secretary of State for Health from advocating that doctors and nurses should learn together as undergraduates, and from questioning the distinction between their roles once they are qualified. Although attractive in breaking down prejudices and reducing 'demarcation' disputes, such an approach seems to go too far. There is a danger that patients will be faced with a pool of generic health workers whose particular skills might be blurred.

Nevertheless, there are examples of where learning with a mixed group of professionals can work well and break down barriers. Practice teams learning together about health promotion (Jones 1990) or palliative care (Eastaugh *et al*. 1998) have been successful initiatives and there is clearly no reason why similar schemes could not be used for learning about mental health issues. One novel approach that appears to have been very successful was a multi-disciplinary Balint group set up for those involved in treating patients with eye conditions (Brook *et al*. 1998). The basis for this group was the fascinating research by Alexis Brook (Brook 1995) into the psychosomatic nature of some eye diseases.

Learning from other professionals is clearly most important in the area of mental health, particularly in dealing with patients with serious mental health problems (see Chapter 13). Such patients are invariably looked after by a multi-disciplinary team and problems can arise if team members do not understand the approach of their colleagues. The frequent clashes between doctors and social workers suggest that a multi-disciplinary approach to education has not yet been adequately adopted. Learning from colleagues is not just important to prevent failures of communication. It is also very useful for doctors to be aware that there are many ways of approaching patients other than the traditional western medical one with which they are familiar.

As well as learning from other professions, an enormous amount of learning can take place from patients themselves, real or simulated. It goes without saying that learning from the consultation is the basis of most training for GPs, but patients can also be used in other situations. Many medical students nowadays have the opportunity to be 'attached' to a family and learn about the effects of illness on the everyday functioning of the family. Patients with particular illnesses can discuss with students or trainees what it means to have such an illness and how it impacts on their lives. Hearing about such experiences at first hand can be profoundly moving for the participants.

Learning about psychiatry in primary care

Attachments to psychiatry departments were the traditional way for undergraduates to learn about mental health issues. As we have seen, Balint showed a long time ago (Balint 1957) that psychiatrists were of little help in dealing with many of the strange symptoms and issues which difficult patients brought to their GPs. And yet GPs *do* come across serious mental illness. They need to gain confidence in diagnosing these illnesses, in talking with extremely disturbed patients and in managing them. Attachment to a psychiatric unit is necessary for such learning. Arguably this need not be for as long as the traditional SHO post of six months. The current pilots of three four-month posts in the pre-registration year could help here, as this is a good time for such training which is useful for all clinicians, not just GPs. Further training for GP registrars could take the form of attachments from general practice. GP registrars could then have an introduction to some of the psychotherapies and learn about psychological approaches and about team working. This experience would help these doctors to understand and form an opinion about the various types of treatment on offer. It would help them to be able to describe and explain to their patients in general practice what referral to a mental health team might involve. Well-trained doctors might also be able themselves to use some of the techniques they had learnt so as to save referrals and enhance their work satisfaction.

Reflective learning

Our education system is being more and more governed by set curricula, examinations, and league tables. One of the risks of this is that doctors in training are so involved in carrying out the prescribed tasks and preparing for the next examination that they do not have time to reflect. Even more worrying is that, at an early age, they lose their natural ability to learn and to adapt to change. These basic skills are absolutely essential to the GP, particularly in these times of very rapid change. Thus, methods used in training GPs that encourage reflection on experience are far more likely to lead to long lasting learning. Experience alone is not in itself of sufficient value. It may just mean accumulated bad habits, but if we reflect on our experience and consider what we did well and what we need to do better, we have a relevant agenda for learning. This should greatly increase our motivation for learning and so is more likely to lead to a successful outcome, to be tested out in our next experience.

In general practice and particularly in dealing with patients with mental health problems, there is another dimension to this process. That is reflecting on ourselves, on the relationships we form with our patients and on the difficulties, the pleasures, the excitements or the anxieties that we encounter in our work. Such reflection can be greatly helped by discussion with others—in a Balint group, with a mentor, or with trusted colleagues. Space for such a process in undergraduate education and vocational training for general practice, as well as being part of continuing professional development for established GPs, seems to me to be essential.

Some would argue that this process of self-growth should go further. Colleagues working in counselling and psychotherapy are obliged to seek supervision in order to have support in their emotionally exacting work and to help them deal with areas of difficulty and blind spots. This sensible approach runs counter to the macho traditions of medical education. It is high time for change. The gains for doctors and for patients would be enormous.

Part III
Mental health thinking in the surgery

8 The practice as an organization

John Launer

Practices lie at the heart of family medicine in Britain. They are the physical and emotional homes for GPs and primary care teams for most of our working lives. Yet almost everything that is written about general practice ignores the work setting itself. There is a *British Journal of General Practice*, but no Journal of General *Practices*. This focus on the content of our work, with a selective inattention to the working context, is telling. It invites comparison with theories of mind that focus on the individual's inner life, while studiously ignoring any background of biographical history or family interaction. In both cases, the narrowness of view leads to an impoverished approach, even a disturbed one.

The separation of content from context is, of course, typical of our wider professional culture. Within medicine as a whole, there is often an assumption that measurable data have a validity that is greater than the personal stories and interactional processes from which they have been extracted. This assumption leads to some peculiar effects. It means that the stories and processes themselves become invisible (or perhaps one should say inaudible). It makes the business of dealing with patients seem a linear, unidirectional one, rather than dynamic and multi dimensional. It also makes the working context seem entirely unproblematic. By talking, for example, about how a practice might 'treat depression', you bypass any distressing thought that general practices, together with the nurses and doctors who work in them, might themselves be subject to depression or to any other states of mind that could impair their function. Such language also carries the implication that doctors, nurses, and practices do not themselves need help in order to help others.

Anyone who has worked in general practice or any other primary care setting will recognize how naïve these assumptions are. They represent typical professional and institutional defence mechanisms, a way of denying vulnerability and one's shared humanity with patients (Obholzer 1994). So a first step in thinking about the world of mental health from a more rounded perspective, and one that does justice to the experience of general practice, is to notice that the background of the picture may deserve every bit as much scrutiny as the foreground. The people who do the treating need to be thought about as much as the people

being treated. This chapter addresses that issue by looking at three intercon-
nected themes. These are:

◆ the idea of the mentally healthy practice;

◆ a view of the practice as a mental health team;

◆ the question of supervision and support for primary care clinicians who deal
  with mental health.

The mentally healthy practice

Every general practice is unique. Each practice could (and perhaps should) write
a detailed and fascinating history, recounting how it attained its current size and
internal shape, and how it formed certain connections with the outside world
and avoided others. Many practices would be able to tell a Tolstoyan story
involving alliances and enmities, love and rivalry, dedication and prejudice.

There is no formal research, either quantitative or qualitative, showing
whether practices that function well in psychological terms are the same ones
that can respond in sophisticated and compassionate ways to patients with
mental health problems. Such research would be welcome. Meanwhile, it
seems reasonable to expect that a practice that is capable of addressing its own
conflicts well enough, either explicitly or by intuition, is more likely to have a
sane and healing encounter with its distressed patients. If this is true, then one
important task for every general practice, perhaps a central task, is to attempt
to model what it means to function with reflectiveness and self-awareness.
Becoming a mentally healthy practice may be a prerequisite for doing good
mental health work in primary care and perhaps good primary care of any sort.

This may be no easy task. In organizational terms, the settings in which GPs
work are diverse and often highly complex. A sole practitioner may only work
with a couple of people—perhaps a receptionist and a part time practice nurse—
but even such a small system is not necessarily a straightforward one in terms
of roles and relationships. At the other end of the scale, a partnership of five or
more principals will be part of a much more intricate system like a set of
Russian dolls. There may be a medical team that includes registrars and assistants, a larger clinical team with practice nurses and health visitors, and a still
larger practice team containing a manager, secretaries and receptionists. There
may also be an extended primary care team involving 'attachments' of various
kinds: midwives, physiotherapists, chiropodists, psychologists, community
mental health nurses, and so on. The team may itself share a health centre with
other practices, health service agencies, or a pharmacy. This list of possibilities
is not exhaustive. It does not cover practices without a partnership base, such as
some of the recent 'PMS pilot' practices set up by the last two governments.
Regardless of the style of practice, however, many GPs today work with
upwards of 30 or 40 other team members on site at different times of the week.

This is very different from the image summoned up in many people's minds when they think of the family doctor. Within such complex settings, the challenges involved in achieving healthy teamwork can be formidable.

Psychotherapists and others who have helped GPs with organizational consultancy have noted two common kinds of tension within the work setting. The first concerns the way that people manage the relationships and boundaries between themselves. For example, a GP partnership is a professional arrangement, but it can also involve personal intimacy and may last over very many years. It is likely to undergo the strains typical of a long-term marriage, yet at the same time it has social and statutory functions to perform. These go beyond the maintenance of the relationship itself. At every turn, decisions have to be made about whether a problem impinges on performance of the task and belongs to the domain of the partnership, or whether it has no relevance to the task and should be left unmentioned or unexamined. These decisions can be particularly difficult at times where illness, mental distress, poor performance, or a mixture of these are at issue. The following case example illustrates this. (This example, and all the subsequent ones, are highly fictionalized. Each one draws on several different cases in order to highlight the themes of the chapter and also to disguise identities beyond any chance of accidental recognition.)

Case A

In a five partner rural practice, one of the older two partners is showing signs of being depressed. He is irascible with staff and seems to avoid seeing unbooked 'extras' who turn up at the end of the surgery. The other doctors know a great deal about his personal life, including recent significant losses and an unhappy marriage. They suspect, but are not certain, that he may be drinking to excess. They feel he should be seeking professional psychological help, but they do not know if he already is. Following a helpful conversation with a psychiatrist trusted by the practice, one of the two women partners agrees to take on the role of 'honest broker' between the flagging doctor and the others. This means that she can open up a confidential discussion with her depressed colleague, offering him an assurance that she will only report back to the other partners if anything has implications on the duties or working arrangements of the practice as a whole.

If partnerships are rarely straightforward, the relationship between GPs and their employees is also an ambiguous one. Doctors and their staff are in theory colleagues, bound together by a shared commitment to the work. Yet they simultaneously operate within the framework of an organizational hierarchy and employment law. This can lead to some serious misunderstandings. A common example is when the partners ask their manager to provide them with overall leadership, but then resist her authority when the style of leadership displeases them. Another example, fraught with strong emotion, occurs when one team member expresses a romantic interest in another. Is this person simply taking advantage of a legitimate opportunity for asking someone out, or is it sexual harassment in the workplace? The debates that centre on these situations in GP practices can go round and round. In terms of communication theory, the participants are stuck in a constantly revolving 'strange loop' (like one of the baffling illusional paintings of M.C. Escher) where no one can decide whether the personal context or the organizational one is the higher (Cronen *et al.* 1982)

The second kind of tension noticed by observers arises from the question: what really *is* the primary task that general practice has to perform? The answer may seem an obvious one, namely to provide general medical services as defined in the national terms and conditions of service (the so-called Red Book). Yet the vast majority of British practices are also constituted in law as profit-making businesses. They are, in other words, structured in the same way as firms of accountants or solicitors. Every human relationship within the organization thus has a financial dimension and every decision made on human or medical grounds will mean that the partners have more or less money in their pockets. Conversely, every financial decision will carry a human price. GP practices have been likened to family businesses. (A minority, of course, are literally so.) They are trying to sustain two different sets of values: family ones and business ones. These sets of values will not always coincide. Sometimes members of the team will have radically different views about which should prevail. Typically, employed staff or attached professional colleagues from other disciplines may regard the doctors' emphasis on the imperative to make money as distasteful or even sickening.

GPs can manage these and other tensions intelligently or unintelligently, maturely or immaturely. Most experienced GPs will probably know times in the practice life cycle when their team is able to face issues openly and with courage, and other times when everyone sinks into a miasma of suspicion, uncertainty and disagreement (see Chapter 6). During these troughs, important things may be said heatedly or they may not be said at all. Without labouring the parallels between intra-psychic life and organizations, it is hard to resist the inference that practices can undergo processes of internal disconnection and integration just like individuals.

The crucial questions are: what promotes internal integration within practices, and what inhibits it? What, in other words, makes a mentally healthy practice? This is another area where research is non-existent, but anecdote and experience provide some indications. One factor seems to be the degree of clarity with which a practice manages *collectively* to think and talk about its own relationships. In some practices, for example, it is possible to talk openly and realistically about power differentials, and how these affect roles and relationships. In others this is denied or avoided, as in the common situation of deadlock when partners tolerate an under-performing nurse or manager because they have always defined her as 'part of the family', rather than conceptualizing her position in terms of her job description and her assigned tasks. By the same token, there are some well functioning practices where people find tactful and appropriate ways of discussing the mental health of practitioners, while in many there are strong unspoken rules that forbid this. There are partnerships and teams where it is possible to talk about the past (including times of conflict and distress), and those that have developed a culture of never referring to certain historical episodes or departed colleagues. Finally, there are practices that regularly review their priorities and find ways of coping with the ceaseless demands of patients and health authorities. Others try to maintain the illusion that there are no limits to their competence.

Another factor in determining the mental health of a practice may be the level and quality of its external relationships. Although there is again no formal research in this area, it is a reasonable guess to think that a practice that is able to identify its problems and seek outside help for them is more likely to be able to perform the same function for its own list of patients. In doing so, it will be modelling exactly the approach that it is recommending to users of its services. The last section of this chapter will consider the appropriate use of support in primary care, but first we need to look at the mental health task itself.

The practice as mental health team

It is no exaggeration to say, as the introduction to this book points out, that GPs and their teams are the principal mental health professionals in Britain (Shepherd *et al.* 1966). Both in terms of the numbers of problems brought to them, and arguably in terms of the range and seriousness of those problems, general practices shoulder most of the burden of mental distress brought to professionals of any kind. Yet this burden is shared by many different people within the practice, not just GPs, clinicians, and those who are formally designated as mental health professionals. It is shared by receptionists, secretaries, perhaps even cleaners and caretakers.

Professor Roger Higgs tells a story that will serve well as an illustration of how the practice functions as a mental health team. It is likely to resonate with anyone who works in general practice:

Case B

One morning, a receptionist came into Professor Higgs's consulting room to tell him that the next patient had arrived, but had been quite distressed at the front desk. She wanted to alert him so that that he could probe further if the patient presented with a trivial problem or underplayed her symptoms, as is often the case. Duly forewarned, he was on his mettle when the patient began the consultation by complaining about some minor ailment. He used a whole repertoire of searching questions and cues, all to no avail. Eventually, he came clean. 'Look', he said, 'I heard you were quite upset out in the waiting room. I wondered what that was all about.' 'Oh, I'm fine now', the patient replied. 'I talked to that lovely lady at the desk and she made me feel so much better!'

Every practice is a community of listeners, each offering to facilitate a different kind of story. Every team member will bring a different context and, perhaps, a different training to their role as listener. The receptionist will probably bring a background as a lay member of the same local community as the patient, but may perhaps bring other roles such as that of an experienced mother. The doctor will bring a framework of biomedical thinking, but also a personal freight of memories and concerns, including the pattern of mental health and distress in his or her own family. Formally trained mental health professionals will bring their own theoretical paradigms and approaches, and their particular histories and prejudices. Each listener will hear the stories brought to them through the filter of their own experiences, beliefs, and preferences. In addition to their various individual approaches, a team that communicates well can bring together the multiple fragments of a family's story, especially when different pieces have been left to reside with different members of the team (Cole-Kelly 1992)

Seeing the practice as a listening community reframes it as something much more collaborative and democratic than is usually the case. It assigns respect to team members who, on account of their social class or lack of formal higher education, might otherwise be seen as having less to contribute than the trained clinicians. It also widens one's view of what general practice is actually offering, so that the reception area, for instance, is no longer just seen as the antechamber to the inner sanctum of the GP's or counsellor's consulting room where the 'real' work goes on, but as a therapeutic setting in its own right.

However, this view of general practice highlights some difficult issues too. For example, it invites the trained professionals within a practice to see their work as a 're-storying' (see Chapter 9) of reality for their patients, rather than a normative process that is meant to assign irreducible definitions to their patients' experiences, in the form of diagnoses or interpretations. The challenge here, especially for doctors, is to see their role in relation to mental health as a more interactive, conversational one that may ultimately be no more effective or privileged than the one the patient has with the receptionist, the local pharmacist or the next-door neighbour. This is a very different view from the positivist one that doctors are imbued with throughout their training, and which is then reinforced by almost everything that doctors read and hear throughout their careers. It invites doctors, but also psychologists, mental health nurses, and other professionals in the practice to take a more irreverent view of their role and their centrality as diagnosticians and decision makers.

Another challenge, which confronts members of other disciplines as much as doctors, comes from the very plurality of stories that can be brought forth by different team members. Faced with the same patient, the GP may offer a conventional psychiatric diagnosis of depression, while the practice psychotherapist interprets what is going on for her in terms of childhood experiences and the secretary thinks the problem would have been avoided if she had continued going to church. These different stories or accounts of the problem may all be true or efficacious in their different ways, but what matters is whether they are offered in a spirit of rivalry or complementarity.

Rivalry can be a serious problem. In the past there have been many descriptions of mental health attachments in general practice suggesting that doctors and counsellors, for example, may see their working paradigms as being in opposition to each other. This can lead to both professions becoming dismissive or even contemptuous of each others' beliefs and working styles. It is very easy for counsellors to stereotype GPs as arrogant, superficial, and paternalistic. It is equally easy for GPs to return the compliment by seeing their counselling colleagues as woolly, precious, or unrealistic (McDaniel *et al.* 1990). What is harder is for GPs and others to work together on noticing what is valuable and mutually enhancing about each others' contributions, rather than just highlighting each others' perceived deficiencies when judged by the standards of the other. This may be equally true where differences exist between the conceptual and technical approaches taken by different mental health professionals in the same primary care team, for example, by those with a psychoanalytic or systemic approach, and those with a cognitive-behavioural one (see Chapter 18).

One framework that can help to unify how one understands the various story-making capacities that are held within the practice is to think of the practice in terms of attachment theory, as a secure base (Holmes 1993). Just as a family provides a context in which a child can both experience dependency and explore independence, a practice can offer an environment in which patients can feel held, while they experiment, as it were, with different attempts to remould their understanding of themselves (Mann 1999). It is no more necessary for the different team members within a practice to offer the same rigidly consistent account each time than is it for all the members of a family to dance to the same tune. Indeed, it can be pathological to do so. What is needed in both cases is a combination of flexibility and containment (see Chapter 6). The practice has to maintain itself as a space for creating meaning, but it also has to be able to behave consistently and with good internal communication in order to protect its own integrity. Only in this way can it offer safety to the people who come to consult there.

Case C

Bruce G is a female-to-male trans-sexual. He has had partial gender reassignment surgery, but is deeply dissatisfied with this. He is aggressive in his requests for further surgical referrals. A local psychiatrist has cautioned GPs against this, saying that he has an underlying personality disorder, which would make him discontent whatever the outcome. Bruce G has been removed from the lists of several other local GPs because of the nature of his demands, and his tendency to make threats to report doctors to the General Medical Council, the health authority, the local MP, and the newspapers. A year ago, the practice agreed to take him on to their list, but made it a condition that he would attend for a regular fortnightly appointment and see the same experienced doctor on each occasion. The first few encounters with his new doctor were very stormy. On one occasion Bruce shouted at him 'You're a fucking waste of space'. He then walked out to the practice manager's office to insist on being reallocated to a different partner. The practice and the GP remained firm, holding to the original contract they had offered. Over a period of several months, Bruce and the GP managed to reach an agreement on a referral to a specialized psychotherapy unit that could offer him psychological support, reassess his wish for further surgery and consider an onward referral to the regional unit for gender reassignment. Bruce is now actively engaged in group therapy.

The role of the practice as a mental health team has particular implications in the area of confidentiality. This takes on quite a different meaning in a general practice context from the one often assumed among other mental health professionals. The kind of confidentiality that operates in the private counsellor's or therapist's consulting room, for example, offers a tremendous amount in that specific context, especially in terms of the trust and sense of safety that it engenders. However, within a complex network of professionals and support staff who are sharing the task of caring for patients, such a purity of approach can be fundamentalist and anti-therapeutic. Furthermore, if the whole range of staff are to understand the nature of mental health provision in its widest sense, even the process of decision making itself may at times have to be shared with many different team members (Launer 1994; Waskett 1999).

This may be self-evident to many GPs, and to counsellors and therapists with a great deal of experience of primary care, but it can be troubling and contentious to people whose training may have assigned an over-arching importance to the notion of privacy, particularly if they are not experienced enough to take risks in this area or to use mature judgement to override their prior education. There are many compelling reasons why confidentiality has to be treated as something much more multi-layered and negotiable in primary care than in most other therapeutic workplaces. For a start, the accessibility of surgery premises, both physically and culturally, means that they are open to people who may not be willing to play by the therapeutic rules, for example by agreeing to attend only at fixed times or to see one particular person. This exposes care workers to risks, including physical danger and verbal or emotional abuse. In addition, the chaotic and unfocused ways in which patients bring their distress into the practice may mean that the team cannot help them without exchanging information in order to translate their complex communications into a more unified story. This exchange of information should not be seen as mere gossip, but as an essential part of creating a therapeutic milieu.

Case D

Mr D is a Kossovan refugee who has experienced unspeakable atrocities at first hand in his own country. Together with his wife and five children, he is receiving considerable amounts of practical, medical, and psychological support from a number of people in the health centre. These include his GP, visiting link workers, a counsellor, and a welfare rights advisor. Recently, he arrived very late for an evening consultation, in fact just at the moment that one of the cleaners was locking the front door. He abused her verbally and then roughly pushed her out of the way, insisting that the receptionists should still fit him in to see the doctor. At a subsequent case meeting of clinicians, everyone agreed that the patient was under excep- tional psychological pressure, and it would be disastrous for his family if he was asked to leave the list and therefore no longer had access to a well resourced GP surgery. One of the GPs agreed to talk to the cleaner and reception staff involved, explaining that there were special reasons for leniency and telling them that the team would prefer to let him off with a strong caution. After hearing enough information to understand why his aggression was not being penalized in the usual way, the receptionists agreed. The cleaner also gave her consent on condition that the practice bought her a personal alarm and also that someone warned her every time the man attended. The doctors also agreed that a male doctor or staff member would always be available to come to the aid of the cleaners if any incident of this kind arose in future.

Seeing the practice as a mental health team also carries implications about over- all issues, such as environment, training, and staff attitude. Practices that are attentive in these areas may be offering better mental health care in the widest sense. If patients attend a practice that has a particular view of certain kinds of behaviour, language, or ways of seeing the world, that view will permeate and perhaps even define how those patients see themselves. To put it bluntly, if there is a paranoid culture where the mentally ill can be discussed as 'nutters', it will influence the way that patients construe themselves. Mental disturbance is not a concrete object, but to a large extent the product of interpersonal encounters. Encounters with primary care are part of this process and for many of the people we see, they may be crucial in the establishment of a mentally healthy or sick identity.

Support and supervision

From the point of view of a sophisticated observer, one of the most problematical aspects of general practice is that the level of training, support, and supervision available is hugely inadequate for the task (see previous chapter). In many cases, there is little or no system, either formal or informal, to support GPs and practice nurses in the work they do. Indeed, the idea of professional 'supervision' is so alien for many GPs that it carries nuances of surveillance and policing, rather than implying, as it should, that clinicians inevitably need space for reflection and the opportunity to exchange ideas with someone independent (Rutt and Batchelor 1998). It is a noticeable irony that front line workers in primary care, who see the most unprocessed and often the most difficult cases in the health service under enormous pressure of speed and demand, have so little opportunity to think about their work, to engage in dialogue about it with their peers or with others, or to monitor and refine their own methods of practice. This irony is in some ways a parallel to the 'inverse care' law that has been noted in relation to deprived patient groups: those who have the greatest need are often those for whom least is provided. In keeping with the same law, a proportion of GPs feel so marginalized that they do not expect, and might not even welcome, any kind of help.

Relationship with secondary care

An important factor in the dearth of help for primary care lies in the nature of its relationship with secondary care. Traditionally, mental health professionals with skills in psychological reflection and analysis have tended to relate to general practices in ways that have deterred, rather than encouraged a culture of training, support, and supervision. First, the conventional system of referral into secondary care usually means that there is a sharp disjunction between the formless, autobiographical narrative that the patient brings to the GP or primary care nurse, and the sanitized formulations of the letter that comes back from out patients. (This kind of interaction between primary care and the specialist services has been called 'the dry cleaning model': an ironic description, but one that is metaphorically precise.) Secondly, when psychiatrists, psychologists, and others have moved themselves physically into surgery premises for a regular session—the so-called 'shifted out-patients' model—the geographical adventure has often disguised a deep conceptual conservatism, so that the work that goes on down the corridor offers no special advantages to the general practice patient beyond the economy of a saved bus fare. Such a shift may not even help to attract the large numbers of distressed and disturbed patients who will not choose to see any professional other than their own GP under any circumstances.

Even the more imaginative 'liaison model', which involves mental health specialists making themselves available for advice and case discussions on primary care premises, may also fail to grapple with some central problems. One of these is the assumed hierarchical superiority of specialist ways of knowing the world above the generalist understanding. Another is the unspoken assumption that generalists should learn from specialists, but not vice versa. Lastly, there is the rule in most of these professional liaisons that the subject material of discussions should be the content of the cases, but not the consulting context itself and how it might be making its own contribution to the construction or perpetuation of the problem (Selvini Palazzoli *et al.* 1980).

Nevertheless, things may be changing (we hope this book may represent a small example of this change). There are all kinds of influences around that may offer opportunities to rewrite the story of specialist-generalist interactions in the health service, especially in relation to mental health. The rhetoric of a 'primary care led health service', first articulated more than a decade ago now, may not in itself change the way that the different sectors of the NHS relate to each other, but it reflects an economic reality (the vast and disproportionate cost of specialist services, and the almost embarrassing thriftiness of primary care) that may well force many more secondary care workers out into the community (Gordon and Plamping 1996). The increased empowerment of consumer groups and users, who inherently see the world in less pathologized and more narrative terms, is also likely to mean that the discourse of primary care is heard more distinctly within the polyphony of voices that define good practice. Most important of all, however, is the emergent issue of *quality*, with its accompanying watchwords: clinical governance, patient protection, continuing professional development, audit, needs assessment, health improvement. These are concepts that have burst onto the health service scene with ballistic speed in recent years. Pushed aggressively by central government, within a framework of primary care trusts and the Commission for Health Improvement, it is these concepts above all other influences that are likely to radicalize the way that primary care and the specialisms connect with each other, and the way that supervision and support happen in primary care.

Changing practices: a general mental health practitioner?

Certain new themes do seem to be emerging in the relationship between the mental health world and primary care. One is the idea that primary care is something to be taken seriously as a specialist field in its own right. This may seem paradoxical, since primary care seems so patently non-specialist, and the general practice sector of it in particular appears deceptively transparent. Indeed, for a naïve colleague from another discipline it may seem obvious what GPs do or are meant to do. Yet for imaginative psychologists, counsellors, or others who take an interest in the field, there is a lot of learning to do in this respect—or perhaps it would be more accurate to reframe this as unlearning, before learning can be effective. Some of the areas for unlearning have already been covered in this chapter and elsewhere in this book: that GP work in mental health is not just with the least disturbed part of the population, but may also be with those who are most disturbed; or that brief consultations may be more effective than they seem.

Other areas of unlearning and learning for mental health professionals may be harder. They may discover, for example, that primary care is not for beginners: contrary to common prejudices, its complexity and unpredictability demand a level of skill and experience that will challenge even the most senior mental health specialists, and will almost certainly exceed the capacity of a novice. Specialists may also find that their cherished professional identities, whether by discipline or by psychological ideology, may be a source of complete mystification or even utter indifference to others such as GPs. How on earth can a practice choose between a cognitive-behavioural psychologist or a psychoanalytic psychotherapist if both speak languages about their work that are incomprehensible to the practice team? What either of these people will be valued for is any capacity to understand the difference of the context and how it might affect the kind of help they are willing to offer.

From this kind of thinking in primary care, the notion of the 'general mental health practitioner' seems to have been coalescing in recent years, even if it has not yet been operationalized in training courses and diplomas. Mental health professionals from various backgrounds have started to see their usefulness to primary care in terms of the question: 'how similar to a GP do I have to become in order to be useful, and how different do I have to remain in order to be effective?' Formulating the question in this way is already perhaps part of the answer. It acknowledges the primacy of the context and the magnitude of the task involved in trying to adapt to it. It represents a dramatic rejection of the traditional discourse concerning 'the need for GPs to have better training' or 'the problem of inappropriate referrals'; such problems are, of course, genuine ones, but the new way of thinking reframes them as problems that belong to the relationship between primary and secondary care, rather than being sited only in the former. It is a healthy move away from the 'patchwork quilt' model of primary care, in which GPs are believed by their outside colleagues to be doing (or meant to be doing) shrunken parts of everyone else's work. It also stands in radical opposition to the simplistic idea of 'relieving the GP's workload' by placing junior psychologists, perhaps with only basic training in one technique, into practices. This is an idea that has gained credibility for obvious economic and political reasons, but which can also be seen as profoundly at odds with the nature and purpose of primary care.

What might a 'general mental health practitioner' do within a practice or primary care team? They should almost certainly be thinking about crossing some of the conventional boundaries between individual and family casework, training, case consultancy, supervision and perhaps even organizational consultancy (Dowling 1994) (see chapter 10). Since the field of primary care is inherently antipathetic to clear categories such as these, attached mental health professionals at least need to be asking questions about how their generic skills can most be useful in the community context, and to be entering into some kind of dialogue with GPs and teams about this. Inevitably, there will always be practices where no one wants anything other than the 'dry cleaning' model. In such places it may be appropriate to offer just that, although perhaps with some graded and tactful questioning about the stresses that led the organization to want such a limited engagement with help. At the other end of the spectrum, there may only be a very few practices wanting to use an outside individual for help with everything from casework to assistance with personnel or partnership matters at the other end. Even in these cases there will be important questions to ask about the exact boundaries of the work and whether it is appropriate to combine several functions in the same person.

Here, it is useful to consider models from the United States, where the Collaborative Family Healthcare Coalition has promoted a staged model of collaboration between family doctors and 'behavioural scientists', ranging from traditional referral models through to integrated co-working on the same site and in the same room (McDaniel *et al.* 1992; Bloch and Doherty 1998). In the United Kingdom, a few practices have already taken journeys along this route (Deys *et al.* 1989; Senior 1994).

Case E

For many years, if not decades, the M Practice had had no connection with local clinical psychologists beyond making referrals and getting letters back from the psychology department. Often these letters stated that the patient would be put on a waiting list for up to 6 months, and almost as often this was followed by a letter about 9 months later saying that the patient had been offered several appointments, but had not turned up. Dr S, faced with a particularly troubling patient with self-harming behaviour whom she felt was most unlikely to go to a psychology department even under the best of circumstances, phoned the new head of the adult psychology team to get some ideas about how to proceed. The timing was propitious since the new person in charge of the team was particularly keen to make contact with primary care and to tailor the service to meet the needs of referrers better than in the past. The psychologist suggested that he would be prepared to come out and see the patient jointly with Dr S at the end of a normal surgery, a proposal that she welcomed wholeheartedly.

An initial joint meeting with the patient to explore his needs was not conspicuously successful, since he declined any kind of further involvement with mental health services, wherever it was sited. However, Dr S found the encounter extremely helpful, since for the first time someone with appropriate qualifications in assessment and supervision had been able to reassure her that she had done her best with this patient and that, in the circumstances, there was no further work she could do without the patient's clear consent and co-operation. Out of this initial piece of collaborative work, however, the relationship between the practice and the department has developed over a number of years and now involves a multi-dimensional service, which has included (among other things) regular attendance by the head of adult psychology at case discussion meetings in the practice, a bereavement group based at the practice, and a monthly session available for families where someone is struggling with chronic or life-threatening illness. In these sessions both the family's GP and a member of the psychology team are present. The practice has also used other members of the department to advise and consult with team issues including tension between the practice nurses and the health visitor. This flexible way of working has now been taken up by the local primary care trust as a model of healthy practice for the locality.

As mental health services and primary care draw closer and as managers look more closely at the best use of human resources, there are likely to be challenges to the belief that GPs just deal with the 'worried well' or that mental health professionals are just in the building to see individual patients behind closed doors. Given all the current changes and pressures on the primary care scene, more innovative and evolutionary models of collaborative working should become the norm. What may be the way of the future is for general practices to be at the heart of mental health care, and for other mental health professionals to be used as resources for thinking and reflection in primary care, and for service development.

9 Systemic family practice in primary care

Hilary Graham and Robert Mayer

We start by quoting from one of our co-authors who has inspired us to introduce family approaches to our general practice work (see Chapter 5):

> I have always envied GPs for being—at least in theory—in a position of picking up problems early...you have to work pretty hard as a teenager to get a referral to a child psychiatrist: attempted hanging or killing the cat, but the rest stays in general practice. I found I could help GPs get at families with teenagers earlier in the story, and encourage parents to take control again. Pathologizing the individual teenager didn't seem to help much and GPs can become good at seeing more than one person at a time. It proved to me how useful the family systems approach can be when it comes to prevention or early intervention—and general practice seems the ideal site for this.
> *(Asen and Tomson 1997)*

The past two decades have seen a rapid expansion in the field of family therapy both in Britain and abroad. The ideas of systemic thinking were proposed by Gregory Bateson whose analysis of communication patterns led him to the awareness that actions become meaningful only through their relationship to context (Bateson 1972; Minuchin 1974; Haley 1976). The crucial innovation of this approach was to emphasize the importance of looking at everything through the lens of relationships. In a family, if something happens to one family member, there must always be consequences in the lives of the others. No human being exists in isolation. We are always acting in relation to others.

Family therapy is a method of treatment that develops this idea of interactions and processes within the family. Rather than dwelling exclusively on problems or symptoms, therapists ask questions that explore how family members relate to each other, and to the problem and its management. Such a 'narrative' approach suggests that families can construct different (better) stories rather than the problem-only story (see Chapter 8) and these stories of old competencies and new possibilities can become lived through being told (White and Epston 1990).

Ideas and practices that have been developed from this include the therapist being 'curious' (see Chapter 5); maintaining a stance of 'neutrality'; acknowledgment of the position of the therapist (and other professionals) in the family system; and an examination of the gender, power, and 'preferred ideas' or 'reverences' as they have been termed by Cecchin (Cecchin *et al.* 1992). Clinical applications of these ideas have been widely used in a variety of contexts: in hospitals, social services and primary health care settings (Christie-Seely 1984; McDaniel *et al.* 1990).

Primary care

The psychodynamic foundations of the Balint school (Balint 1957) had a profound influence on undergraduate and postgraduate education for general practice, and are based on an interpersonal understanding with an awareness of transference and countertransference in the consultation (see Chapter 7). Family therapy ideas add the extra dimension of 'interactively recursive' relationships and processes within the family or larger system. This interactive perspective, is applicable in consultations with individuals as well as whole families (Jenkins 1989; Jenkins and Asen 1992). Our experience suggests that much clinical interaction between doctor and patient still lies in a paternalistic model (Launer and Lindsay 1997) with the doctor attempting to transfer or even impose his view of medical treatment, health education, or even behaviour on to the patient or family.

Although GPs are often in the privileged position of knowing individuals in a family very well and often over a long period of time, there is a curious reluctance among GPs to see working directly with whole families as a core part of their job. Possibly with the doctor's traditional role to reach a diagnosis and to reach it quickly, there is a fear of confusion and loss of control— the idea that a *family discussion* about the symptom might be the cure could seem very strange! Most family problems (school refusal, eating problems, soiling, etc.) are referred to specialist services—although many such referrals never materialize because families are often reluctant to accept the need to see a mental health worker. Nevertheless, there is an increasing interest among primary health care professionals in translating principles derived from family therapy into their every day practice (Deys *et al.* 1989; Launer 1994). Medical educationalists in the USA have led this process, both in dealing with families and professional systems (McDaniel *et al.* 1992), and a parallel process has occurred in this country (Asen and Tomson 1992, Tomson 1990).

At the time these ideas were gaining momentum, a group of GPs at the Highate Group Practice were trying to move away from the idea of individual diagnosis and towards a focus on family relationships. Our experience can be described under four main categories:

♦ The adoption of a systemic approach in ordinary surgery consultations and in discussions about cases in the practice.

♦ The development of a Family Therapy clinic *within the practice*.

♦ The growth of a body of primary care professionals working together to develop ways of 'thinking families' as an integral part of their daily work with patients.

♦ Experience gained in teaching—at undergraduate and postgraduate level— the usefulness of ideas from family therapy in managing difficult problems with patients.

The authors have been part of a family team in a general practice for 10 years (Carpenter and Treacher 1993). The team was formed partly because of a perceived dearth of child and adolescent mental health services in the area, but also as a result of interest within the practice in family therapy ideas. The practice had been a venue for a course in these ideas and had subsequently become 'infected' (Asen and Tomson 1997).

The family clinic

Since its establishment the Family Clinic has been held on one half-day a fortnight, in a large practice common room that is usefully 'different' from the rest of the surgery and has the benefit of a video link to an observing room. Referrals are from other clinical members of the practice team (usually GPs or practice nurses, but also the practice counsellor and health visitors). Referrals also often arise from the regular multi-disciplinary practice meetings, where difficult families are discussed. Responses to referral include (but are not limited to) the offer of a formal appointment for the family. Frequently, discussion with a clinic team member results in the referrer being able to continue managing the case or to holding a network consultation that includes the referrer. This may be particularly helpful with 'heartsink' patients, a phenomenon well described in general practice (Douglas 1992); where helping the dysfunctional doctor–patient relationship (as described in Chapter 5) may be the most useful approach.

Mr Williams

Mr Williams, age 55, a government researcher who lives alone in an old Victorian house has been a patient of the practice for 25 years. At the time his GP consulted the team he had been bed-bound for 3 years. His doctor was summoned by the patient, his carer, and his neighbours with escalating frequency. They were desperate for a convincing diagnosis and treatment that would get him back to work. Over the years the GP had tried hard to understand his troubles and had investigated him thoroughly, seeking opinions from physicians and the psychiatric team. The GP felt at a loss about how best to be helpful. She consulted the team members in a practice meeting. The meeting felt that a network meeting might help her to feel less stuck, but was sceptical about being able to improve her patient's condition. The doctor said that even discussing the case with the team, did indeed make her feel less stuck—particularly helpful to the GP was the idea that, although they may not be able to improve Mr Williams' medical condition, they might be able to help the patient/doctor/carer/neighbour system. At the meeting, all participants were able to voice their concerns and clarify their positions and responsibilities.

The clinic has five members—three GPs, a counsellor with family therapy and social work training, and an external therapist, who has been funded on a trial basis by the Health Authority. In addition there is usually a student on placement for a year from one of the Family Therapy training centres.

This clinic in the practice has proved useful to both the practitioners and the patients. One study showed that:

> There was a high level of satisfaction among GPs referring patients. The clinic proved to be highly acceptable for clients, with 90% agreeing that it was easier to attend a clinic at the practice than at a hospital. Eighty per cent of the patients felt that the problem had improved at the time of follow up. Where the problem had not improved, 60% felt that they were dealing with it better. Almost all of the patients felt that the family therapy clinic should become a permanent part of local services.
> *(Graham et al. 1992)*

The clinic provides a continuing base for teaching medical students, GP registrars (Mayer and Graham 1998), and trainee family therapists. Although the majority of family problems have concerned children and young people, the oldest client approached the practice when he was 96, concerning his and his wife's anxieties and their communication about his inevitable death. (Louden and Graham 1998).

Other primary care teams have been working with family therapists or using these ideas in their day-to-day work, and a group of interested professionals (social workers, GPs, counsellors, and nurses), have been researching and working together for a number of years. They have watched each other at work, videoed consultations, and been active in teaching students, GPs and GP registrars, as well as publishing (Launer 1996; Mayer and Graham 1998), and running workshops and conferences.

How do we create space for thinking about families?

In our practice, the primary health care team meeting (a multi-disciplinary meeting where cases are discussed) has a long history as a 'thinking' space

(Smith *et al.* 1983; see Chapters 6 and 8) and has become part of the structure of the practice. The model that informs the meeting has evolved from one that was psychodynamically based and paid attention to group processes, to one that was more systemically orientated. This model had first developed from a pioneering social work attachment from the Tavistock Clinic in the 1970s (Graham and Sher 1976), following an earlier initiative (Brook and Temperley 1976) to bring psychotherapeutic thinking out to practices in ways that were *useful to them*. It had served the practice well in helping the professionals understand the conflicts that are sometimes enacted within the healthcare team and the professionals' own feelings that can be aroused. However, the overall mood of working in this way could often be gloomy and allow (sometimes unintentionally) a 'patient-blaming' focus to develop. We found that the interest that we have in systemic ideas gave a different and frequently more positive flavour to the team meetings and allowed for a better way of working systemically, understanding our own and each others postions in relation to the problem; (McDaniel *et al.* 1992) between the patient, the family, and the professionals involved.

Thus, we listen to the various stories that emerge around a patient's illness, while attending to the biopsychsocial context (Engel 1997). For professionals working in less pressured therapeutic settings, this thinking space may seem unremarkable, but for GPs who are used to 10-minute consultations, it is an 'essential luxury'.

Thinking processes in the practice system may be thought of as flowing in several parallel circuits. Beyond the consultation, a simple loop would be the 'gossip' or casual conversation between GP partners or with practice nurse, health visitor, or counsellor, all of which could provide feedback to a question, doubt, or dilemma. The meeting provides a space for these information streams to be connected, examined, and reflected back. Thus, a GP may find that an anxiety presented by a parent is mirrored or confirmed, or perhaps reassured and lessened by a health visitor's contact with the children. A picture emerges more in keeping with a view jointly developed by all the parties concerned and hopefully with better definition to guide the action of all the participants.

In our practice, we have the option of our family clinic, but this is not always chosen, representing, as it does, an unusual concentration of thinking for a primary care context. More often, discussions at the meeting allow the practitioners to continue their work feeling more enabled to carry on themselves, possibly to invite a colleague to join the in a consultation or visit, or to permit him to to acknowledge that a resource outside the practice is required and appropriate, rather than to soldier on unsupported.

How do we 'think families'?

Opportunites for thinking about families are frequent in our interaction with patients—we see parts of families all the time—and we have a repertoire of questions relating to family interaction and process that is as much part of our core way of working as a prescription for antibiotics. Such questions are non-blaming and generate a benign curiosity which is comfortable for both patient and practitioner (Cecchin 1987; see Chapter 5). For example, we have for many years incorporated a genogram on the front sheet of our records as a prompt to information gathering and hypothesis generation that starts when patients first register with us. This family tree not only gives important medical information, but in a pictorial way discloses family events and 'connections'. We can become more interested in how 'hypothesizing' leads to discoveries of new stories and ideas in our conversations with families, rather than concentrating on getting ' right answers'.

Clinical examples

Mrs Roberts brought her son Paul (age 11 years) to the surgery. He was increasingly naughty, difficult to control, and she was at her wits end. Whilst trying to understand what was going on, the doctor constructed a genogram with Paul and his mother. This 'illustrated' that his father had left the family after violent behaviour and that this was the case also with his paternal grandfather. Mother thought he was going the same way as they had, and could say little positive about him. The doctor (through the genogram) discovered that there were 'good' uncles on mother's side and got her to speak of some the good times that Paul had had with them. They discussed the possibility that further contact with these men might help Paul. Mother thought these ideas were helpful and began to tell more positive stories about her son.

Requests for help with problems in our surgeries may be covert or relatively straightforward. Here is something close to home in which the relevant part of the 'toolkit' is the idea of asking the questions around family interaction and process in the form of a ' diary task' for the family to participate in.

Here are some typical opening gambits that might lead on to a family-orientated approach:

Well Mrs Jones, David's hearing and eyesight are both fine. I've examined him carefully and can reassure you that there's nothing serious going on with these headaches. You don't think he's worrying about something?
Of course not Doctor, everything is perfectly all right at home—his father would tell you just the same. It's time this got sorted out; you've got to do something!

and this;

She just gets into these moods, at anytime; there's nothing we can do to stop her. It's upsetting the little one and getting between Jim and me. We've no idea what's causing it.

The rhythm of general practice is based around working in relatively short time slots. GPs face problems where we sense we need more time. However, the problem is often presented in such a way that, even with time, we are not sure how to tackle it and we experience a feeling of being cornered. We are looking for more information about the problem and, if we are thinking about family process, for more understanding of the relationship between the problem and the functioning of the family.

It is probably not feasible to invite the whole family into the surgery and it may be difficult to question an anxious patient who may be feeling the doctor is trying to get at something that he or she is not ready to or is unwilling to talk about.

Here using the idea of a diary can be very helpful. For example, in the first scenario:

- A diary allows the GP to ask questions indirectly and without prejudice, e.g. 'I'd like to know more about David's headaches. Perhaps you and your husband could keep a diary of exactly when and how they start—and perhaps any ideas you may have either at the time or later about things that may have made them worse or helped them to become any better.'

- The doctor can explore coping strategies: 'Could you keep a careful note of what you do to try to help him, and what sort of effect that has?' or 'What was the most helpful thing that either of you has done so far?'

- If the GP feels that one of the parents is more preoccupied with the problem than the other, she could ask: 'Would you like to do a diary together so that I can hear about your shared ideas?' Or, if she suspects that they share a fixed idea, perhaps ask: 'Maybe each of you could keep a diary separately of what you observe or think may be affecting his headaches and we could look at it together when you come next time . . . ?'

Such strategies are respectful: the doctor is honestly asking to know more in order to try to be more helpful. The parents are empowered in that it will be their own observations and their ideas that they bring back to share with their GP. The child will be closely observed, perhaps a little differently, more compassionately, rather than ignored or criticized. Probably the solution, as is most often the case, will be found by the parents, but if not, these ideas are unlikely to have been unhelpful and may give you useful information.

Not uncommonly, a parent will bring a child to the surgery as 'the problem'. What is generally meant is that an aspect of the child's behaviour has become a problem, but by the time the consultation occurs, the identities of the problem and the child have become merged. This is usually unhelpful and leads to parents viewing their children negatively.

Techniques which we find helpful include *reframing*, by which is meant ascribing an alternative meaning or intent to the behaviour that is more positive, and *externalization*, in which the identities of the problem and the child are separated through questioning (White and Epston 1990). For example, the doctor might ask a child brought in by a distressed parent because of tantrums, 'Have you ever caught Tantrum napping? How did you manage to disobey him?'

Through questioning of this kind, children can discover agency in areas that have become disabled by the problem. It is often helpful for someone who is being viewed with hostility, to become the subject of more benign attention. Family-centred questions (like the diary questions), offer manoeuvrability in situations where one is feeling stuck. They allow for neutral questions and can have a lightness of touch or playfulness, which can lessen the tension around a problem. Often, families have their own 'solutions' to problems. Stimulated by the family-based interview with the doctor, they make their own explanations of the symptom's meaning and find novel ways of approaching how they solve it: 'My wife took him to a homeopath and there's been a great improvement' or 'It's been a lot better since we stopped him having Coca-Cola'. Or again, 'My doctor has this funny idea about keeping a diary; we knew she'd been missing school dinners, so we've sorted it out with her teacher'.

Sometimes a family problem can present as an emergency.

The Smith family

Mr Smith came to see one of the partners in the Saturday morning emergency surgery to tell her that his 15-year-old son Philip had tried to hang himself after a family row. She established that Philip was physically unharmed and negotiated how the parents could guarantee his safety over the weekend, by mounting a 'suicide prevention watch'. She contacted one of the partners in the family team and an emergency family session was arranged for Monday morning. Two of the family team joined the GP for a brief session at which the seriousness of the situation was acknowledged and some of the anger and frustration that preceded the suicide attempt was aired. The focus of this session was to keep the boy safe. Over the next 6 months the family was seen in the practice family clinic for a total of five sessions. Philip's behaviour became more 'normally adolescent'—according to his parents he was becoming bloody-minded. The clinic team and the family doctor helped the parents cope with their difficulties around dealing with a teenage boy. They both had childhood experiences that had left them frightened and ill equipped for setting limits and coping with fears around violence. Father had experienced a violent childhood and when faced with having to control his son's teenage rebelliousness, was 'paralysed' by the fear of his own potential violence, whereas his wife, who had sisters, felt safe with daughters, but 'completely at sea in dealing with boys'. Philip seemed uncontained and uncontrolled, and his behaviour moved between being very miserable, frightened, and unsafe and therefore very difficult. Some time later Mr and Mrs Smith reported that they were working together as a couple better than ever and father was coming to terms with the disagreeable business of setting limits—there were no further suicide attempts.

Some colleagues have expressed concern over the management of this case by a family practice, since it falls into the category of cases, which usually earns psychiatric involvement. We believe that the *swift* and supportive response from the GP and the practice team contained a potentially tragic situation, and allowed the parents to change the way they dealt with adolescent rebellion. Referral to a specialist would have taken much longer and may well have been less acceptable to Philip and his family—they had decided that they could manage overnight and wanted to talk with their trusted family doctor in the morning. Furthermore, in that consultation, they were able to convince their doctor that they had the ability to protect their son at least until the emergency family clinic meeting. Therefore, the GP who was well aware of the inadequacy of the local acute adolescent services (from previous experience in the practice), felt that the support offered by the presence of the family team allowed them to take the risk of letting the family deal with the situation over the weekend without recourse to a formal psychiatric assessment.

An anxious GP was able to know she had a quickly responding resource at hand and could take what otherwise might have seemed to be a risky decision in allowing the family to 'hold on' and ensure their son's safety. (The mention of this case to various mental health colleagues has in fact produced much anxiety and criticism. One is, however, reminded that patients in secondary care settings are still able to harm or kill themselves. GPs have to manage many primary/secondary interface crises, not necessarily connected to mental health problems, where moving to a secondary referral may be actually less appropriate or even more dangerous, in spite of first appearances.)

The family clinic team as a resource

One of the partners may keep the 'family resource' in mind as in the next case:

A rather shy and private woman came with her daughter Susan. Both were anxious and depressed and consulted their GP together. Susan could scarcely leave her mother and felt unable to go to school. Her parents were both ill. Her father had had a pulmonary embolism a few years previously and remained very breathless; her mother had a benign cerebral tumour and was found unconscious on the floor shortly after her husband's embolus. She made a slow but good recovery after brain surgery, but became very depressed. Susan had started her 'A' levels but her attendance at school was very erratic; she was becoming a protective child rather than a young adult and seemed unable to separate and become more independent.

The GP spoke to one of the family team and suggested a family meeting which was hesitantly taken up—it was acceptable because the family knew two of the GPs who were members of the family team.

Susan and her mother came first on their own. They said that they didn't think father would come because he would not want to show his feelings. He did come to later sessions however. The family believed they could not change their nature and would not stop worrying, but were able to talk about their worries for each other. Conversations about their strengths and skills gave a picture of a family that could cope with major problems. Susan heard and possibly believed a little more that her parents could manage without her and that none of the feared disasters would necessarily arise. Similarly, she started to believe that she might have the resources to live a little more independently.

A year and a half later Susan has finished school and still lives at home, but has a full-time job. She is still anxious, but the family is calmer. She now consults her doctor on her own, when necessary. Her mother is no longer so depressed.

None of us, not least her GP, believes that stories like this end in complete cure, but the ongoing nature of the general practice relationship allows the doctor to remain available when required.

This family would have been difficult to help without the opportunity to develop new ideas about themselves both as individuals and members of a family system, which included conversations about their strengths and abilities. They would have been unlikely to take up a referral to a hospital-based adult mental health team. It was important to them that they felt safe with the doctors they knew (particularly father). It was also important that the referring GP could exchange information with team members.

Adolescent eating disorders as an example of systemic work in general practice

One initially surprising result of our involvement with systemic ideas has been the ability to venture into areas that previously would have been deemed too difficult, or worrying, but for which no satisfactory service existed. Adolescent eating disorders are increasingly recognized as relatively common problems, which are under-diagnosed (see Chapter 12). Because the sufferer is often likely to be the last person who seeks help, the GP may expect worried contacts from parents or concerned others. The use of neutral, but empathic questions ('curiosity'), for example 'If it were your mother rather than you that had this problem, what would your concerns be?' This allows for a more constructive engagement with the problem, rather than unhelpful confrontation or, worse, the risk of false reassurance ('It's just a phase'):

Jane was a 16-year-old who presented to her GP with a 3-month history of amenorrhoea, weight loss, and food restriction. She was doing well at school, the elder of two children in what the GP knew as an otherwise untroubled family. Although, at one stage, she had been a little plump, both she and her mother had been pleased with the results of her diet. She had a good relationship with her (female) GP who had become concerned when her mother attended describing Jane's increasingly worrying behaviour, moodiness, and social withdrawal. Jane's GP invited her to attend with her parents. She was sullen and denied any problems despite looking very thin.

Her GP, rather than confront Jane, became 'curious' (Palazzolli *et al.* 1980) about whether Jane could describe what worries her parents might have about her; she responded to this, albeit rather grudgingly. This allowed her to hear her parents' concerns arising from a position of care, rather than interference, and together they were able to map the domains where anorexia was taking over and spoiling her life. Her doctor was able to negotiate a physical examination and the necessary investigations to allay her own anxieties. Following this she talked with Jane's parents with Jane present about what sort of diet a 16-year-old might need to allow weight gain to occur and how they might ensure she received it. The meeting ended with an agreement that Jane would keep a food diary, meals would be eaten under parental supervision, and that Jane would return for follow-up weighing with the practice nurse, before being seen again.

The diary confirmed that little change had taken place, with inadequate calorific intake and restriction of food types. Her doctor asked the practice dietician to comment on it. The comment to the effect that diet contained adequate calories for an adolescent's basal metabolic needs and no more was put into a concerned letter to Jane and her parents suggesting that if they could not negotiate a better diet with the anorexia, then Jane would need to stay in bed, since her intake did not allow for any extra energy expenditure.

This rather alarming and strategic message (strategic in the sense that the intention was not to confine Jane to bed, but to raise anxiety about the potential seriousness of her position and certainly the seriousness with which her doctor regarded it) had the aim of helping Jane's parents help her fight the anorexia more effectively.

When they met next, Jane seemed to have turned the corner with regard to weight and within a few weeks had regained her lost weight. Although she harboured some resentment against her doctor for seeming to have ganged up with her parents, she felt able at a later stage to ask for help with underlying problems of low self-esteem, which led her into useful work with her school counsellor.

The work in this case occurred without referral to the family clinic although the GP at various points discussed 'tactics' with a member of the family team. As a piece of early intervention in what may have progressed to a serious eating disorder, it demonstrates the potential value of family approaches even in areas not usually regarded by general practitioners as lying within their area of competence.

Conclusion

These cases show different aspects of family work within our general practice. Practitioners themselves, in their surgeries, may use information from genograms or ask slightly different sorts of questions in order to understand processes within the family, rather than become 'saturated' with the details of a problem (as in the first two scenarios). In the third case, the in-house team was used as an adult mental health resource that was accessible and unthreatening. The fourth case shows how the interested GP can (albeit with support) utilize strategies from formal family therapy in the surgery to provide a powerful piece of early intervention. Despite drawing some examples from our clinic casework, many of the strategies discussed have been deployed by us and our colleagues in ordinary general practice consultations and in inter-professional conversations.

The current changes in the NHS seek to place General Practice, through the instrument of Primary Care Groups and Trusts, at the centre of the health care system in terms of thinking about patient's needs and the commissioning of services. It is too early to know whether this huge experiment in delivery will be more successful than the one it replaces. The current imperatives (described by key phrases such as 'evidence-based', 'cost-contained', and 'outcome-driven') place great emphasis on what General Practice can deliver, but one consequence of this change may be to devalue the task of *creating space for thinking*—with the patient, their family, colleagues, or even self-reflection. These activities are necessarily harder to measure and to justify, but we believe they are essential nonetheless. The lack of opportunity for the space in which to practice in this way produces burnout, dissatisfaction on the part of patients and professionals, and ultimately a degraded form of practice, which is less creative and relies more on secondary care, rather than less. We believe that a systemically-informed family medicine can help overcome this disaffection and help the key players in Primary Care Trusts work together for the benefit of patients.

10 Therapists and counsellors in primary care

Mary Burd and Jan Wiener

Most counsellors and psychotherapists enjoy working in primary care. Because such therapists have not been recognized by any of the NHS pay scales, their independent contractor status has enabled GPs to employ them directly and so tempting opportunities for work have been more available, especially for people who do not have a core professional background in psychology, medicine, or social work. Such posts, when advertised, attract large numbers of applicants, all apparently rushing to the front line to work with patients in distress at the site where they most commonly first present themselves. There are now about 3000 part-time counsellors employed in practices across the country, amounting to 1300 full-time posts (Mellor-Clarke 2000). At the same time, there is also a tradition of other NHS employed staff, such as clinical psychologists and CPNs working in primary care.

While there is a fertile literature that evokes the character of a GP practice as an environment in which to practice counselling or psychotherapy (East 1995; Burton 1998; Wiener and Sher 1998; Pietroni and Vaspe 2000; Keithley, Bond and Marsh 2002), there is less focus on the particular skills, training, and personality that are likely to best equip such therapists to work effectively in primary care. The effect of the present political atmosphere of profound and rapid change in mental health service provision has had significant implications for the employment structures and practices of the counsellors and therapists who work there, what could be called the *headland* of the work. However, when pragmatic or economic considerations are uppermost, it is easy to neglect the *heartland* of the work, its pleasures and subtleties, which make it both necessary and therapeutic for patients as well as potentially satisfying for the professionals involved. In this chapter, we try to interweave the headland with the heartland into a tapestry from which to evolve a picture of what therapists need to know to work in surgeries.

Employment Trends in Primary Care

Recent government policy has set in motion a reorganization of the overall commissioning and delivery of health services with power moving away from Health Authorities to new Primary Care Trusts. Alongside this has evolved the development of large Mental Health Trusts, particularly in inner cities and the requirement to integrate health with social care. The introduction of the National Service Framework for Mental Health (Department of Health 1999a) and the NHS Plan, both of which form the basis for the provision of high quality services consistent across the country, means that primary care mental health services are coming under pressure to review their current provision.

Although some primary care teams see themselves as having responsibility for providing a comprehensive mental health service from the practice premises, traditionally only selected practice-based treatments have been available for patients and the question of who works in practices has been largely a matter of chance factors, propinquity, cultural and social trends of the time, and government policy (Sibbald 1993, 1996a,b; Dammers and Wiener 2001). This is now changing. As Bell states:

> contemporary health services are a Benthamite world of objectives, outcome measures, evidence-based medicine, foci and formulation. The introduction of this culture was seen as a necessary tonic to the sleepy world of self-serving professionalism that preceded it. (Bell 1996)

Bell's comment sheds light on recent shifts away from haphazard and individual employment practices of mental health professionals towards the growth of managed schemes that employ and place counsellors, psychologists, and psychotherapists (from here on, we will use the term therapist to include counsellors, clinical psychologists, and psychotherapists, except where stated) in surgeries. An evidence-based approach to psychological treatments has lead to a healthy questioning of the roles, training and skills of therapists working in a primary care setting and provides an opportunity to consider the particular context and meaning of the surgery as a base from which to offer patients psychological help. However, his 'sleepy world' implying as it does a less self-critical approach to work, provides a necessary containing space for robust reflection about clinical issues with patient and staff dynamics in mind.

The original source of funding practice staff through General Medical Services has enabled surgeries to employ therapists directly, often in a self-employed capacity. However, current National Health policy is supporting the introduction of Personal Medical Services (PMS) in which staff, including the GPs, may become salaried members of the new Primary Care Trusts. It is predicted that this employment practice will be implemented in up to 60% of general practices within the next 5 years. In spite of this trend, the self-employed counsellor is still in evidence. In some surgeries this works extremely well and therapists develop rewarding attachments to their practice and the staff within it, permitting collaborative work of a high standard. In others it can lead to conflict when colleagues from different disciplines cannot find a common language or when GPs make stringent stipulations about therapeutic activity, numbers of sessions available for patients, and which other services they can access. In these cases, it is easy for the self-employed therapist to feel isolated or marginalized.

Managed schemes

In contrast to and perhaps in recognition of some of the above problems, many more managed schemes are developing, usually from NHS Trust clinical psychology services. An example of one such service is the Tower Hamlet's Primary Care Psychology and Counselling Service. This service has on-site psychologists and counsellors at 22 practices (70% of the practices in the area). There is also a small centralized service for those surgeries that are not part of the scheme. From a population of approximately 160,000 patients, about 120,000 have access to the service. In most cases, therapists become core team members, at least for the time they are working at their surgeries. They can attend practice meetings and take part in other activities. All members of the team are employed by the local PCT, and have access to the many employment benefits and opportunities that an NHS Trust provides. Apart from contracts of employment, they have opportunities for continuing professional development (CPD). This is an important part of the clinical governance agenda and can include further training, attendance at relevant conferences with some funding from local education confederations. Management and supervision is an integral part of their CPD with some specialized clinical supervision provided externally. The overall negotiations with practices including funding are the responsibility of senior members of the team. Individual practices and the therapists themselves tend to decide how to manage the day-to-day organization of their work. For a description of other schemes see National Service Framework (Department of Health 1999a).

With the development of managed schemes has evolved a preference for equity and rationing where practices are offered an equal number of counselling hours with recommendations for a fixed number of treatment sessions. These formal procedures, while potentially ensuring standards of good practice that may be implemented across primary care trusts, run the risk of sacrificing quality, flexibility, and the value of specialist skills. Equity and quality are not necessarily companionable bedfellows.

There is still much debate as to whether a model of work where therapists are directly employed by the practice is preferable to one in which mental health professionals are employed outside the practice. There are many instances of well-trained and well-supervised therapists who are self-employed and who do become valued members of the practice multi-disciplinary team. There is more potential to feel as if they are part of a 'nuclear family', with their professional 'home' sited within the practice. Relationships with patients and practice staff can be more rewarding, certainly closer, and provide the benefit of real shared care. Patients seen by therapists in a primary care setting often feel contained by the idea that there are two (or more) parent figures—GP and therapist—taking care of them.

In the current context, with the introduction of PMS (see above) and the possibility of changes in the independent contractor status of GPs, there is an inevitable pull towards managed schemes provided by Hospital Trusts, PCTs, or a range of independent organizations. Such schemes permit a greater clarity of thought about standards, modalities of work, and management style. Therapists are more likely to be perceived by patients and practice staff as part of the 'extended', rather than the nuclear family, in other words a more distant relative, as their professional family is more likely to be within the managed scheme, rather than within the surgery. This is clearly the evolving shape for future therapy services in primary care, but it is difficult to avoid some sense of loss for the greater freedom to evolve a more personal attitude to therapeutic work with patients that is suited to an individual practice that self-employment affords.

Irrespective of future trends in employment practices, the issue of qualifications, training, knowledge, and skills that therapists will need, and what it is that makes primary care an exciting yet different setting from other services, takes us to the central theme of this chapter. It is the place where headland and heartland meet, where a fulcrum supporting the more impersonal questions of standards of practice and the personal, less easily observable requirements of the job can be held in a delicate balance.

What kind of therapy is practiced in a primary care setting?

David Shapiro in his introduction to Roth and Fonagy's (1996) book, 'What works for whom? A Critical review of Psychotherapy Research', states in no uncertain terms that 'there is ample room for improvement in the efficacy of psychological treatments in mental health' (Shapiro 1996). With particular reference to primary care, Roth and Fonagy highlight 'the need for further standardization of mental health care provision in primary care settings and the rigorous periodic audit of these services by an independent agency'. This is now well under way (Ward *et al.* 2000, Sibbald *et al.* 1996a, Sibbald *et al.* 1996b). However, at present, inter-professional rivalries between counsellors, psychotherapists and clinical psychologists about who offers the optimum services to GPs can lead to defensive debates. It seems more important to delineate what exactly therapists *should* be doing and then to try and define and describe the range of *skills they will need* and their usefulness to the patient population referred to them in a practice setting. Whilst there has been much recent research to explore the validity of counselling and psychotherapy in primary care (Ward *et al.* 2000), as far as we know, there has been little, if any, work to try and map out the prerequisite skills and training requirements for a therapist employed to do effective therapy in one or more local surgeries.

Strupp (1978) defines psychotherapy as:

an interpersonal process designed to bring about modifications of feelings, cognitions, attitudes and behaviour which have proved troublesome to the person seeking help from a trained professional.

Implicit in his definition is an emphasis on a relationship that will be therapeutic, some idea of an evolving process in the work, and explicitly, that the therapist is trained. What is left out of his definition is any reference to the context in which the therapy is taking place, the *role of the setting*, and its effect on the process and the relationship. Also left out is the role of the *model of mind* influencing the therapist's techniques and aims. However, within Strupp's definition, it seems that many different kinds of intervention could be described as psychotherapeutic.

The aim of any therapy of whatever modality is to help patients—via a therapeutic alliance—become more self-aware and less anxious. Different models involve *listening in different ways* to what patients bring. Different ways of listening influence what is heard, and what is heard depends, in turn, on the preferred model of the mind used, which then affects treatment aims and techniques used. The question then arises as to which forms of listening are likely to be the most effective for therapists in primary care? This is an environment where audit and evaluation are becoming more of a priority (Pietroni and Vaspe 2000) and short-term interventions are the most common practice. We agree with Pietroni and Vaspe (2000) when they comment that:

there are no 'easyfit' counselling approaches that we know of to meet the range of need with which we are confronted. That is why we have developed a menu of counselling services and use it flexibly but with rigorous scrutiny and debate.

A number of writers (Holmes 1998; Kernberg 1999; Tuckett 1999) are sensitive to the effects of the changing culture on the conceptualization and practice of different therapies. In our view, a steadfast and rigid application of psychoanalytic principles and techniques to therapeutic work in primary care is neither realistic nor suitable (Wiener and Sher 1998), although an *analytical attitude* to the activities that take place in the surgery, including an understanding of unconscious dynamics between patients and staff, is invaluable. Holmes (1998), describes the overall aims of psychotherapy as follows, 'to set in train the unfolding of a developmental process, either within the therapy itself if it is prolonged, or as a catalyst that can augment potentially benign experiences in 'real life', in brief therapy'. His remarks apply equally to analytic and non-analytic therapies. Holmes (1998) also makes a useful distinction between *outcome goals*, the overall strategic aims of therapy (e.g. the reduction of symptoms, fostering maturation, better quality intimate relationships) and *process*

goals, the session-by-session objectives, and the means by which these objectives are achieved (e.g. fostering a working alliance, maintaining boundaries,
making interpretations). This distinction between *outcome* and *process* brings
us closer to the issue of how best to describe the skills of therapists working in
primary care; what can be made more explicit (outcome) and what is equally
important, but more likely to be implicit (process).

Core requirements for therapists working in primary care

General practice demands generic skills and for any professional therapist who
comes to work in a practice irrespective of core training (see Chapter 8), there
are several overarching basic requirements:

◆ A need for a thorough understanding of the nature of the primary care
setting and how primary care is delivered.

◆ An ability to carry out mental health assessments often in collaboration with
the GP, to decide which patients may be contained or treated in the practice,
which are suited to short-tem interventions and which should be referred out
of the practice for specialist psychological or psychiatric treatment (see
Chapter 18).

◆ The capacity to contain and work with some very disturbed patients.

◆ The capacity to work collaboratively as a member of a multi-disciplinary
team.

◆ An ability to manage sensitive issues such as the appropriate sharing of
information with other professionals and the maintenance of sufficient space
to reflect together on work with patients.

◆ An understanding of how primary care connects up with local secondary and
tertiary mental health services.

Expanding on some of the above requirements will help to bring alive the
context in which therapy in primary care takes place.

Understanding primary care

Primary care as a setting for psychotherapeutic work has very particular
characteristics. Therapists are likely to see a broader cohort of patients than in
specialist psychology or psychotherapy departments, which will tax the extent
of their assessment skills. Working on site in a surgery also makes therapists
porous to the influences of their GPs and the ways in which they organize their
work. Practices can be chaotic places as GPs lead busy lives, need to make quick
decisions and often find it difficult to create sufficient space and time to reflect

on the work they do. Wiener (1996) has used the metaphor of a *souk* to describe the atmosphere in a GP surgery:

> an Arab souk or bazaar, where everything is potentially available, is like a practice, where GPs have to maintain a gate-keeping function with often limited resources. GPs have to cope with whoever walks through the door and must decide what is treatable and what must be borne or managed.

Such an environment stands in stark contrast to the more familiar strong-walled *citadel* mentality adopted by many psychotherapy and psychology departments who exercise tight control over referral and entry procedures:

> the erection of a citadel may be the only means by which therapeutic integrity can be maintained, however such an active gate-keeping function involving stringent referral procedures, long waiting lists and often minimal communication with GPs, will not necessarily help to foster good relationships between these services and primary care. (Wiener 1996)

Working in the souk actually requires a very high level of knowledge, skill, and experience. It is not an easy option, as some therapists and GPs think, and it is certainly not for the faint-hearted. Wiener and Sher (1998) have described the attractions of the work, emphasizing in particular the rewards of participating in a process at its inception—*at the coalface*—where therapists can work with problems when they are fresh, presenting real opportunities to prevent reactive disorders from becoming chronic:

> while the coalface inevitably brings a dirty, darker side with many pressures to do the most in the least possible time, primary care is 'the real world' of mental health problems, where counsellors are forced to learn how to use all the psychodynamic and management skills they possess appropriately and flexibly. (Wiener and Sher 1998)

The setting of primary care has its own particular *rhythms*, its patterns of functioning. For GPs some of these rhythms remain constant, for example, a more or less fixed schedule of consultations per session, each lasting about 10 minutes. Other rhythms are constantly changing and the rhythmic structure can be highly complex (see Chapter 3) to accommodate for urgent home visits, the need for speedy decision-making, and longer appointment times for some patients. However, the use of deputizing services, co-operatives, and within the surgeries, practice nurses who run their own clinics and sometimes triage patients who request urgent appointments, can reduce this burden.

Adaptation is required for therapists coming to work in this setting, who may be more familiar with hospital or private practice with their slower, steadier rhythms. This is a two-pronged task. First, to learn about the rhythms of the particular surgery in which they are working and second, to find a way of adapting their own personal rhythms to the setting without losing their professional identity and value systems. For example, therapists accustomed to regular supervision for their work and a space to think about what they are doing will probably identify with the nineteenth century Italian composer, Busoni, who wrote of the tense silence between movements as music itself and more elastic than sound. Many busy or over-worked GPs may have neither the leisure nor the inclination to make the most of the 'spaces between'. When there is pressure from many referrals, GPs, though respecting a different model of work, can become quite envious of what they see as the luxury that therapists have to control the flow of patients they see, to choose whom to see and to see them for session times of up to an hour:

> Mrs Birch, who is well known to various members of the primary care team, comes to see the practice therapist in an anxious and depressed state. Her husband has left her to set up home with another woman. She is self-contained and does not talk easily about her feelings. Because the marriage had been unhappy for some years she is surprised to be reacting so strongly. During the course of three assessment interviews, she comes to see that her feeling of abandonment is part of a re-enactment of an earlier trauma, when she felt emotionally abandoned by her mother. She was pushed out into the cold and this has probably contributed to her impression that others—including her husband—see her as a cold and distant person. She never knew her father and is an only child. Mrs Birch's capacity for psychodynamic psychotherapy is immediately evident and she and the therapist discuss the possibility of a further referral. However, she returns to say that since she had made good contact with the therapist, she would like to carry on with sessions in the surgery. She knows that the therapist is a relatively scarce resource and feels that occasional sessions every few weeks would suit her well. The therapist enjoys working with Mrs Birch and they meet occasionally for nearly 2 years, during which time she works through much of her grief, both about the loss of her husband and of any good relationship with her mother. She begins to adjust to life alone and is encouraged by the return of her enthusiasm to pursue a long-held interest in academic study and travel.

Assessment and treatment

The day-to-day work of therapists in primary care has been well documented (Burd and Donnison 1994; Wiener and Sher 1998; Pietroni and Vaspe 2000), and includes mental health assessments and short-term treatments for patients, as well as consultation, support, and education about the psychological care of patients to other members of the practice team. Sometimes therapists work with the whole practice team when there are conflicts of interest or between different personalities. This requires knowledge of the individuals involved and also a sensitive understanding of the unconscious and systemic processes constellated.

In our view, this is a very different role from that of the non-specialist mental health facilitator described by Bashir *et al.* (2000).

Although some GPs are knowledgeable about the whole area of mental health, research shows that there are wide disparities between individual GPs and between practices in their ability to identify patients with common mental health problems (Paykel and Priest 1992). The issue becomes more complex if we consider how the personal psychology of GPs can affect their decisions as to whether a patient should be treated in the practice or referred to a specialist. To a certain extent, a clinician's capacity to identify a psychological problem may depend on whether they feel able to deal with what they find. If, in addition, the possibility of referral on is limited due to a paucity of local secondary services, GPs may choose to work with the patient in the primary care setting. Many GPs build up relationships with their patients that includes a depth of understanding about psychological difficulties. There are GPs, however, who lack the confidence to become involved with their patients' emotional problems and they are likely to refer these patients on to secondary care services.

Goldberg and Huxley (1992) describe a stringent filtering system, demonstrating that only a small proportion of patients identified with mental health problems are referred on to secondary services. Most will remain in the surgery under the care of the GP and even with a therapist on site, the number who are assessed and treated by the therapist will not be great. However, for every patient seen, as many as six others could be the focus of discussions between the therapist and members of the team either individually or in the more formal setting of clinical meetings.

Therapists are better equipped to do this kind of work in primary care if they have had a core mental health training. High-level assessment skills are required, as well as a wide knowledge of possible interventions. Treatments known to be effective are cognitive behaviour therapy, interpersonal therapy and brief psychoanalytic psychotherapy (Roth and Fonagy 1996; see Chapter 18), as well as focused counselling interventions (Ward *et al.* 2000)

Links with secondary mental health services

Therapists should understand how mental health services are provided in their own locality, as some patients may need shared management with local psychiatric services and the community mental health team.

Familiarity with local social services and any voluntary sector provision is important and can open up the possibility for patients of access to other supportive therapeutic facilities, particularly when specialist services such as psychotherapy and psychology have long waiting lists for outside referrals:

Dr Hollis refers Mr Johnson for treatment for his depression. During the initial session, the therapist explains that she works as part of the primary care team and that she will not, in general, disclose confidential information without the patient's consent. However, when she has concerns about the patient harming himself or others, she will, with the patient's knowledge, need to share this information with his GP. About a month into the treatment Mr Johnson comes to a session full of suicidal thoughts and graphically describes how he intends to kill himself, begging the therapist not to take this information outside the consulting room. He is adamant that he will not accept a referral to a psychiatrist as it will go on his medical records. The therapist finds herself with an ethical dilemma. Will discussing the situation with the GP undermine the possibility of future therapeutic work and communicate to Mr Johnson that she, the therapist, cannot contain the patient's depressed and dangerous feelings? She is clear, however, that she cannot carry this knowledge alone because the patient (being in his late fifties and single) falls into a high-risk group for potential suicide. The therapist's relationship with the GP is such that she can arrange a three-way meeting with Mr Johnson and Dr Hollis. This would have the aim of thinking together about the best way to work with this situation. After being reassured by the therapist that she will continue her sessions with him, Mr Johnson agrees to the meeting. The outcome is that the GP is sufficiently concerned about Mr Johnson's mental state to encourage referral on to the psychiatrist who is well known to the practice and has worked with the therapist with other patients. Mr Johnson agrees to an appointment with the psychiatrist at the practice who advises medication and the possibility of admission if his distress escalates. He offers the patient appointments at his monthly clinic at the practice. The therapist continues to work with Mr Johnson on a weekly basis and all feel contained by the input from the secondary care team. Mr Johnson is also referred to the local MIND drop-in centre where he receives informal support by attending various daytime activities.

Here, the therapist has demonstrated to her patient that the members of the primary care team work in partnership, both with each other and with him. This is only possible where both the therapist and the GP are committed to the ethos of collaborative work, including shared principles about confidentiality. This vignette illustrates how care can be offered both inside and outside the practice and the complementary roles of secondary care services and voluntary agencies.

Interpersonal collaboration

Where professionals are working under pressure and in close proximity, the individual skills and personality of the therapist need to be in keeping with the practice style and the personalities of the other members of the team, as well as with the characteristics of the local patient population. As in an individual therapy relationship, there should be 'a fit' or therapeutic alliance between the therapist and the practice team. For the therapist, this depends on a well worked out ethical attitude (Wiener 2001) and a good grasp of boundaries. Therapists should know when to hold firm and when to be flexible, as well as having a good understanding of organizational dynamics and the capacity to work in partnership with others whose roles and models of patient care may be very different. In the words of Rimmer-Yehudai (2001) 'to hold the mind and body as a whole in primary care, sometimes requires more than one body and one mind'. As Burd (1996) suggests 'a partnership model means that liaison and joint work continue after referral, beyond assessment and through to discharge, providing an essentially nurturing environment':

> The health visitor attached to the practice expressed her concern both to the GP and the practice therapist about a young mother she had visited at home. Anne Thorne was having difficulty in coping with her new baby and appeared to lack the confidence to carry out simple and appropriate childcare tasks. She also seemed very slow to react to her baby. The health visitor wondered if she was severely depressed. The GP thought the therapist who had a wealth of experience of mothers with post-natal depression, should assess Anne Thorne. Because Mrs Thorne was anxious about leaving home, the health visitor and therapist made a joint visit to see her at home. They used the Edinburgh Post Natal Depression Scale as part of their assessment and from this and their more general assessment, decided that Anne Thorne was, indeed, suffering from postnatal depression. They discussed with the GP whether or not to refer her out of the practice to secondary mental health services. The GP then arranged to see Mrs Thorne himself. He felt that anti-depressant medication would be helpful and encouraged her to attend sessions with the practice therapist. Mrs Thorne was relieved to receive some support. Because of the level of concern about her in the practice team, the health visitor continued to maintain regular contact throughout the first few sessions of her therapy and there were also regular meetings between the GP, the health visitor and the therapist to review her progress.

We hope that this picture of life and work inside a surgery puts paid to the assumption that therapists with a basic training and qualification in one orientation can then simply transfer their knowledge to primary care without first undergoing further training focusing on the texture and specific characteristics of the setting. Several authors (Wiener and Sher 1998; Pietroni and Vaspe 2000; Dammers and Wiener 2001) have emphasized the need for the adaptation of core practice to the different rhythms of the primary care setting and the value of regular supervision to facilitate this process. However, therapists working in primary care are not always well supported and supervisors and managers may not themselves have an adequate understanding of the impact of a surgery on therapeutic work. Posts may founder if there are insufficient training and support structures to help therapists manage their workload, and the inevitable conscious and unconscious pressures that accompany this taxing work.

Integrating the 'headland' and the 'heartland' of the work

Headland

The NHS as a whole is starting to address the question of how to integrate different psychological therapies (see Chapter 18). In the National Health Service Executive (NHSE) Review of Psychotherapies (1996), the statement is made that:

> psychological therapies are an important part of the mainstream NHS mental health care. They are one of the two main approaches to the treatment of the mentally ill (the other includes physical treatments such as medication and ECT) (see Chapter 16).

The review recommends that each region provide a comprehensive, coordinated and cost-effective psychological therapy service. It divides the therapy services to be made available into three types:

◆ Type A (*integral*): general psychotherapeutic skills provided by any mental health worker within a multidisciplinary care package.

◆ Type B (*generic*): a complete (stand alone) and clearly delineated psychotherapeutic intervention informed by a range of different models, tailored to individual goals.

◆ Type C (*formal*): a complete (stand alone) and clearly delineated psychotherapeutic intervention based on clear theoretical underpinnings with implications for the use of different treatment interventions to achieve different aims. These would include cognitive, behavioural, psychoanalytic and systemic therapies (NHSE Review of Psychotherapies 1996).

This review and political developments since its publication, seem to be giving impetus towards a partnership between psychological therapies in primary, secondary and tertiary services.

Applying this model to psychotherapy in primary care, the relevance of Type A (*integral*) is relatively easy to comprehend and is likely to include listening skills, and the capacity to empathize and to carry out supportive counselling.

Hopefully, all members of the primary care team, GPs, health visitors, practice nurses, and receptionists, and not just therapists will be competent at this level. Type B (*generic*) implies a training that leads to skills in using more than one kind of intervention, for example, analytical therapy *and* cognitive behavioural therapy (CBT), as well as a capacity to choose appropriately between modalities depending on what patients want and are able to use. Most practice-based therapists will use Type B skills, which by implication requires competent assessment skills. It remains an open question as to how many have the necessary skills in different modalities to make expert distinctions between them to suit individual patients. Type C (*formal*) implies a core training and qualification in *one* specific modality, for example, psychoanalytical psychotherapy, cognitive behaviour therapy, or family therapy. It involves the capacity to work in a modality in depth and to be able to put it into practice in a work setting.

Types A and B together constitute the heartland of therapeutic work with patients in a surgery. It is doubtful as to whether Type C is appropriate for primary care since most therapists are employed for a limited number of hours and, in today's NHS climate, these approaches belong more comfortably in specialist and tertiary settings.

Organizations such as the British Association of Counselling (BAC) and Counsellors in Primary Care (CPC) have been working to establish standards of practice for counsellors working in surgeries (CPC 2000). However, counsellors do not necessarily have a core profession to equip them with the broad base NHS experience necessary as a background to work in primary care settings. They usually come to a surgery 'cold' and need special further training. Some can work flexibly in different modes and are often extremely competent at working with patients from ethnic minority groups. They bring expertise with specific patient groups—HIV counselling, sexual problems, bereavement, and abortion counselling. However, they often have limited experience of making mental health assessments and knowing when to refer on to specialist services.

For the most part, psychodynamic psychotherapists do not practice long-term formal psychotherapy in a surgery and usually do not have skills in different modalities of therapeutic work. However, they do bring the possibility of good quality assessments and an analytic attitude that offers a depth of understanding about the therapeutic process, including transference and counter transference dynamics, especially useful with very disturbed patients.

Clinical psychologists have provided sessions in primary care for over 25 years (Day and Wren 1994). Originally they worked out of hospital settings, but now, as in the Tower Hamlets service described above, they are often based in health centres and work as part of the primary care services. There is now a special interest group within the British Psychological Society for psychologists working in Primary Care. With secondary mental health services, particularly community mental health teams restricted to working with patients with severe and enduring mental health problems, clinical psychologists working in primary care teams tend to be offering interventions for patients not considered appropriate for CMHTs, but, nonetheless, with severe and complex needs.

There is a place for counsellors, psychoanalytic psychotherapists, and clinical psychologists to work in primary care. In an ideal world, a mixture of professionals working on site is probably the best way to ensure that primary care teams, and their patients are offered the most effective and accessible service. This is an unlikely scenario at least at present, highlighting the immediate need for those involved in the recruitment and training of therapists to remain vigilant about the strengths and weaknesses of their students and employees, in particular the limits of their skills. The requirement for postgraduate training that is context-specific points to content which is geared towards the provision of Types A and B skills.

Heartland

In our view, the three types of skill described above are insufficient to account for the full extent and potential of the therapeutic endeavour that takes place in the surgery. While they *are* more amenable to description and observation, they fail to do justice to the subtle processes and relationships between therapists, GPs, and other practice staff. These constitute the essence and, indeed, the pleasure of work in primary care, and are the 'music' that gives form and shape, rather than the words or libretto. If understood, these processes and the meanings attributed to them, permit true collaborative work and better quality therapy for the patients in the practice.

As a central thesis of this chapter, we suggest that there are *unseen levels of skill*, usually dependent on good training and supervision that is context-specific, and that broaden the employment brief for Trusts and Managed Schemes looking to hire good quality therapists. Such skills are essential, we believe, because in the 'real world' as opposed to the 'perfect world' of recommended service provision, therapists are likely to have to manage far more than is stipulated in their contract. For example:

◆ Brief work, often a six-session model, is usually recommended as the optimum treatment length with the possibility of further referral to specialist services, such as psychology or psychotherapy departments. *But why only six sessions one could ask?* Although more recent guidelines suggest that optimal outcomes cannot be achieved in less than eight sessions (Department of Health 2001), in our view, a fixed and well-defined approach such as this is unrealistic for two reasons. First, referrals to secondary services often involve waiting lists of up to a year raising the question of what is to happen to patients during the waiting period. Secondly, different patients may ask, directly or indirectly, for different kinds and amounts of therapeutic attention. To treat everyone the same runs counter to one of the

basic aims of any therapeutic intervention and counter to the basic philosophy of general practice, to value the individuality of each person. For the
most part, therapists and GPs on site in the surgery have to find creative
ways of managing patient distress.

◆ Many complex and disturbed patients are referred back to the practice as
inappropriate for secondary care services. There is some evidence to suggest
that patients seen in primary care are as disturbed as those seen in specialist
units (Tata 1996).

◆ Some patient groups for example, elderly patients, adolescents, or children
in emotional distress can be neglected in primary care. GPs often don't pick
them up as they may not always be aware of these patients' psychological
needs or find them difficult to work with.

Therapists and GPs, if they can work together, have to find ways of containing
and working with a wide range of patients in difficulty, a truly heavy load. The
weight of the burden will only be manageable through collaborative work. This
involves flexibly *adapting the recommended therapeutic strategies*, and understanding in psychodynamic and systemic terms, the therapeutic processes
between professionals from different disciplines working with patients in the
practice. It is here that what we are calling the unseen levels of skill become an
essential prerequisite for effective therapeutic practice.

The skills here may be divided into three main types:

Understanding patient narratives

Understanding how patients relate to their practice—often a kind of home to
which they return, as if through a revolving door, at different points in their
lives. The structure of the system means that therapists will often need to take
more account of the circumstances of the referral, not just the patient:

A GP referred a woman for an assessment to the therapist in the practice.
The GP said that he 'wondered if she might benefit from psychotherapy?'
The patient turned out to be unsuitable for referral. She was unapproach-
able, angry, at times showed psychotic behaviour, and shouted at the therapist throughout the session. The therapist was puzzled by this referral from
a doctor who seemed to be behaving out of character, as she usually referred
patients thoughtfully after some preliminary groundwork. Because the
therapist knew this GP well, she was able to discuss the referral with her.
It emerged that this was a patient who had been asked to leave a number of
practices in the area, as GPs could not bear her relentless demands.
Unconsciously, the GP needed the therapist to know what a difficult time
she was having. On realizing this, the therapist could then offer the GP
a service where she could support some of the 'difficult practice patients'

for a time as a way of relieving the over-burdened GP with a welcome rescue operation.

Understanding practice narratives

A grasp of how what is happening politically, socially, and personally in the practice is affecting patient care and the personal relationships among the staff:

A senior partner in the practice, Dr Maygrove, begins to send formal letters of referral to the therapist. Previously, he has followed the model of referral used by all the partners, where patients are encouraged to book an appointment for themselves through the receptionists. The therapist is asked to set up an immediate appointment with the patients, as, in Dr Maygrove's view, they require a speedy intervention. The implication is that a valuable opportunity for a productive intervention could be lost. The therapist, caught up in Dr Maygrove's anxiety, obediently struggles to fit two patients into her already well-filled diary: a depressed freelance designer who has had no work for a year, and an anxious young dancer with an irritable bowel and what appears to be a potentially serious eating disorder. Both attend the first session, but then fail to turn up for their second and subsequent appointments. The therapist wonders why the GP has become so precipitously anxious about these two patients, as in many ways they are typical of the people she usually sees for assessment. She reflects that Dr Maygrove's change in referral patterns from the usual informal mode to a more formal mode, reminiscent of referrals to outside special-ists, is an unconscious communication to her that his own usual capacity for containing the anxiety of his patients is under stress. It emerges when they talk together later that Dr Maygrove is overworked and feeling hurt that his colleagues are expressing resentment about his work outside the surgery. They consider this to be limiting the amount of time and energy he is putting into the development of practice services. The therapist has the capacity to understand the meaning of unconscious communications and has developed a 'good enough' working relationship with Dr Maygrove to be able to approach him to discuss inter-professional difficulties.

The therapist's self-understanding

The interpersonal skills of therapists should include the capacity to adapt to the setting and the individuals they are working with, and to build collaborative working relationships that take account of differences in training ethos (Truax and Carkhuff 1967).

As Wiener and Sher (1998) put it 'they may have to struggle to maintain a delicate balance between flexibility in terms of work style (the *souk*) and firmness in order to maintain a space to retain their own identity (the *citadel*) so that the assessment and treatment process may develop satisfactorily':

In a practice meeting, Dr Doyle (a young female GP) was talking about her difficulties in working with two or three older patients who demanded seemingly high proportions of her surgery time, but did not improve. The therapist, with an interest in elderly patients offered to see them, also commenting in the meeting that the patients in question could well be contained in a helpful way by regular meetings with Dr Doyle, even though a 'cure' was unlikely.

She saw Mrs Hutchins, a 75-year-old woman who had had a stroke and suffered from angina. She had difficulty in walking any distance. Mrs Hutchins seemed less preoccupied by her physical symptoms than with obsessive rumination about her husband's long-term affair with another woman. The affair had ended some years ago, but recently a child of this liaison was visiting the family home, and she was finding herself furious with her husband and resentful of 'his' son's presence. They were squabbling all the time. It quickly became clear to the therapist that the problem was in the marriage and she suggested that Mr Hutchins come with her to the next session. Mr Hutchins, also aged 75, was similarly disabled by two small strokes, but was trying his best to please his wife and make amends for his past misdemeanours. He felt that nothing he could do would make any difference. It seemed unlikely that they would separate at their stage of life and the therapist offered them four joint sessions of focused work to look at ways in which they might understand each other better and find ways of tolerating their differences. Mrs Hutchins found the sessions particularly helpful and asked the therapist if she could come back for occasional one-off sessions if she needed to. The therapist agreed. At a practice meeting some weeks later, Dr Doyle thought she now understood that the Hutchins' physical disabilities had been blinding her to their emotional needs and alerted her to her prejudices about older patients who were reminiscent of her own ailing parents.

These unseen skills demonstrate the importance of attending to unconscious processes, both in terms of the effect patients have upon the professionals they come to work with, and in terms of the power and impact of the setting on staff relationships, and the therapeutic process. The question arises—whether the capacity for effective collaboration is a personality attribute or whether it can be taught? Are team workers 'born' or 'made'? Probably, both are true. The therapists who work better alone in the more rarefied atmosphere of their own consulting rooms are unlikely to be drawn to the collaborative approach which is of the essence in primary care.

Conclusion

In this chapter, we have emphasized that the time is now right to pose the question: who can do best for whom in primary care? We have tried to map out the essential skills and attributes necessary to equip therapists to work effectively in a surgery, as well as some of the specialist options and their potential benefits to practice patients. Our hope is that this will help future employers, PCTs, GPs themselves, or the administrators of managed schemes, to know what they are looking for, how to evaluate which candidates of the many who apply to work in primary care they should employ and what kinds of special training they are likely to require. Therapists from different disciplines who come to work in primary care have different levels of ability and experience and there is scope for effective work in different modalities. Which orientation is preferable will depend on the psychological skills and expertise of the practice team, the particular needs of the local patient population, and the existing secondary care and voluntary services in the area.

While it is possible to map out the skills required in primary care in terms of levels advocated by the NHSE, what might be described as the *headland* of the work, there are several significant unseen levels of skill, more representative of what we find to be the *heartland* of the work. They are complementary, not mutually exclusive. The first are easier to evaluate; the second more difficult to measure as they embody not just the training, core profession, and skills of the therapist, but also personality attributes, as well as personal flexibility and the capacity to reflect about the processes involved in the work.

It may be that no one profession can offer all the interventions appropriate in a primary care setting and that where resources are available, the primary care team could contain a mixture of professionals. Clinical governance is becoming increasingly important in all areas of clinical work. This, together with the continued discrepancy between need and resources in mental health, makes the requirement for clear recommendations about good models of mental health provision in primary care, all the more essential. If 90% of patients with mental health problems remain the responsibility of a primary care team that may include an on-site therapist, then surely, we have a responsibility both to secure posts for those therapists who are best qualified to do the job, as well as funding any supplementary training they are likely to need to adapt successfully to this most rewarding work setting.

Part IV
Perspectives from secondary care

11 Postnatal depression

Maret Dymond, Lynne Murray and Peter J Cooper

Postnatal depression is one of the more common mental disorders faced by general practitioners and other primary care professionals: a number of studies show that 10–15% of women are affected (Cox *et al.* 1993; O'Hara and Swain 1996). This figure is even higher under adverse social and economic conditions (Cooper *et al.* 1999). Not only is postnatal depression extremely distressing for the mother and those around her, it is also well established that it is a risk factor for adverse child emotional and cognitive outcome (see review by Murray and Cooper 1997). For example, children of postnatally depressed mothers have been shown to have significantly raised levels of emotional disturbance when adjusting to school (Alpern and Lyons Ruth 1993; Sinclair and Murray 1998) and, at the same age, are more likely to be reported by their mothers as having behavioural difficulties at home (Murray *et al.* 1999). In addition, in high-risk groups, there have also been reports of poorer cognitive development in children of mothers who have had postnatal depression (Cogill *et al.* 1986; Sharp *et al.* 1995).

Notably, these links between postnatal depression and later adverse outcome in the children have been found to hold even when account is taken of subsequent maternal depression. It is important to bear in mind, however, that although such risks are increased by postnatal depression, relationships between depressed mothers and their infants are highly variable, and it is by no means inevitable that such sequelae will occur.

Postnatal depression and health care use

Women's failure to recognize and report symptoms of postnatal depression

Postnatal depression is phenomenologically similar to depression occurring at other times in life. It is typified by pervasive low mood, or loss of interest and enjoyment, in combination with a range of other symptoms. These include sleep disturbance (unrelated to being woken by the baby), lower energy than would be expected given the parenting demands on the mother, an inability to concentrate, an increased or decreased appetite, and feelings of worthlessness or guilt. In spite of the incapacitating nature of postnatal depressive illness, it is striking that a substantial proportion of those who experience the condition are either unaware that they are depressed or else reject a medical description of their experience. Depression is an isolating disorder, and the very nature of the illness itself means that sufferers may believe that nothing or no one could alleviate their feelings. It is, therefore, common for sufferers of major depressive disorder to be unwilling to discuss their situation or they may even conceal the way they are feeling. One study based on interviews conducted with women suffering from postnatal depression, found that, although 97% reported that they felt worse than usual, only 32% believed they were depressed (Whitton *et al.* 1996). Furthermore, over 90% of the women had not reported their symptoms to any health professional.

The most common reason given by these mothers to explain why they had not recognized that they were suffering from postnatal depression was that they had thought their symptoms were not sufficiently severe to warrant diagnosis. Another study of a postpartum sample, McIntosh (1993) found that, of mothers who had reported feeling depressed, more then half (53%) had not sought help from any source. Many of these women claimed that this was because they felt that professional help would not be relevant, since they attributed their depression to external, social pressures. In addition, many women recounted that they had not sought help because of a fear of being labelled as mentally ill and unfit to care for their children, with a small number even believing that their baby would be removed from their care. It is evident from this work that women's perceptions of postnatal depression, as well as of the manner in which it is viewed by the medical profession, are misguided. In particular, women do not seem aware that effective treatments are available and are appropriate to their needs.

A number of factors have been found to be associated with the mother's failure to recognize that she may be depressed and with the reluctance to bring her experience to the attention of relevant professionals. Primiparous women, for example, are less likely than those who are multiparous to recognize that they are suffering from postnatal depression, presumably because they have no previous experience with which to compare the way they are feeling (Whitton *et al.* 1996). Strikingly, Whitton and colleagues noted that women of higher social classes were also less likely than working class mothers to recognize that they were suffering from postnatal depression. Evidence from our own research confirms this finding and suggests that this may be because middle class women may not associate the possibility of depression with their own favourable living conditions (Dymond, in preparation).

Finally, evidence has also suggested that teenage mothers are particularly vulnerable, not so much because they do not recognize that they are depressed, but because they are frequently unaware of the professional support systems available to them (Irvine *et al.* 1997).

Detection of postnatal depression in primary care

The fact that many women do not realize that they are suffering from postnatal depression or are worried about the consequences of reporting such feelings, coupled with the isolating characteristics of the disorder, may go some way to explaining why many cases of postnatal depression are not identified by the primary care team. Additionally, unless the mother volunteers how she is feeling, or she is specifically asked, health care professionals may not always identify depression from the mother's immediate clinical presentation. As noted previously, depression can manifest itself in many different ways. A mother who has anxiety symptoms along with depression may experience feelings of agitation that cause her to speak quickly and not appear depressed. This can seem very different from the classic picture of the melancholic depressed woman, who is tearful and listless, that it is perhaps not surprising that primary health care professionals may miss the underlying disorder. The fact that anxiety is frequently co-morbid with depression makes the need for diagnostic training particularly pressing.

A number of studies have attempted to estimate the scale of failures of detection. Thus, Briscoe (1986), Seeley *et al.* (1996) and Murray *et al.* (2000), all examined GP, health visitor, and/or midwifery records concerning maternal mental health in the postnatal period, and compared rates of health professional-identified depression with independent assessments. In each case, as many as 40% of those who were independently assessed as being depressed were not identified as being so by the relevant health professionals.

The reluctance of many depressed mothers to reveal their condition and the relatively poor rate of detection of the disorder is reflected in the pattern of health care access and use. Seeley and colleagues (1996), for example, found that depressed mothers, many of whom were undiagnosed, received no more visits from their health visitors than well women, and were rather less likely to attend the health visitors' mother and baby clinics. Murray and colleagues (2000), similarly found that women who were depressed in the first 2 months postpartum had no more GP or health visitor contacts than did well women. In cases where depression was detected, by contrast, the number of contacts substantially increased. Whether these were initiated by the women themselves or by the health care professionals is not entirely clear, but there were certainly suggestions that, once depression was identified, primary health care workers adopted a range of measures to care for the mother and infant.

Although the overall number of contacts with primary health care professionals does not appear to differ between depressed and well women in the first 2 months, there is evidence to suggest that depressed mothers may bring their infants to health care professionals more than well women during this period. In fact, a number of researchers have reported that infants of mothers who are postnatally depressed are more easily distressed and difficult to manage than infants of non-depressed women (Field 1984; Field *et al*. 1985, 1988; Whiffen and Gotlib 1989; Cutrona and Troutman 1986). Earlier conceptualizations of the link between infant distress and maternal depression tended to assume that depressed mothers' poor caretaking may have caused the difficult infant behaviour (Field 1992). More recently, however, research has shown that difficult infant behaviour, such as early persistent or excessive crying, is quite unrelated to insensitive parenting (St James-Roberts *et al.,*1998). Rather, there is evidence to suggest that such behaviour may be caused by foetal exposure to high levels of maternal anxiety or depression (Diego and Field 2000; Glover and Gitau 2000). In addition, individual differences in infant characteristics can exert an effect on the experience of parents. Indeed, prospective research has shown that certain behaviour patterns in the neonates of non-depressed women were strongly predictive of postnatal depression at 8 weeks (Murray *et al*. 1996). Thus, having an infant who was classed as 'irritable' or as having a relatively poor motor regulation, substantially increased the risk of subsequent depression.

The association between difficult infant behaviour and postnatal depression is reflected in patterns of health care contacts. Mandl and colleagues (1999), for example, found that women with high levels of depressive symptoms made multiple, infant problem-orientated visits to the GPs as well as increased emergency department attendance for their infant. Similarly, Murray *et al*. (2000) found that postnatally depressed mothers were significantly more likely to attend GP clinics for infant crying problems than were well women.

Taken together, these findings suggest that, in the context of reported or observed difficult infant behaviour, primary health care professionals should be alerted to the increased risk of maternal depression, particularly in cases where the mother has poor social support (Murray *et al*. 1996).

Improving the detection of depression

In view of the difficulties outlined above in the detection of postnatal depression, many health authorities have introduced routine screening for postnatal depression by health visitors, using standardized tools to make systematic enquiry, such as the Edinburgh Postnatal Depression Scale (EPDS, Cox *et al*. 1987). The EPDS is a 10-item self-report questionnaire with well-established validity (Murray and Carothers 1990), the administration of which, by health visitors, has been shown to be an extremely valuable and effective way of identifying those with postnatal depression (Seeley *et al*. 1996). The growing evidence base in favour of postnatal screening for depression forms a convincing argument for those health authorities that have yet to implement such a policy. It is important to note, however, that such a screening procedure is only constructive if it is administered and managed correctly. Since the postnatal period is a time of increased stress and anxiety, it is imperative that women receive a sensitive explanation of the procedure, privacy whilst completing the questionnaire and adequate time for follow-up discussion, as well as reassurance regarding confidentiality and potential outcomes. This type of approach is, of course, in turn more likely to foster the new mother's trust in the primary health care team, thus encouraging openness and honesty in the relationship and facilitating the role of the health professional.

Postnatal screening alone, however, may not identify all of those who are suffering from postnatal depression. For example, women who are too frightened to admit to feeling depressed may not always give honest answers to questionnaire items. One way in which the health authorities and Primary Care Trusts might address this problem is by making use of the evidence described above regarding patterns of health care use. For example, future research could be targeted to addressing the issue of whether the monitoring of neonatal health care use can improve the detection of postnatal depression. Similar work could also be carried out to investigate the effectiveness of directing extra resources towards following up women who fail to attend for routine mother and baby clinic appointments.

Antenatal screening to identify those at high risk for developing postnatal depression might also be an effective means of identifying those to whom careful attention should be paid in pregnancy. Cooper and colleagues developed a predictive index for postnatal depression the PDI (Cooper *et al.* 1996) for this purpose. Although the PDI will not identify all women who go on to develop postnatal depression and, of those whose scores on this measure are high, not all will develop the disorder, the use of such tools can undoubtedly assist the primary health care team in identifying mothers who merit careful monitoring. An individual's score on such a measure, moreover, considered in combination with postnatal risk factors (e.g. difficulties with infant feeding or temperament), may well increase detection of risk for postnatal depression (Cooper and Murray 1997).

In attempting to improve the detection of depression, as well as instituting screening in pregnancy and the postnatal period, there is an important role for improvements in public education concerning emotional adjustment following childbirth. Whitton and colleagues (1996) note that antenatal classes are, potentially, an ideal venue for raising awareness of postnatal depression and increasing the understanding and acceptance of available treatments.

Recent surveys of women's use and perceptions of antenatal classes suggest, however, that considerable restructuring of these programmes is required. Newburn and Singh (2000), for example, in a survey involving a representative population of mothers of infants, found that only 40% had attended antenatal classes. Apart from multiparous women who reported that they felt little need to attend, others reported that they were uncomfortable about attending, feeling that they would not fit in with other women, and many of these women would have preferred to see someone individually. These mothers were more likely to be primiparous, young, of low socio-economic status, and from ethnic minority groups. The survey also showed that, even for those women who did attend classes, substantial numbers reported that they would like to have been told more about postnatal depression and care of the infant (e.g. management of sleeping and crying). These findings are also reflected in a recent Royal College of Midwives report based on focus group meetings (Royal College of Midwives 2000), and in our own research involving interviews with women who were identified antenatally as being at raised risk for depression. In this latter study (Dymond in preparation), half the mothers interviewed reported that they had felt unprepared for having to care for the baby.

Together these findings suggest the need for education programmes in pregnancy to be made more acceptable and relevant to parents, and particularly those who may be vulnerable. A review of antenatal education does, therefore, seem appropriate in order for health authorities (and PCTs) to ensure the maximum effectiveness of this service provision. Empirical research is also needed, investigating progressive means of increasing awareness of postnatal depression, such as having presentations by mothers who have previously experienced the disorder themselves.

Treatment of postnatal depression

A number of randomized controlled trials have found that home-based psychological support, delivered by health visitors or nurses on a weekly basis over a period of 6–10 weeks, is generally effective in bringing about remission from depression (Holden *et al.* 1989; Wickberg and Hwang 1996; Cooper and Murray 2000a). In each of these studies, the recovery rate of women who received the intervention was significantly greater than that for women receiving routine primary care (recovery rates in the intervention groups ranged between 65 and 80%, compared to 25–38% in the routine care control groups).

Where different kinds of psychological support delivered in this way have been compared, for example, counselling versus cognitive behaviour therapy, there is little evidence to favour one of these psychological treatments over the other (Cooper and Murray 2000a). The common component of giving the mother consistent, committed emotional support over a number of weeks appears to be the key ingredient. This kind of treatment can certainly be delivered by health visitors who have received additional training. Not only has it been found to be helpful in alleviating the mother's depression, in one of the studies (Murray and Cooper 2000), which involved follow-up to 5 years, there was also benefit in terms of the mothers' reports of difficulties in the relationship with the infant and in the child's development, with fewer behavioural problems being reported by teachers for children whose mothers had received the early support.

Recently, such treatments have been extended to include the infant, aiming to help the mother understand her particular infant's characteristics and needs (Brazelton 1992; Murray and Cooper 2000; Murray and Andrews 2000). In this kind of intervention, it is hoped to prevent the mother from slipping into feeling guilty about her handling of the infant or feeling resentful of the infant's demands. This approach is based on the findings described above that individual infant characteristics, such as 'irritability', or the tendency to become easily and inconsolably distressed, increase the risk of mother becoming depressed.

In contrast to psychological treatments for postnatal depression, there is rather little evidence regarding pharmacological interventions, only one randomized controlled trial having been conducted. In this study, Appleby and colleagues (1997), compared counselling to pharmacological treatment (fluoxetine), and found counselling to be just as effective as the medication. No additional benefit of fluoxetine, over and above that conferred by counselling, was found. One striking finding of this study was the fact that many mothers refused to take part in the trial because they were unwilling to take antidepressant medication. Interviews carried out with women suffering from postnatal depression by the same research group (Whitton *et al.* 1996), noted that 81% would not consider pharmacological treatments, the main reasons cited were fear of addiction and the belief that the depression would pass without drug treatment.

Rather than being the routine first line of treatment, therefore, this evidence suggests that medication may be most appropriate for those whose symptoms fail to remit with supportive home visiting or used as an adjunct to initial supportive counselling in those whose symptoms are particularly severe.

Prevention of postnatal depression

In recent years there has been increasing interest in the question of whether episodes of postnatal depression might be prevented by giving support to vulnerable mothers during pregnancy. A number of studies, using the model of routine antenatal classes, have attempted to deliver such support to high-risk mothers in group settings; typically, such interventions have been started in the third trimester of pregnancy, with some extending into the early postpartum period (e.g. Stamp 1995; Buist *et al.* 1999; Brugha *et al.* 2000; Elliott *et al.* 2000). While the rationale for such interventions is sound, including the notion of helping to build up support networks and increasing the awareness and understanding of depression, none of these group interventions has been successful in bringing about a significant reduction in the rate of depression. In addition, each of the studies has encountered substantial problems of compliance. Similar disappointing results have also emerged from programmes delivering support to high-risk women on an individual basis, in some cases in their homes (Marks *et al.* 2000), including our own research on the possible benefits of early health visitor intervention (Cooper and Murray 2000b). Notably, however, in each of these studies, as in those employing a group design, the intervention was structured and brief. In contrast to these interventions, other studies have delivered longer term, more broadly-based support to vulnerable mothers in their homes (Olds and Korfmacher 1998; Armstrong *et al.* 1999; Heinicke *et al.* 1999), and these have met with more success.

Thus, it is evident that brief time-limited therapy may well not be appropriate for many women vulnerable to postnatal depression (Cooper and Murray 2000b). In our health visitor preventive intervention study, the health visitors providing women with extra support found that many of the mothers faced circumstances of an overwhelming nature. The health visitors also found that it was difficult to enlist the involvement of some mothers in the therapeutic process. These mothers often seemed uninterested in the health visitor's presence and would fail to become emotionally engaged, avoiding eye contact or otherwise distancing themselves from the health visitor's efforts to be supportive. It seems likely, therefore, that for such women, a brief limited therapy would be insufficient to permit the establishment of a trusting relationship between the mother and the therapist, without which therapy might be unlikely to succeed.

The potential role of adult attachment in health service contacts

Challenges to effective intervention

It will be apparent from the previous discussion that a substantial proportion of mothers, often those who are most vulnerable, fail to make full use of or gain access to the health care services set up to meet their needs. This applies to attendance at antenatal and postnatal groups, to the question of whether women feel able to disclose their experience of difficulties, including depression, to individual health care professionals, and to their engagement and co-operation with treatment programmes. It is also evident from the findings outlined above, and in particular from the reasons women give for their failure to participate fully in health care, that a core dimension of their experience that might help to explain such processes of self-exclusion concerns their perceptions, beliefs, and feelings about interpersonal relationships. Thus, in general, women who fail to enlist health care professionals' support are often suspicious and mistrustful, or worried that they will meet with unsympathetic responses. In seeking to understand why some individuals may be more responsive to intervention than others, recent research has begun to examine the role of the individual's capacity for engagement in the therapeutic process.

Adult attachment style

Research addressing the role of adult attachment in interpersonal functioning leads to the suggestion that attachment difficulties may be a key mechanism preventing some women from benefiting from the therapeutic relationship. In the last two decades research has extended Bowlby's (Bowlby 1982), and Ainsworth's (Ainsworth *et al.* 1978), work on infant–caregiver attachment to look at adult attachment style. This research is based upon the premise that adults, like infants, possess an internal working model, constructed from prior relationship experiences. This model shapes an individual's emotions, behaviour, and beliefs about the self, as well as continuing to exert an influence over their relationships with others, thus forming a pattern or style of attachment.

Several different measures of assessing internal working models of attachment in adults have been developed. These include interviews about the way in which childhood relationships are represented [the Adult Attachment Interview (AAI), George *et al.* 1985; Main and Goldwyn 1991], as well as current adult relationships [the Attachment Style Interview (ASI), Bifulco *et al.* unpublished manuscript]. All of these measures of attachment generally distinguish between three different styles or patterns of attachment, namely secure, avoidant, and anxious. In brief, these are characterized as follows: securely attached adults find it easier to get close to others and are more comfortable depending on them; insecure, avoidantly attached adults are uncomfortable being close to others, and find it hard to trust them; and insecure, anxiously attached adults see others as reluctant to get close to them.

Previous research into adult attachment

Many studies have demonstrated that adult attachment patterns continue to exert an influence on an individual's ideas and relationships throughout their lives (e.g. Hazan and Shaver 1987; Feeney and Noller 1990; Kobak and Hazen 1991; McCarthy 1999). Indeed, attachment style is now considered to play a central role in human relations. Recent work has, therefore, moved towards examining the relationship between attachment style and the therapeutic relationship. It has been demonstrated empirically that a client's attachment style influences both the responses of therapists (Hardy *et al.* 1999), and the client's response to psychotherapy (Fonagy *et al.* 1996).

Furthermore, a relationship between adult attachment style and psychopathology has been established (Mickelson *et al.* 1997; Sroufe *et al.* 1999; George and West 1999), particularly in relation to depression. Mickelson and colleagues (1997), for example, in a study using a large, nationally representative sample, found an association between insecure attachment and depression. Similarly, Bifulco and colleagues (2002), found that non-standard (insecure) attachment styles were significantly more prevalent in women at high-risk of depression due to adverse childhood experience or adult vulnerability factors, than in an unselected comparison group. In addition, women with non-standard attachment were twice as likely to become clinically depressed than secure women. In support of such findings, preliminary analyses of the authors' current work also suggest the emergence of a similar relationship between postnatal depression and attachment style.

The results of these studies examining adult attachment have important implications for patient behaviour around childbirth in the context of primary care. They suggest that, since attachment style influences both mental state and an individual's relationships with others (including primary health care professionals as well as their family and friends), many of the women who are in need of help may be effectively prevented from benefiting from it by their attachment style. This suggests that first time mothers' individual attachment style might hold valuable information for health care professionals, which may help to guide their interventions. In particular, it is likely to be the case, as researchers into postnatal depression have noted, that several attempts are often necessary in order to secure an initial meeting with high-risk mothers.

Such difficulties in treatment research experienced by Egeland and Erickson (1990), led them to stress the need for practitioners to spend time building up trust with their clients. This is especially important with high-risk women who have often experienced abusive or exploitative relationships. Egeland and Erickson describe how, upon completion of their STEEP (Steps Toward Effective Enjoyable Parenting) preventive intervention programme, some of the mothers described their 'initial scepticism' towards the programme. Some of these mothers also claimed that they ' "tested" their facilitator in various ways by missing appointments ... or trying to shock her with stories of outrageous things they had done'. These difficulties of engagement, trust and non-presentation are, of course, not unique to research work. Members of the primary health care team are faced with such obstacles on a daily basis. This is particularly relevant to any professionals who do 'outreach work', and who are at the front line of treatment, since they often find themselves having to work especially hard to earn the respect and trust of high-risk clients in order for the therapeutic relationship to succeed.

The results from studies concerning attachment suggest that a measure of attachment style, administered antenatally, might eventually be a good method of targeting which soon-to-be mothers might benefit from special clinical attention and might need more time to build an effective therapeutic alliance. This would ensure effective and efficient use of scarce resources and time. Research might also be usefully directed to establishing whether particular kinds of interventions are effective for individuals with different kinds of attachment style. In the mean time, it is undoubtedly the case that in order to address current difficulties in delivering effective care to those mothers who are most in need, at a time of immense importance for the establishment of the mother–child relationship, flexible practices will be required that are tailored to the individual, psychological needs of clients.

Conclusion

The issues discussed in this chapter have important implications for primary health care professionals working with mothers in pregnancy and in the early postnatal months. First and foremost, it is important for health care professionals, when they suspect that a mother is depressed, to take account of the fact that she is likely to be experiencing feelings of isolation or hopelessness that may make her unwilling to discuss her experiences, or even to conceal her true feelings. In addition, the fact that the mother may be unaware that she is suffering from postnatal depression should also be considered. In such cases, health professionals should have supportive strategies in place to help the mother understand the significance of her symptoms, particularly in cases where the mother rejects a medical description of her experience or holds the belief that treatment is not appropriate to her situation. It is also important for the health professional to bear in mind that diagnosis should not rely on the mother's general demeanor because women suffering from postnatal depression commonly make special efforts to appear to be cheerful in public.

When postpartum depression is detected, primary care support is provided. However, given that the detection of postnatal depression is often problematic and given the associated adverse outcomes for the children, it is important that primary health professionals identify women most at risk of postnatal depression. For example, special attention should be paid to those in high-risk groups, such as teenage mothers, women with high rates of infant referral, and women who fail to attend routine postnatal checks. In addition, routine postnatal mental state screening, administered sensitively, should also be considered as a method of improving the detection of postnatal depression.

Treatment for postnatal depression via home-based psychological support delivered by health visitors has been shown to be effective for the majority of cases. Although more studies of pharmacological treatment of postpartum depression are required, it seems, at this stage, that health professionals would do well to consider that treatment by medication might be appropriate only for those whose symptoms fail to remit with supportive home visiting, and as an adjunct to psychological support for those whose initial symptoms are particularly severe.

Further research is necessary, in a number of areas, such as in examining the value of antenatal screening to identify those at a higher risk of becoming depressed postpartum, and in evaluating the content and structure of parental education programmes to maximize learning and alleviate concerns. Further studies are also needed to investigate whether improvements in preventive intervention programmes produce a lowering in the incidence of postpartum depression. Furthermore, research is also needed to determine whether variables can be identified (such as maternal attachment) to enable a targeting of resources and to establish the preferred type of intervention. Research carried out to date, however, on the management of postpartum depression, highlights the enormous importance of both the therapeutic relationship and the consideration of an individual's personal characteristics and circumstances, in both successful identification, and in treatment.

Acknowledgments

The Reading preventive trial (2000) was supported by the UK National Health Service Executive. The audit of primary care contacts (2000) was supported by the UK Department of Health. Maret Dymond is supported by a studentship from the Medical Research Council of Great Britain.

12 Eating disorders

Ulrike Schmidt

Let us start with a problem. We are bombarded daily by images of emaciated supermodels and other media images of thin women; unsurprisingly, weight and shape concerns, and dieting are the norm among young women. This preoccupation with appearance provides a fertile breeding ground for eating disorders, in particular for bulimia nervosa (British Medical Association 2000). The incidence of bulimia nervosa presenting to primary care has recently tripled (Turnbull *et al.* 1996), whereas that of anorexia nervosa has remained stable. The average general practitioner in the UK will have about two patients with anorexia nervosa and about 18 patients with bulimia nervosa on their list, but that does not mean that he or she will necessarily be aware of these cases. In primary care-based surveys of eating disorders the GP was not aware of the diagnosis in up to 50% of cases discovered by the researcher (King 1989; Whitehouse *et al.* 1992). Yet individuals with eating disorders consulted their general practitioner significantly more frequently over the 5 years prior to the diagnosis of the eating disorder than control subjects (Ogg *et al.* 1997). These patients presented to their GPs with a variety of symptoms, including psychological, gastrointestinal, and gynaecological complaints. In many cases, the earlier consultations had been prompted by complications of the eating disorder, but the diagnosis was missed.

There are multiple reasons for this poor case detection rate. For example, eating disorders get overlooked in ethnic minorities, individuals from lower socio-economic classes, and in men, as doctors don't expect these groups to be affected (Noordenboos 1998). Moreover, many of the cases presenting to primary care are partial cases and are therefore more difficult to pick up than full cases. Individuals with bulimia nervosa typically are ashamed of their disorder and have difficulty confiding in others, including their general practitioner. Those with anorexia nervosa actively tend to hide their disorder by wearing baggy clothes, so milder cases may be difficult to identify. Communication difficulties between doctor and patient may also play a part. In a survey of members of the Eating Disorders Association 43% of 1638 respondents said that their initial consultation with a GP was unhelpful (Newton *et al.* 1993). Female patients may especially expect their male doctors not to understand their problem or be sympathetic about it.

Does it matter that there are diagnostic delays in many cases? Research on the long-term outcome of anorexia nervosa suggests that early identification and intervention seem to improve prognosis (Zipfel *et al.* 2000). Most general practitioners have not had the opportunity to attain the management skills needed for these patients and prefer to refer them on. However, the NHS Research and Development Strategic Review into Primary Care (1999) concluded that 'we cannot afford specialist referrals for all of these patients', and this review and the National Service Framework for Mental Health (1999) emphasize the need for training in the detection and management and the development of primary care based interventions for women with eating disorders.

The patients

Health professionals often fail to appreciate that anorexia nervosa is a severe mental illness (Goldberg and Gourney 1997). The mortality rate of anorexia nervosa is 20 times and the suicide rate 200 times that of the general population. The mortality rate is twice that of other psychiatric inpatients (Nielsen *et al.* 1998). In addition, there are high levels of medical co-morbidity, related to starvation and/or weight-control measures (e.g. self-induced vomiting or laxative abuse), and psychological co-morbidity, like depression, anxiety, or obsessive compulsive disorder. The median duration of anorexia nervosa is 6 years (Herzog *et al.* 1997). There is evidence that the course of the illness has become more severe in the last few decades, as indicated by increasing admission rates (Munk-Jørgersen *et al.* 1995) and rising mortality from anorexia nervosa (Møller-Madsen *et al.* 1996). Whilst bulimia nervosa does not have a high mortality, it too is often a chronic disorder and the quality of life of sufferers is markedly impaired (Keilen *et al.* 1994).

Clinical presentation

The typical sufferer from anorexia nervosa will be a teenage girl brought to see her GP—against her will—by her concerned parents. She may be shy and withdrawn, avoiding eye contact and will deny that anything is the matter. She will appear thin, pale, and clad in multiple layers of clothes. Her hair may appear lank and thin. The parents may report that their previously 'perfect' child who was quiet, well-behaved, and totally devoted to her school-work has turned into a 'stubborn monster' who is moody and withdrawn, avoiding, or putting up fights over family meals, studying relentlessly, always on the go.

In contrast, the typical bulimia nervosa sufferer will usually be in her late teens or early twenties, and will consult her general practitioner by herself. She may report that she was chubby as a child or adolescent, and that she was repeatedly teased because of this. She may recount that she went on her first successful diet a few years ago, leading everybody to compliment her on her appearance and her self-discipline. Her efforts to loose weight having re-doubled, she then found herself increasingly unable to keep up her strict routine. Episodes of binge eating set in, which she experienced as her worst nightmare coming true and self-induced vomiting seemed like the perfect answer. Now, several years later she may feel that she is locked into a vicious cycle that she cannot escape from and which affects all areas of her life, including her physical and psychological well being, her relationships, and her work.

As mentioned above a proportion of patients will not volunteer that they have an eating disorder. Physical symptoms or problems that should prompt enquiry into a possible eating disorder, especially if they occur in a young woman and in the context of marked weight change, are listed in Table 12.1.

The families of sufferers

The families of anorexia nervosa patients are usually very concerned and will want the general practitioner to take rapid action to refer their daughter to a specialist, so that she doesn't die or come to serious harm. Family therapists like Minuchin *et al.* (1978) have described the families of anorexics as 'over-involved', but many experts thought that this over-involvement simply was a 'side-effect' of having an anorexic family member. However, recent research has shown that unresolved grief is common in the mothers of anorexics (Ward *et al.* 2000), as is a history of obstetric losses (Shoebridge and Gowers 2000), both of which may contribute to a high-concern over-involved parenting style, predating the onset of the eating disorder.

Table 12.1 List of presenting physical problems in patients with eating disorders

Problems	Presenting features
Reproductive problems	Menstrual, fertility and pregnancy difficulties
Gastrointestinal problems	Salivary gland hypertrophy, irritable bowel syndrome, constipation, upper and lower intestinal tract bleeding
Cardiovascular problems	Palpitations, syncope, hypotension
Renal problems	Nocturia, renal stones
Metabolic	Hypoglycaemia, liver dysfunction, hypercholesteraemia, hypothermia, dehydration, hypokalaemia, hyponatraemia
CNS	Tetany, fits

In contrast with the rather stifling family atmosphere common in anorexia nervosa, the families of those with bulimia nervosa often are more disorganized with neglect, abuse, or serious family discord occurring in about 60%. Families often do not know about the sufferer's difficulties or if they do may be critical of her 'disgusting' habits, and of the fact that vast amounts of food disappear and are seemingly wasted.

Very little is known about the impact of chronic severe eating disorders on the family. One study examined the burden of care giving in patients with hospitalized anorexia nervosa and found that the degree of burden was as high as that for carers of individuals with psychosis (Treasure *et al.* 2001).

Parents often blame themselves for their daughter's eating disorder. They may also have lots of practical questions as to what to do so as to not make the situation worse. The GP has an important role to play in educating families and helping them not to blame themselves or their daughter, both of which are counter-productive. There are a number of excellent books that address most of the common questions family members ask and may assist the general practitioner in their task (Crisp *et al.* 1996; Palmer 1996; Treasure 1998; Bryant Waugh and Lask 1999). Parents might also be encouraged to join the Eating Disorders Association (website: www.edauk.com), which runs a number of carer support groups. When meeting with sufferers of eating disorders and their parents the GP has to be careful not to side with either parents or patient, and instead to acknowledge that both have valid positions and concerns.

Assessing and engaging the reluctant patient

Interactions with a sufferer of anorexia nervosa never leave the clinician unaffected. Seeing a young patient with a potentially life threatening illness, which to some extent is self-inflicted, who seemingly plays games to avoid help, can be infuriating and terrifying for the general practitioner. Being confronted with exhausted and worried parents who urge you to get their daughter admitted to hospital adds to the pressure. Occasionally, it may be the school or university that raises the alarm bells, and the general practitioner may be presented with a young anorexic who assures him that, although her weight is extremely low and falling, she '*has to continue* with her studies'. She may be supported in this by her family and if the GP decides to take the situation seriously, he alone is made to feel responsible for the sufferer's unhappiness. Thus, either the GP will feel compelled to 'heroic' action or is left feeling guilty, helpless, and increasingly anxious.

In bulimia nervosa, the GP often feels overwhelmed with the patient's distress and their woeful tales of neglect, abuse, and being alone and misunderstood. Her vacillation between wanting help for her bingeing yet being adamant that if treatment involved the slightest risk of any weight gain she'd 'rather be dead' may be irritating, at the very least.

Ironically, there is no other psychological disorder other than anorexia nervosa, which is so 'positively valued' by those affected (Vitousek *et al*. 1998). The anorexics' premise is that they do not wish to give up what has served them so well, makes them feel special and 'safe', and helps them to avoid difficult thoughts and feelings. Evidence-based therapeutic techniques exist to address this ambivalence and reluctance to change (motivational interviewing; Miller and Rollnick 1991). These have been adapted for use in eating disorders (Treasure and Ward 1997; Treasure and Schmidt 2000) and in primary care (Rollnick *et al*. 1997), and have been incorporated in patient and therapist manuals (see Table 12.2).

Physical assessment and investigations

A physical examination including measurement of weight and height, blood pressure, and pulse should form part of the assessment of an eating disorder. A full blood count, and urea and electrolyte measurement are usually sufficient as base-line investigations, unless there are other indications. A bone scan may be indicated in those with well-established anorexia nervosa of 1–2 years duration, especially if the body mass index is below 16 kg/m^2. Feed-back about physical abnormalities, especially about loss of bone mineral density, can be very motivating for patients, but needs to be done sensitively.

Current knowledge about treatment of eating disorders

Much more is known about the treatment of bulimia nervosa than that of anorexia nervosa. Two systematic reviews (Bacaltchuk *et al*. 1999; Hay and Bacaltchuk 2000) summarized the evidence base for psychological and pharmacological treatments of bulimia nervosa as follows:

◆ Cognitive behavioural therapy of 16–20 sessions is the treatment of choice and produces recovery rates of between 40 and 60% of cases.

◆ Other out-patient psychotherapies, e.g. interpersonal therapy, are less well studied, but also hold promise.

◆ Antidepressant medication alone (e.g. fluoxetine) is less effective than CBT, but combinations of the two may be superior to psychological treatment alone.

Many general practitioners like to use antidepressants as a first line treatment for bulimia nervosa, however, most bulimic patients prefer and are more compliant with psychological treatments in the first instance, so it may be best to reserve the use of antidepressants for those cases where psychological treatment has failed to help or only led to partial improvement. The use of brief psychological interventions for use in primary care is described below.

Table 12.2   Principles of motivational interventions

General principles

◆ Systematically direct clients toward motivation for change by getting them to express the arguments for change and strategic empathic reflection on these

◆ Avoid confrontation or arguments

◆ Resistance is seen as interpersonal problem between therapist/client, not seen as client problem

◆ Resistance flags up need to change gear

Specific examples of how to translate motivational principles into dialogue with the patient

◆ Respect for patients, e.g. acknowledge their reluctance to come, e.g. 'I appreciate that it was not an easy decision for you to come today'

◆ Affirmation, e.g. 'I have been very impressed with how openly you have talked about what are very difficult issues'

◆ Focus on eliciting the patient's *own* concerns, e.g. 'your mum has brought you here and is clearly concerned. Are you worried at all about having lost some weight?' Or 'It seems you have lost quite a bit of weight since I last saw you. How is that affecting you? (Probe for effects on physical and psychological well being, ability to study/work, relationships with parents, peers, boyfriends)

◆ Enquire about and acknowledge the positive aspects of the disorder, e.g. 'What are the good things about your anorexia? How has it helped you?'

◆ Explore goals and values, e.g. 'If you compare where you are now in terms of how life is going and five years ago, what are the differences?' 'If everything went well for you, how would you like life to be in five years time?'

◆ Empathic reflection is used selectively to reinforce the patient's concerns and positive self-talk, e.g. 'it sounds like the anorexia has really affected your life in very major ways'

◆ Emphasis on personal choice, e.g. 'what would you like to happen as a result of our meeting today?'

◆ Offer advice and feedback about health risks/problems where appropriate, without lecturing or threatening. You may need to ask patient's permission for this, e.g. 'I have seen a number of young women with eating difficulties not dissimilar to your own—would you like me to tell you about the kinds of difficulties people with this type of problem tend to run into and what they have found helpful?'

◆ Seek to create and amplify the client's discrepancy in order to enhance motivation for change, 'You are pleased about being so good at keeping your weight down, it feels like a major achievement to you, yet there also is a price to pay … in that you are unable to study and have lost interest in seeing your friends'

◆ Support self-efficacy and optimism, i.e. get client to mobilize own resources to change, e.g. 'What do you think might help you change things if you decided to do so?' 'It is clear that you have been very determined in pursuing your studies, despite the fact that the more weight you have lost the poorer your concentration has become. That determination and staying power will be a great asset, should you decide to make some changes'

> ◆ Give menu of change options, e.g. in a case of bulimia nervosa: 'One option we
> have is to refer you to our practice counsellor to look at some of the issues we
> discussed in some more depth. Another option is to prescribe some medication,
> which might be helpful. Which option would you prefer?'

Current knowledge about out-patient treatment of anorexia nervosa can be summarized as follows: in adolescent anorexia nervosa family therapy is superior to individual therapy both as first line treatment, but also for relapse prevention (Russell *et al.* 1997; Robin *et al.* 1999). Family counselling, where parents and the affected adolescent are seen separately, seems to be as effective as conjoint family therapy (Eisler *et al.* 2000), but the latter may have advantages in situations where there is family conflict and expressed criticism. In adult anorexia nervosa, a number of studies have shown that different psychotherapies (cognitive-behavioural, psychodynamic, cognitive analytical) are effective both in the acute phase of treatment and as relapse prevention, and are superior to generic out-patent support or dietetic treatment alone (for review, see van Furth 1998).

No clear guidelines exist as to when to admit a patient, e.g. in continental Europe patients often get admitted as soon as they fulfil the diagnostic criteria, in the US-American guidelines a body mass index of below 15 kg/m^2 qualifies patients for admission, whereas in the UK patients get admitted if their weight falls below 13 kg/m^2 (see referral guidelines, Table 12.3). There is some suggestion that in-patient treatment is associated with a worse outcome and compliance with in-patient treatment is poor, so where possible it should not be used as first-line treatment.

Brief interventions suitable for use in primary care

A number of studies have addressed the issue of how evidence-based treatments for bulimic type disorders can be adapted for primary care, e.g. by delivering brief formats of CBT (Waller *et al.* 1996) or using psycho-educational groups, which focus on symptom management (Davies *et al.* 1990). Several studies have evaluated the use of cognitive-behavioural self-help (Cooper 1993; Schmidt and Treasure 1993; Fairburn 1995). The findings from this research can be summarized as follows (Treasure *et al.* 1994, 1996; Carter and Fairburn 1998; Thiels *et al.* 1998; Banasiak *et al.* 2000): pure self-help with a book leads to recovery rates in bulimia nervosa of 20%, i.e. is roughly as effective as treatment with an antidepressant like fluoxetine. If a patient is given a self-help book in addition to some sessions (up to eight) with a therapist either concurrently or after having worked through the book on their own, the outcome can be as good as that with full cognitive behavioural treatment, even if the therapist is not

Table 12.3 Protocols for eating disorders for primary and secondary care (adapted from J. Treasure, personal communication)

Treat in primary care

◆ Mild anorexia nervosa (BMI > 17 kg/m²): treat with information (Palmer 1996; Treasure 1998; Bryant-Waugh and Lask 1999), exploration of the 'good and not so good' aspects of their problem and weight monitoring

◆ Mild to moderate bulimia nervosa (i.e. bingeing and vomiting less than daily, no severe co-morbidity like diabetes or impulsive behaviour) or binge eating disorder (binges without compensatory behaviour): treat with self-help book (e.g. Cooper 1993; Schmidt and Treasure 1993; Fairburn 1995)

Guidelines for referral to Eating Disorder Unit

◆ Patient fulfils the criteria for mild anorexia nervosa (BMI > 17 kg/m²) or mild to moderate bulimia nervosa (no additional co-morbidity or impulsivity) or binge eating disorder, and has failed to respond to treatment in primary care as outlined above within 8 weeks → routine referral

◆ Moderate anorexia nervosa (BMI 15–17 kg/m²) and no evidence of system failure → routine referral

◆ Severe anorexia nervosa (BMI < 15 kg/m²) or rapid weight loss and evidence of system failure (e.g. bone marrow, circulation, kidneys, salt/water balance, proximal myopathy) → urgent referral

◆ Severe bulimia nervosa, e.g. purging daily with significant electrolyte imbalance or co-morbidity like diabetes, severe impulsive behaviours, self-harm, shoplifting → urgent referral. If alcohol or drug dependent refer to addiction service first. If self-harm/suicidality is a major problem refer to CMHT first. Most of these patients will need joint management between CMHT and EDU

Guidelines for admission to In-patient Eating Disorder Unit

◆ BMI < 13 kg/m² with signs of major systems failure or psychiatric risk, or failure to halt weight loss with out-patient intervention

◆ Failure of full course (1 year) of out-patient treatment (BMI < 15 kg/m² with physical or psychosocial co-morbidity after out-patient therapy and follow-up)

---

a trained cognitive behavioural therapist (Cooper *et al.* 1996; De Zwaan *et al.* 2000). Thus, GP counsellors may be able to deliver these interventions, irrespective of their theoretical leanings.

Management of the chronic anorexic patient

About a third of sufferers of anorexia nervosa become chronically unwell (Sullivan *et al.* 1998). After 12–15 years of chronic anorexia nervosa full recovery is rare (Ratnasuryia *et al.* 1991). Many of these cases will have had repeated admissions to psychiatric units with a 'revolving door pattern' of losing and gaining weight, often admitted under the Mental Health Act. As a result, their trust in mental health services may be extremely limited. Others have avoided any contact with services, and only present to their general practitioner when some late complication arises. The general practitioner is an important advocate for these women who often are very isolated. In these cases the most realistic therapeutic option may be to help the patients to survive at a low—but stable—level of body weight and to work on enhancing their quality of life, rather than to continue to force the issue of full recovery. However, the GP needs to remain open to the possibility that some limited change may be desired by the patient, perhaps when there is a change in her life circumstances. The GP also needs to be watchful and to look out for evidence of deterioration, especially when the patient faces additional stresses. This is a delicate balancing act for the general practitioner trying to stay clear of either collusion or coercion. It may be helpful, in discussion with a local specialist unit, to agree with the patient a minimum weight below which the patient will have to be admitted. Most patients do comply with monitoring of their weight and general health under these circumstances.

The Mental Health Act and anorexia nervosa

Compulsory treatment of anorexia nervosa has been a controversial subject, largely because of concerns expressed as to whether anorexia nervosa constitutes a mental disorder. However, there is clear guidance from the Mental Health Act Commission (4th Biennial Report 1989–1991) to say that anorexia nervosa falls within the definition of mental disorder in the Mental Health Act. Therefore, treatment of anorexia nervosa necessary for the health or safety of the patient, including involuntary feeding and maintenance of hydration, is permissible in patients whose anorexia is causing serious concern. A further reason for the controversy surrounding the use of the Mental Health Act in anorexia nervosa is that some critics have equated compulsory treatment with coercive or punitive treatment (Treasure and Ramsay 1997). However, if treatment under the Mental Health Act is given in a specialist unit by a skilled team the patient usually experiences the detention as something that makes her feel safe and contained.

General practitioners are often concerned that if they do become involved in a Mental Health Act assessment this will destroy their therapeutic alliance with a patient. However, the majority of anorexic patients, who have been detained compulsorily, are later grateful that someone stopped them from self-destruction (Serfaty and McCluskey 1998).

13 Management of serious mental illness

Christine Wright and Tom Burns

Serious mental illness is rarely an isolated episode. A diagnosis of schizo-phrenia, bipolar affective disorder, or recurrent severe depressive illness, is, at best, a lifelong vulnerability and, at worst, a continuous chronic condition with serious associated disabilities. Like many physical chronic diseases, such an illness demands of the individual and those closest to them acceptance of a highly unpalatable diagnosis, adjustments in lifestyle and life expectations, and the often unwelcome realities of long-term treatment and service involvement— if relapse and long-term disability are to be minimized. As with other chronic diseases, the organization of care needs to include a greater emphasis on certain key elements. These include:

♦ helping patients to own and manage their illness;

♦ more intensive follow-up;

♦ optimal drug management;

♦ more explicit and pro-active approach to the tasks of patient management whether carried out in primary care by GPs themselves, or other members of the primary care team, or in conjunction with secondary care (Davis *et al*. 2000).

Care giving can also be psychologically, as well as practically, challenging to the GP concerned. Acute psychosis may be personally disturbing and threaten-ing. Serious mental illness demands a balance between empathy for the patient and over identification; between recognition of the severity of the illness and stigmatization; between anxiety and over-involvement, and distancing or dis-missing the person. These challenges may interfere with the care a GP can offer—as they may also for a psychiatrist!

The term serious mental illness incorporates a range of conditions— schizophrenia, affective bipolar disorder, severe recurrent depression and obsessive compulsive disorder, and others. The following discussion will be weighted towards schizophrenia, but it is important to bear in mind the broader range of conditions from which patients may suffer.

Pathways

The patient's pathway

No serious mental illness is static, and neither are its consequences. The initial episode may be followed by a period—long or short—of health. There may be relapse at times of stress—so that at life's most difficult times, the individual also suffers increased vulnerability to further psychiatric breakdown. In addition, the illness (and therefore the needed care and interventions) changes over time. Schizophrenia, for instance, usually does not deteriorate further after the first 5–10 years and the 'positive symptoms' (hallucinations and delusions) of the acute illness become less. However, the deeply disabling and life-limiting residual damage of 'negative symptoms' (loss of drive and determination, emotional unresponsiveness, apathy), as well as depression, still require intervention and support. Significant cognitive impairment is present in three-quarters of those with schizophrenia (Palmer *et al.* 1997), affecting social and functional outcome. For all those with serious mental illness there are also the secondary effects of loss of education and employment, marginalization, and stigma—effects that will often become more marked over time.

Each of these disorders may also be associated with other problems: physical ill health, or other psychiatric disorders related to drug and alcohol misuse, or personality disorder. Schizophrenia and depression are themselves closely related, with more than half of first episode or drug-free schizophrenic patients experiencing depressive symptoms, and about 25% developing depression in the first six months after discharge for an acute episode (Johnson 1981). Illness patterns may thus be complex, and complicated by secondary social effects.

The pathway of contact with primary care

> *Vignette*
>
> Ben's father saw his GP for back pain, but also wanted to talk about Ben, then 19. He and his wife had been increasingly concerned, over the past year about their middle son, who he described as moody, withdrawn and irritable. Ben had dropped out of college, and was now staying in his room a lot, playing music loudly. He looked anxious and preoccupied, and expressed vague fears that his college tutor was troubling him in some way. The GP agreed with Ben's father that he would write to Ben, offering him an appointment. Ben did not respond.
>
> Four months later the police were called one night when Ben was shouting out in the street. His parents took him to A & E where he was seen by

a junior doctor who called a psychiatrist to come and see him – but Ben left before they arrived. Ben's older brother phoned the GP the following morning, angry and upset that Ben was not receiving treatment. His GP called at Ben's home the same day, and found him to be withdrawn, complaining of pains in his legs, and probably deluded. He arranged a home visit by a psychiatrist from the local CMHT 2 days later. She agreed Ben was psychotic and prescribed medication which Ben took for $3\frac{1}{2}$ days and then stopped. She did not find Ben to be sectionable at that time. Ben was not willing to see her again, despite several attempts. Three weeks later he threatened his father with a knife, the police were called and he was admitted to hospital under Section 2 of the Mental Health Act after an assessment which included his GP.

From the GP and the practice's point of view the profile of service contact will also change greatly over time. Onset of illness varies. It may be acute, but typically a young person's behaviour changes insidiously. There may be increasing social withdrawal from friends and family, loss of drive and interest, and subsequent failure to complete education or stay with a job. There may be the development of odd interests or habits and routines: drug or alcohol use may increase. During this initial period of deterioration (often unrecognized by the individuals themselves), distressed relatives may make multiple contacts with the practice wanting advice and intervention. The receptionist will be the point of first contact. Symptoms presented may be vague and the relatives struggle to explain the reason for their concern—increasingly desperate to convince others that 'something is wrong'. At a later stage recognition is easier when it becomes apparent that there are other symptoms—delusional ideas or hallucinations—and the person's behaviour becomes more disturbed and bizarre. This first contact is critical to early recognition and intervention, and there is now evidence of its relationship to better longer-term outcome (McGlashan 1996).

This first episode presents dilemmas for the GP. Is it really more than an adolescent developmental crisis, maybe related to drug use? What can be done if the individual resists care? The re-active patterns of response usual in primary care will not be sufficient—pro-active approaches, such as an unsolicited (by patient) home visit, may be needed. Crises may occur. Police may be involved. There will then be issues of diagnosis and prognosis for the family, and the individual and therefore for the GP. Family members may well consult the practice for the effects on their own health. This will be a stressful and difficult stage of involvement for the GP, and early liaison with local mental health services is important. This may lead to formal referral and attempts by the CMHT to effect contact and engagement. It also allows for crisis plans to be agreed in advance by the GP and secondary care.

After the initial crisis, ongoing monitoring, support, medication, and rehabilitation into normal routines and responsibilities are required. Secondary care should continue to be involved wherever possible, for at least the first one to two years. Over this period and the subsequent years the GP remains of pivotal importance. She is responsible for physical care, usually the first point of call to anxious family members, and is closely involved with psychological care, prescribing and monitoring alongside secondary care, and sometimes the only medical point of contact acceptable to the patient. There may be other members of the individual's family also in need of psychological or psychiatric care. Other practice members will be involved—the receptionist, other partners, possibly the practice nurse, or health visitor—and will need to be aware of each other's roles. There are communications with other agencies to maintain and manage—mental health services, housing, children's agencies, and benefits agencies. As with any chronic illness, prevention of further episodes is key, and where subsequent crises do occur the GP will often be the first professional to know about them.

Epidemiology of serious mental illness in primary care

Prevalence and consultations

All GPs have patients with long-term mental illness on their lists. The estimated prevalence of schizophrenia and affective psychosis combined is 3–10 per 1000 population (Department of Health 1992). There are approximately 15 new cases of schizophrenia per 100,000 population per annum, characteristically in early to mid-adulthood (18–45 years), and equally common in men and women.

An average GP list of 2000 patients could be expected to contain between 6 and 20 patients with schizophrenia and affective psychosis. In SW Thames in 1991, two-thirds of GPs had 10 or less patients with schizophrenia on their list, but the distribution was uneven. They were more common in practices located in Greater London, and in those that had a large mental hospital within a three mile radius, or had a visiting psychiatrist. 40% of these patients had had no contact with secondary mental health services in the preceding year. There was a high rate of consultation with GPs by this group of patients with a mean of 8.1 consultations per year, compared with 2.8 for the control patients (Kendrick et al. 1994). Other research has also shown that up to a quarter of patients with schizophrenia are cared for *only* by the family doctor (King 1992). However, this may be quite appropriate in that they are those who have become more stable, with less symptoms, and better social functioning and quality of life (Kendrick et al. 1999).

Many patients with severe mental illness (who in the past would have remained in long-term hospital care) now live with relatives in the community or in supported or independent housing. In a study following their de-institutionalization in the early 1960s, two-thirds of patients with schizophrenia were seen by their GP in the first year, with the bulk of day-to-day care, as well as care in crisis, being handled by the GP (Murray *et al.* 1962). Little has changed. In 1991, a year after discharge, 57% of patients with schizophrenia had seen their GP within the past 3 months, while only 52% had attended psychiatric outpatients (Melzer *et al.* 1991).

Co-morbidity

The co-existence of either physical illness or drug and alcohol abuse will influence the role of primary care with these patients. Overall mortality rates among patients with schizophrenia are about twice that in the general population. Some of this is related to increased suicide and violent death, with about 10% dying by suicide, usually in the early years of the illness (Miles 1977), and about one-third self-harming (Johnstone *et al.* 1991). However, most is related to physical disease (Allebeck 1989). One study judged 44% of long-term day psychiatric facilities users to have medical problems requiring care (Brugha *et al.* 1989), and found that much physical ill-health goes undetected or untreated. A significantly higher incidence of obesity, smoking, and hypertension than in the general population contributes to this (Kendrick 1996).

A significant proportion also abuse alcohol or drugs. Sometimes this is to self-medicate for distressing symptoms or to counteract the side effects of the medication, such as sluggishness or tremor. Lifetime rates of substance use disorder among people with severe mental illness are currently around 40–60% in the US (Cuffel 1996) and 36% in the one London study (Menezes *et al.* 1996). This is likely to be an increasing problem. Treatment outcomes such as hospitalization rates, symptom levels, functional status, and housing stability, are worse in this group than in those with single disorders (Drake *et al.* 1998). Current thinking is for care to be integrated—that is, for the same clinician(s), whether GP or specialist, to tackle the mental illness and substance misuse simultaneously, providing consistency in approach. Many patients are poorly motivated early in treatment, not seeing their drug use as a problem, so a long-term perspective (from both GP and specialist) is needed. Standard substance misuse treatment approaches (e.g. requiring explicit motivation, inflexible appointments, confrontation, rapid withdrawal of the drugs, discharge for non-attendance, etc.) are inappropriate in this group. A longer-term approach emphasizing support and harm reduction is the aim, and relies heavily on achieving trust and engagement (Osher and Kofoed 1989). GPs and PHCT members are particularly well placed to further this process when seeing the patient for other reasons.

Principles for primary care of the severely mentally ill

There are four essential principles for effective primary care of those with serious mental illness—a long-term relationship, a holistic approach, a systems view, and a chronic disease management model.

An effective, long-term, working relationship

First, an effective long-term working relationship is needed with both the patient and their family that takes account both of their changing needs over time, and of their agendas and priorities. Chronic disease management research in other patient groups confirms that taking patients' views into account is associated with higher satisfaction, better compliance, and greater continuity of care. The same principles apply in the care of those with serious mental illness. Patients and carers need information about the illness, its risk factors, and its management—as do any other patients with chronic illnesses. They also need to participate in and contribute to every treatment decision. They need to be able to discuss their diagnosis and their experience of treatment—especially adverse effects of treatment. A diagnosis of serious mental illness does not preclude any of this. The timing of giving of information, especially in regard to diagnosis, will of course be an important clinical decision, and depend on the patients and carers' wishes also; but education about the illness and its treatment is a fundamental part of good care in serious mental illness. Informing patients of the possible side-effects of antipsychotic drugs does not lead to reduced compliance (they soon get to know of them anyway), more often the opposite (Chaplin *et al.* 1999).

People with severe mental illness, not surprisingly, give higher priority to having sufficient money to live on, reasonable accommodation, and a meaningful daily schedule, than to medical care (Shepherd *et al.* 1994). To engage them successfully requires recognition and discussion of these issues during consultations—along with the medical tasks of assessment, review, advice, and medication.

There are particular issues about consistency of care and relationship in larger practices. A system is needed to ensure that, wherever possible, appointments are with the same GP. When this is not possible, communication back by other partners must be reliable. This consistency is particularly important at times of early relapse, where individual patients show reasonably predictable patterns of symptoms for a period of a few days or even weeks prior to each relapse ('early warning signs'). These are patterns that the family and the GP, as well as the individual, usually become familiar with, despite the symptoms often being fairly non-specific. Although the progression on to relapse then depends on many factors, prompt, and effective therapeutic intervention, including increased antipsychotic medication, when these symptoms emerge can be effective in reducing this progression (Herz and Lamberti 1995; Norman and Malla 1995; Herz *et al.* 2000). Thus, an important therapeutic activity for both mental health worker and GP is to help the individual (when better) and their carer to specifically identify relapse symptoms, and their order of appearance over time. Discussion can then take place as to what needs to be done at each stage of relapse to prevent further deterioration—by the individuals themselves (e.g. reducing alcohol or drug use, restarting or increasing medication, extra rest, etc.), by the carers (e.g. encouraging the patient in these, contacting care co-ordinator, etc.), and the services (e.g. urgent review, daily monitoring, increase in medication, etc.).

A long-term relationship between patient and GP is the ideal, but not always practically possible. In particular transient populations in urban areas and temporary residents present GPs with particular challenges—especially when the first contact is at a time of crisis.

Holistic approach to the individual's health

A holistic approach to the individual's health is also essential. With this patient group, however, it is the reverse of the usual emphasis, as it requires the recognition of physical health issues and needs, as well as mental and social ones! As outlined above, there is considerable evidence that people with long-term mental illnesses suffer increased physical health problems. In addition to mental health management, there is a vital primary care role in physical health care and health promotion as well.

Patients with schizophrenia consult their GP almost three times as often as same-aged controls (Burns and Kendrick 1997) and this rate of consultation is unaffected by contact with psychiatric services. This high rate of GP consultation provides GPs with the opportunity for an enhanced role in monitoring all aspects of the patient's treatment. Regular screening for hypertension, checks for weight gain and its possible causes, and advice regarding smoking and regular exercise are all important. Primary care can play an important role in both primary and secondary prevention of ischaemic heart disease and hypertension in this group of patients (King and Nazareth 1996). The vast majority of GPs are willing to share the care of the long-term mentally ill, including responsibility for the patient's physical health care (Kendrick *et al.* 1991), but the care provided is usually unstructured and reactive. Why much physical health need in this group goes undetected or untreated is unclear, but the individual's way of presenting to their GP and their own, often low level of awareness of their health needs, may be significant factors. Screening for physical disease in patients with long-term mental illness requires a systematic approach to regular physical health checks, as it does for any other risk group, e.g. diabetics—either through existing health clinics, opportunistically when patients consult, or using computer-aided reminders. The possible benefits of targeted fees for such checks in this patient group are being explored (Burns and Cohen 1998) and are currently implemented in a few PCGs. The use of case registers to facilitate this is discussed later. In group practices, identifying a 'responsible' GP for each patient with serious mental illness also allows improved continuity of care.

A systems view

A systems view is needed that is able to take account of the role of the wider family and social environment. This is a view that primary care is uniquely able to hold for many patients, caring not only for the individual, but also for others within their family and community. About half of those with severe mental illness live with family or friends, and many others also receive support from them.

The patient's family or other carers will often consult on behalf of the patient, and need ongoing support and education about the illness. They often feel responsible for the patient's illness, and certainly this will be a common view that they have to face from others. It is important to understand and, where necessary, confront some of the mistaken assumptions held about the causes of the illness and the family's part in it. The important message is that they are not responsible for the illness, but that there are things that they can do to help or, indeed, to hinder their relative's progress. The underlying need is for the relationship between GP and carers to be a long-term and honest one, where the reality of the patient's illness and needs can be openly addressed. Finally, the health effects on carers of patients with any long-term illnesses are well known and may result in stress-related appointments of the carer with the GP.

Confidentiality can be a problem when carers request information that the patient might not wish to be shared. Judgements have to be made as to how to handle this. Often, the care of those with serious mental illness involves several groups of people and much more information sharing is necessary than in physical illness. It is not possible, nor correct, to exclude family members from this: they also need to know about the patient's illness and their involvement will affect its outcome. There may be specific areas of information, perhaps in regard to drug-taking, for example, that the patient does not want shared. Where possible, after assessing any risk to the carers, this can be respected, while encouraging the patient to reconsider this.

Mental health services now have an obligation to offer carers an assessment of *their* needs—leading to a care plan for them if necessary. The National Service Framework for Mental Health (Department of Health 1999a) requires this. It expects that GPs will prompt carers to request this from mental health services, as well as themselves checking carers' physical and emotional health at least annually. Where a GP has concerns about the effect of caring on the carer, this should be communicated to the secondary services. GPs need to be aware of what carer support is available locally and to pass on that information. A plan by Social Services for the carer may include arrangements for short-term breaks, advice on income or housing, or assessment and treatment of their own mental health needs by mental health services.

A systems view is also required in regard to the network of professionals involved in the patient's care. Practical issues need addressing, such as difficulties in contact and communication ('he's in a meeting', 'she's out on visits'), as these are decisive factors in the quality of co-ordinated care a person receives. Professionals with differing backgrounds and approaches, e.g. GPs and social workers, often need more understanding of each other's roles and of their complementary nature. A crisis involving serious mental illness often puts a strain on professional relationships, and these issues need to be explored and clarified in less stressful times. A regular liaison meeting between practice and CMHT staff allows for this.

Chronic disease management approach

A chronic disease management approach to the care of those with severe mental illness is needed. The key management strategies are given in Box 13.1.

Case registers

Disease or case registers have been used increasingly by GPs to provide more regular, pro-active care for those with chronic conditions, such as diabetes, hypertension, or asthma. Usually linked to management guidelines, they aim to promote more systematic follow-up, earlier intervention, and prevention of relapse or complications, increased patient satisfaction, and more effective

---

Box 13.1 **Components of a chronic disease management approach**

- Formation of case registers
- Regular, systematic assessment and review, including medication monitoring and review of side effects
- Patient and carer involvement and education
- Avoidance of precipitating factors where possible, with a focus on relapse prevention
- Explicit delegation by the primary care doctor of particular tasks of care to other members of the primary care team—especially practice nurses
- Shared care by primary and secondary services, with explicit roles for each

collaboration with secondary services. In mental health care, introducing a disease register and a regular, modest, comprehensive structured assessment has also been found to improve the overall process of care (Kendrick *et al*. 1995).

The establishment of registers involves firstly determining *who* should be included, and for this a definition of serious mental illness needs to be agreed in the practice, with consultation locally. Diagnosis, duration, and disability have all been used in definitions (Bachrach 1988), while noting that the need for support is related more to disability than to diagnosis (Wing 1990). Disability may be defined by inability over 2 years or more to hold down a job, care for oneself and one's personal hygiene, do necessary domestic chores, or participate in recreational activities as a result of specific types of impaired social behaviour (e.g. withdrawal and inactivity, responses to hallucinations or delusions, bizarre or embarrassing behaviour, or violence). Diagnoses may be varied. Ongoing inclusion in a register will result from consideration of all these factors. For instance, a patient on long-term psychotropic medication for schizophrenia may remain on the register even though back in employment.

At least 90% of those with serious mental illness in individual practices can be easily identified through practice records, i.e. recorded diagnoses of psychotic illness, psychotropic drug prescriptions, and a review by the GP of recent appointments and home visits' lists. In addition, receptionists and practice nurses should be asked for their input. The ease of this process is obviously affected by the level of IT development in the practice and Primary Care Trusts can help the process especially for single-handed, inner city practices with high levels of serious mental illness, by supporting such IT development for them. A further check with local psychiatric services' and social services' caseloads only identifies a further 10% (Kendrick *et al*. 1994). Thus, starting with a relatively simple in-house identification and then adding

Figure 13.1 Case register

Case register Updated 20.11.2000						
Patient	DOB	GP	Date last medication review	Date last physical check	Care Co-ordinator	Psychiatrist
Ben Smith	01.06.76	Dr Jones	25.10.00	7.4.2000	John Andrews	Dr Brown

opportunistically as patients present, soon produces a comprehensive functional register (see Figure13.1).

As with other chronic disease management, the register allows both for recall and review of patients within the practice, and for the structured review of patients in shared care between primary and secondary services. Within the practice annual physical health checks can be encouraged, and psychotropic medication can be monitored for dosage, missed prescriptions, and side effects. Care plans can be checked for implementation with the patient.

A register also facilitates a systematic approach to discussion and review between GPs, other members of the primary health care team (PCHT), and the corresponding community mental health team (CMHT). Liaison meetings between psychiatrists and general practitioners are now well established in many areas usually also involving other CMHT and PHCT members. One study (Midgley *et al*. 1996) found high attendance rates among professionals—over two-thirds of the professionals attended. Over 90% of the discussion focused directly on patient care, with two-thirds relating to patients already in shared care. Psychotic patients accounted for a high proportion of these discussions. Registers of those with serious mental illness can be the backbone of such joint meetings, allowing a comprehensive but quick means of review of all those patients in shared care.

There are contentious issues of confidentiality in regard to the use of psychiatric registers, given the stigma and prejudice experienced by those with mental illness. MIND suggests a policy that includes data being held confidentially, patients being informed, and data for service planning and audit being anonymous (MIND 1993).

Assessment and review

Regular structured review is routine practice in some chronic medical complaints. Few practices, however, have implemented similar policies for long-term mental illness—and repeat prescribing may occur over long periods without review (Holloway 1988). Item-for-service payments to GPs for monitoring long-term mentally ill patients were effective in recruiting practices and ensuring assessments (Burns and Cohen 1998). Where incentives for pro-active disease management are in place, this has been associated with an increase not only in the clinical care, but also in the extent of continuing professional development undertaken in the topic. This approach is now in place in several areas of the country.

The style of interviewing advised for eliciting emotional problems in primary care (open-ended questions with the patient determining the content) is not appropriate for patients suffering from long-term mental illnesses. Low self-esteem and confidence, apathy, poverty of speech and thought as consequences of the illness, associated depression, or lack of insight militate against a spontaneous expression of current problems. Significant deterioration can be missed where an unstructured approach is exclusively used (Wooff *et al.* 1988). A different interview approach from that for common mental disorders is therefore required. In a more tightly time-restricted primary care assessment, it is doubly necessary that a targeted approach be used.

What should be covered in such an assessment interview? Obviously the patient's mental health status, and any problems or side effects to their

Figure 13.2 Structured assessment

Questions	
I have a set of questions to ask you. I am interested in changes in how you have been since we last met. *Anxiety* Have there been times lately when you have felt very anxious or frightened or tense? (More than before?) *Depression* Have there been times lately when you have been very depressed or sad or tearful? *Delusions* Have you had the feeling lately that people are talking about you or plotting about you or trying to hurt you? Is there anything special about you that would make anyone want to do that? *Hallucinations* Have there been times lately when you have heard noises or voices or seen strange things when no one else was about and there was nothing else to explain it? *Physical symptoms* How have you been feeling physically? Have there been times lately when you have had trouble sleeping? Have you had any pains anywhere lately? Have you developed any lumps anywhere lately?	*Daily occupation* Do you have somewhere that you go out to most days? *Social support* Is there anyone that you can really count on for help in a crisis? Is there anyone who really counts on you? Is there anything else I can do for you? **Observations** *Bizarre behaviour* Postures, grimaces, flippant remarks, loss of social restraint. *Slowness and under-activity* Sits abnormally still, moves very slowly, says very little. *Hostility* Irritable, verbally or physically aggressive. *Self neglect* Clothes, hygiene, nutritional state. *Incoherence of speech* It is difficult to make sense of what the patient says. *Side effects of drugs* Tremor, rigidity, orofacial dyskinesia, akathisia.

Figure 13.2 (*continued*)

PATIENT CODE NUMBER

Tick box(es) to indicate problem(s) found

Date				
No problems found				
Anxiety				
Depression				
Delusions				
Hallucinations				
Physical symptoms				
Daily occupation				
Social support				
Bizarre behaviour				
Slowness/under activity				
Hostility				
Self neglect				
Incoherent speech				
Side effects of drugs				

medication, but also their physical health, and their general life-style and daily routine. Kendrick and colleagues (Kendrick *et al.* 1995) tested the impact of teaching GPs to carry out structured assessments of their long-term mentally ill patients. They used a structured assessment card that fits onto the Lloyd George envelope (Figure 13.2), with specified questions on each area. Training was provided over two sessions, each of 2 hours duration. The first session highlighted the problems of those with long-term mental illness and the principles of structured assessment. It included a videotape of a young man with schizophrenia interviewed twice: first using open-ended questions, and later with specific targeted questions. The second session was for the GPs to report on their experience of using the assessments and addressing any problems encountered. The format of the card can, of course, be adjusted to A4 or paperless patient records as required.

Three-quarters of the GPs trained in this study used the structured assessment, and they demonstrated increased involvement in the care of these patients, with more changes of treatment and referrals over the 2-year follow-up period. While they found the structured assessments easy to use and acceptable to patients, about half found them too time-consuming for routine surgery consultations. This suggests that special sessions may be necessary, with practice nurses or community psychiatric nurses in support, as in asthma and diabetes clinics.

Patient and carer involvement and education

General practice has an important role to play in educating the patient—and their carers—about their psychotic illness and in motivating both to ensure adherence to medication, and where relevant to decrease street drug use.

Maintenance on antipsychotic medication will significantly reduce the relapse rate in schizophrenia (Davis *et al.* 1980), and non-adherence to medication is an important predictor of relapse. Asking about adherence, side effects, and satisfaction with prescribed medication need not be time-consuming, and needs to be part of each consultation. Side effects such as weight gain and sexual dysfunction may be embarrassing for the patient, and a powerful reason for non-adherence. Most patients, however, react very positively to the GP broaching these issues. It legitimizes them as concerns and confirms the doctor's broad interest in them as an individual. At its simplest level, it provides the vocabulary for discourse. Information and negotiation about dosage or alternatives will be necessary, so that the patient can make an informed choice about adherence. Given the GP's status with most patients her role in this process can be very effective.

A critical or over-involved family atmosphere, and stressful life events, are known to increase relapse rates in severe psychiatric disorders, particularly schizophrenia. Helping reduce the level of criticism, through focused family interventions, or the time spent in direct contact with each other within such families, has been shown to decrease relapse rates (Kuipers and Bebbington 1988). Support for the family in their care of the patient, and education about the illness and the effects of criticism has been shown to reduce relapse rates (Leff 1994). GPs are often the first port of call for support and advice by relatives and other carers of those with schizophrenia. They can increase the carers' understanding of the illness, and this usually allows them to be less critical and hostile. Knowing that the GP is providing care to the patient ought to reassure carers and reduce family tension. Certainly, GPs in a London study (Nazareth *et al.* 1995) recognized that consultation with the carers or families of patients with schizophrenia was a significant part of their work with such patients.

The role of practice nurses

The role of practice nurses in the primary care of those with serious mental illness demands special mention. They are often involved not only with the patients themselves, but also indirectly through contact with relatives and carers, although only 30% have received recent mental health training (Gray

1999). Most of such training concerned depression, counselling skills, stress, and anxiety management. Nurses frequently give depot antipsychotics, despite feeling inadequately trained and supervised in this role (Sutherby 1992). Of the 61% of practice nurses in a national survey (Gray 1999) who administered depot antipsychotics at least once per month, only half monitored patients for side effects. Given that the majority of practice nurses already have a role in working with those with serious mental illness, there is an urgent need to support and develop them further in this role, and to provide adequate training.

A near replication of the SW London GP study of systematic structured assessments was conducted with practice nurses for their care of patients receiving depot antipsychotic injections (Burns *et al.* 1998). Assessments were repeated every 3 months for a period of 1 year. Practice nurses were predictably more successful than GPs at completing the assessments. Over 80% of patients were assessed and over a third on all four occasions during the year. Disappointingly, there was no impact on the care process (e.g. referrals, health promotion, medication change). This may reflect the nurses' lack of confidence in their knowledge of schizophrenia (Millar *et al.* 1999) or that no advice was given to them on what to do if they detected abnormalities. To achieve health gains both nurses and GPs probably need to be involved, and more extensive training is needed for the nurses.

What are the implications for such training of practice nurses? Training needs to include the nature and treatment of serious mental illness, the social impact of the illness, the use of depot neuroleptic medication, identification and management of its side-effects, psychiatric assessment (preferably using a checklist) with a protocol for what to do if abnormalities are detected, review with the GP, and subsequent referral mechanisms to mental health services and local resources. Updates are required after initial training. Supervision from the employing GP and local mental health professionals is a necessity. Agreements can be made between the practice and local mental health professionals to provide training. While this may seem demanding, the alternative is to continue to try and provide an essential treatment by staff who, loudly and clearly, state that they are inadequately trained for the task.

Shared care—how do we achieve it?

The majority (60–80%) of those patients with serious mental illness known to the GP will also be under the care of secondary services. We use the term 'shared care' to refer to the co-ordination of care across primary and secondary services for this group. It is important that both primary and secondary care hold the same understanding of what 'shared care' needs to involve in the context of serious mental illness—and what it does not. For instance, it *does* require clearly understood roles for each service—different, but complementary. It does *not* involve alternating appointments for the patient with each service, as might occur in antenatal care. Arrangements for shared care need to be realistic about the time constraints of both services and yet be adequate for effective care, including risk management.

Most CMHTs cover populations of between 35,000 and 60,000, which means that a number of practices will be relating to the same CMHT. The development of Primary Care Trusts with a corporate commissioning role may strengthen a co-ordinated approach to the relationship between primary care and a particular CMHT. Many CMHTs have re-configured to be co-terminous with a number of practice populations. Each consultant psychiatrist will relate to at least 15–20 GPs, and nationally there is one CPN between 5–10 GPs.

A number of models of shared care have been used, falling into three broad categories (Strathdee and Williams 1984; Burns and Bale 1997):

◆ regular consultation between GP and psychiatrist in the practice setting about difficulties experienced with a patient;

◆ out-patient consultations, between psychiatrist and patient held in primary care settings (shifted out-patients);

◆ liaison attachment.

Of these the liaison attachment is now the most widely used. It consists of regular meetings between primary and secondary care teams—often combined with a named CMHT link member for communication and co-ordination. This worker can also help to ensure that shared care registers are kept up to date. The shifted out-patient model is less favoured, but there are many mental health professionals, most commonly psychologists or community psychiatric nurses, who see patients in the surgery setting on a sessional basis.

A number of recurring problems are recognized in shared care. The most serious arises when both teams think the other is performing some agreed task and neither are doing so. This may be particularly likely with follow-up arrangements, provision of repeat prescriptions, and monitoring of blood lithium levels. For example, who will monitor whether a patient asks for their prescriptions? If a patient defaults from follow-up to one service, or if the GP or psychiatrist adjusts a medication dose, will the other be informed? If one is aware of specific risks, how is this information shared?

Despite the potential problems, there are real gains from such a co-ordinated approach. To achieve it initial attention is required to some structural issues and procedures outlined in Box 13.2.

An ambitious long-term possibility is that service agreements between primary care and mental health services will allow co-ordination of patients' care to be built into commissioning. Clinical guidelines that are developed locally, and agreed between primary and secondary care can clarify respective roles and build trust.

Box 13.2 **Establishing conditions for successful shared care of those with severe mental illness**

◆ Agreement locally on criteria for referral to and discharged from secondary care

◆ Clarify roles—who is responsible for mental state and medication monitoring? Who prescribes the medication? Who is responsible for checking lithium or other drug blood levels?

◆ Case registers held in the practice of those with serious mental illness in shared care

◆ Structured consistent communication: regular liaison meetings between the primary care team and relevant members of the CMHT, using the case register for systematic review of those in shared care. This also provides an opportunity for advice and review of medication. A named link worker agreed for each practice

◆ Agree and write down arrangements for out-of-hours access, with mechanisms in place to ensure that locums, deputizing staff, etc., are aware of them

◆ Agree arrangements for crisis care, with written contact points and procedures for locum staff

◆ Agree arrangements for level of engagement with CPA reviews, mechanisms for primary care professionals to feed in information if not present

◆ Introduce some regular audit of chosen key aspects of mental health care

Alternative models of care: home and hospital

In the majority of England and Wales Community Mental Health Teams (CMHTs) provide services to all patients living in their area (Johnson and Thornicroft 1993). Recently, however, there has been increasing interest in alternative models of care, such as home treatment teams, assertive outreach services, crisis teams, and others. These may mean that patients can continue to be cared for outside hospital, even at times of high levels of illness, and in this situation the GP retains medical responsibility. The most common alternative model, encouraged by Department of Health policy, is the assertive outreach service. Such teams have staff with lower case loads than in a routine CMHT, allowing for more intensive care for the patient in their usual environment—sometimes even visits on a daily basis. Patients find such services very acceptable, and some clinical and social function gains have been reported (Marshall and Lockwood 1998), although UK studies do not find the same substantial reductions in hospitalization as have been reported in the US. The effect of these services on the primary care contact with these patients is not yet known, although anecdotally GPs report satisfaction with the increased levels of care.

At present the question of alternative models is a developing area, very much in flux and with little evidence of consistency between services bearing the same title. Over the coming decade there will, no doubt, be consolidation of the better models, but currently it is important for a primary care team to know how their own local service works, and what functions local teams fulfil.

Use of the Mental Health Act

In serious mental illnesses there are occasions when in-patient care becomes necessary. Sometimes this will be against the wishes of the patient and assessment under the Mental Health Act may be necessary. This can raise uncomfortable issues for the patient's GP. However, honesty and decisiveness are needed. GP involvement ensures that the decision pays due regard to the patient's unique history and can often bring a better understanding of subtle deteriorations in the patient's condition. The different relationships of the GP and the psychiatrist with the patient can themselves be helpful in these situations. The GP may have more personal authority with the patient and their family, and be a source of comfort to them at what is usually a very distressing time.

The important issue is the protection of the patient and any others at risk and the provision of sorely needed care. Failure to use the Act's powers may lead to far worse consequences than any immediate distress or anger. Patients rarely hold a grudge against their GP (or even psychiatrist) when they recover. It is perfectly possible to sustain a respectful and even warm relationship despite compulsory treatment. At worst, if a Section has been used wrongly it can be promptly lifted and an apology given. Failure to apply a section when it really is needed may result in catastrophe, with no second chance.

The Mental Health Act is currently under review and there will be a new Act within the near future. Any technical or detailed advice will soon be out of date. The local Approved Social Worker (ASW) is the expert and it is helpful for GPs to keep informed about ASW practice, through an annual CPD meeting or other forum locally

Hospitalization

Care programme reviews in the community are now the critical points in care planning for a patient and there are more possible care alternatives to inpatient care than were available in the past. None the less, admission to hospital remains a very powerful experience for the patient when it occurs and is a vital component of care when required.

The GP will often be involved in the admission and the value of maintaining some contact during the hospitalization should not be under-estimated. If the GP can attend the pre-discharge care planning meeting, this is particularly useful, although in reality is not often possible. Where it is not possible, there needs to be a clear protocol about the communication of the plan to the GP within an agreed time, e.g. faxed within 24 hours of discharge.

Conclusion

The role of primary care in the care of serious mental illness has often been under-estimated in the past and given little focused attention. In part, this has related to the much larger numbers of patients who present to GPs with common mental disorders. In part it has also reflected a lack of awareness of the chronic disease management approaches required to adequately provide primary care to this group of the most severely ill patients. They are, however, an important group of patients, whose care often causes their GPs considerable stress at times of crisis and who themselves value their relationship with their GP highly.

This emphasis on 'systems' and 'structures' in this chapter should not blind us to the essentially human and creative nature of the therapeutic relationship between a person with a severe mental illness and their doctor. This can offer a refreshing opportunity to see the world from a different angle, and experience a different set of priorities and values. It also draws on our capacity for empathy—for all the normal problems of everyday patients that are experienced particularly frequently by this group—grief for a lost future, loneliness and rejection, stigma, and exploitation. Empathy is also needed for their other, less usual, experiences—the terror of panic, the undermining doubt of paranoia, the self-criticism of depression. In working with the full range of such experiences—as courageously as we can—we strengthen ourselves as doctors.

14 Suicide, deliberate self-harm and severe depressive illness

Jonathan Evans

Those who work in primary care could be forgiven for thinking that suicide is a rare event, which is difficult to predict and therefore difficult to prevent. It might be thought that those who are going to kill themselves do not consult their GP before doing so and that if they do they will be unlikely to disclose their intent. It is difficult enough to predict suicide amongst high-risk groups within secondary care (Pokorny 1983) and so the challenge in primary care should not be under-estimated.

Associations with suicide

A number of associations with suicide have been reported and are shown in Table 14.1.

While social deprivation is associated with poor health in general, suicide often takes place in the context of social fragmentation. This was first observed by Durkheim towards the end of the 19th century. Examining suicide rates across different regions of France, he discovered that suicide rates were higher in those areas where social integration was poor and called this 'anomic suicide'. His influential work meant that for many years suicide was considered to be a social phenomenon that could only be prevented through broad social change. His findings have received support from contemporary epidemiologists. Whitley *et al.* (1999) found an association between suicide and an area-based measure of social fragmentation. This measure consisted of the proportion of: privately rented accommodation, single person households for those aged under 65 and, mobility in the previous year. This was independent of the association between suicide and measures of social deprivation. It seems that communities where there is some stability, where families remain together despite poverty and poor housing, are relatively protected from suicide compared with more socially fragmented areas. However, although environmental factors such as

Table 14.1 Associations with suicide

- ◆ Male
- ◆ Unemployed
- ◆ Social deprivation
- ◆ Social fragmentation
- ◆ Marital status—single, separated, or divorced
- ◆ Mental illness
- ◆ Previous attempted suicide
- ◆ Substance misuse
- ◆ Recent discharge from psychiatric hospital
- ◆ Immediate access to lethal means

these influence suicide rates, there is no doubt that individual constitutional vulnerability also plays an important role.

Suicide and mental illness

The link between suicide and psychiatric disorder is indisputable. Psychological autopsy studies involve interviewing the relatives or other close informant of those who have died by suicide so that a retrospective diagnosis can be made (Barraclough *et al.* 1974; Foster *et al.* 1997). These studies have suggested that 95% have a diagnosable mental illness, the most common being depressive disorders (35%), alcohol dependence (25%), and schizophrenia and related psychoses (11%). Viewed the other way round, all psychiatric disorders carry an increased risk of suicide, especially substance abuse disorders, depressive disorders, anorexia nervosa, and bipolar affective disorder (Harris and Barraclough 1997).

The neurobiology of suicide

There is a growing body of evidence indicating that both suicide and suicidal behaviour have a neurobiological basis independent of any psychiatric disorder. Numerous studies have reported associations between various indices of reduced serotonin function and suicidal behaviour (Asberg *et al.* 1976; Lester 1995). Serotonin may be important in controlling impulsive and aggressive behaviour (Coccaro *et al.* 1989) and provisional associations have been reported between these traits, suicidal behaviour, and genetic polymorphisms of the serotonin system (Nielsen *et al.* 1994, Evans *et al.* 2000). These personality traits, in part determined by genetic inheritance, may then predispose individuals to act to take their own lives in the context of psychiatric disorders and social adversity.

Epidemiology

There are wide variations in the suicide rate between different countries. The highest rates are found in former Eastern block countries and amongst women in rural China. There are, however, differences in the recording of suicide, which make international comparisons difficult. Although the incidence of suicide is lower in the UK than many countries it remains a leading cause of mortality, particularly when measured as life years lost, as it includes the young, as well as the old.

The suicide rate in the UK is 11 per 100,000 of the population and accounts for around 5000 deaths annually in England and Wales. For a general practitioner with a list size of 2000, there will be, on average, one patient who dies by suicide every 4–5 years. There are considerable regional variations in suicide with up to a three-fold difference in age-standardized rates between Health Authorities. There are both rural and urban areas with high suicide rates and no evidence of clear patterns to regional variation in suicide rate across England and Wales, although suicide rates are particularly high in Scotland. Social class has a U-shaped relationship with suicide; the highest risk is for those at either end of the social class spectrum, amongst those with professional occupations, unskilled manual workers and the unemployed. Males are twice as likely to take their own lives as females and there has been a consistent pattern over the last century, whereby suicide risk increases with age. From 1980, however, there has been a marked rise in suicide by young men, such that they are now at greater risk than middle-aged men. Similar trends have been witnessed in a number of other developed countries. There is no clear explanation for this rise, but risk factors such as unemployment, and drug and alcohol use may be important. Another explanation is that young men have been unable to adapt to changing gender roles within developed countries and live in a social vacuum often with little purpose or meaning in their lives (Hill 1995).

Prevention

Prevention of suicide is an important, but difficult challenge. Targets have been set for suicide reduction within the UK and suicide rates have been adopted as service performance indicators. The government white paper *Saving Lives: our healthier nation* aims for a 20% reduction by the year 2010 from the baseline rate in 1995–97 (Department of Health 1999b). A number of other national governments have set targets to reduce suicide. Although many of the associations with suicide such as unemployment, debt, and divorce are outside the power of health services to change directly, the role of a contemporary public health service is to advise policy makers on social policy that might improve the physical and mental health of society. Furthermore, the strong association with treatable mental illness implies that the health service does have a major part to play in suicide prevention.

Role of the GP

It is unknown how effective health professionals are at preventing suicide (see Chapter 1). It is not possible to identify for certain when a clinician has been successful in preventing the suicide of an individual, but only when they appear to have failed. Those who go on to commit suicide will often have consulted their GP beforehand, 30% in the 4 weeks before their death. Many of these individuals will already be in contact with psychiatric services. It would seem there is a modest opportunity for GPs to intervene at this stage, although on average GPs will be consulted by a patient shortly before they go on to kill themselves only once every 8–10 years. One study examining the content of the final consultation before suicide reported that consultation patterns for those without a psychiatric history were little different from controls and that few cases (3.3%) were recorded to have expressed suicidal ideas during this final consultation (Matthews *et al.* 1994).

In the light of these difficulties it has been argued that given the strong association between affective disorders and suicide, then improving the recognition and treatment of depression would have the effect of reducing suicides. This approach gained momentum when the results of a study undertaken in Gotland (an island off the Danish mainland) were published (Rutz *et al.* 1989). The intervention, consisting of a broad educational package on the treatment of depression, was followed by a reduction in suicide. This reduction, however, was not sustained, suicide rates were steadily falling anyway, which may have accounted for the effect and the study had no control group. A large randomized trial of a practice guideline and practice based educational package in the recognition and treatment of depression, the Hampshire Depression Project, involving 60 GP practices in the UK, found no effect of this intervention on either recognition or outcome of depression (Thompson *et al.* 2000). This result is disappointing for those who are enthusiastic about preventing suicide through GP education, coming nearly one decade after the launch of a joint initiative between the Royal Colleges of General Practice and Psychiatry (Paykel and Priest 1992). A potential shortfall of the study was that the practices recruited were self-selecting. Only 60 from 224 eligible practices were recruited: a bias that may have reduced the power of the study as it is likely that participating practices will be interested in mental health, and already be skilled at detecting and managing depression. Furthermore, evidence for the effectiveness of pharmacological interventions or counselling for minor depression in primary care is limited (Kendrick 2000).

Despite these drawbacks, suicidal patients will still consult their GPs, and attempts should be made to identify those at risk and ask about suicidal ideas.

The consultation

A variety of risk factors for suicide have been identified (Table 14.1). A case control study based in general practice examined consultation patterns, diagnosis, treatment of mental illness, and recording of risk factors for suicide (Haste *et al.* 1998). This study found that, a previous history of attempted suicide, serious mental illness untreated in the previous year, recent marital problems, alcohol abuse, and frequent consultations were all independent risk factors for completed suicide.

The actuarial approach to predicting suicide has considerable limitations when it comes to managing the risk. Most of the risk factors predict the likelihood of suicide over the next year. During the consultation, the clinicians concern will be with the risk of suicide within the next few days. It is important to ask about suicidal ideas in anyone who presents with psychiatric disorder, but particularly when additional risk factors are present. There is a myth that asking about suicide will lead patients to think of suicide for the first time. The contrary is likely to be the case; sharing these frightening ideas with a professional is often a relief, particularly if the disclosure is heard sympathetically. Suicidal ideas are common in the general population. One study reported a lifetime prevalence of between 10–18% across different countries (Weissman *et al.* 1999) and some patients will volunteer these suicidal ideas. It is also a myth that those who talk of suicide do not kill themselves. Some individuals may fear that the disclosure of such ideas would lay them open to being considered 'mad' and having their autonomy removed if they are taken to hospital, although this course of action is only necessary in a minority of those with suicidal ideas. It is important to avoid premature reassurance as this may leave patients feeling they have not been understood or to suggest that suicide would be morally wrong. The latter would simply amplify the guilt and self-blame which are important components of a depressive illness. Asking a series of questions starting with 'does life not seem worthwhile at times' through 'have you felt like harming yourself in any way?' to clarifying any suicide plan and whether it has been initiated will be the most important way of establishing risk. Having encouraged the ventilation of suicidal ideas it is helpful to gently challenge feelings of hopelessness. Identifying what to do when suicidal ideas escalate, such as contacting the Samaritans, other crisis line, or making telephone contact with a member of the primary care team can be helpful. Offering an early follow-up appointment can be an effective way of maintaining hope and keeping contact to review risk. Concern about suicide risk is one of the most common and appropriate reasons for a referral to secondary mental health services.

The consequences of suicide

Suicide is a tragedy for the individual, family, and others left behind. It is hard to think of a death more difficult to accept for parents than the loss by suicide of a young adult son or daughter. The grief of sudden loss is often compounded by the experience of stigma. The usual supports following bereavement may diminish as friends and colleagues of those left behind may be frightened by suicide, not know what to say and actively avoid contact with the bereaved. Health professionals may feel guilty and fear the anger of relatives, but the GP has an important role in meeting with relatives, and providing information openly and promptly. Those left behind may suffer intense guilt and continuously question why they had not been able to prevent the suicide. They may blame themselves about a single argument or particular problem. It is important to explain what is known about suicide, that an interaction of factors, rather than one single explanation is likely to be the cause. There may be intense anger towards the deceased or they may be idealized. Anticipating these reactions and gently challenging some of the more extreme or unhelpful beliefs may help achieve some level of acceptance.

Case example

A 35-year-old man lived alone in a privately rented bedsit. He had recently been discharged from psychiatric unit where he was admitted following an overdose of benzodiazepines. He suffered from heavy alcohol dependence secondary to underlying social anxiety. He was separated from his wife and had not seen his children for over 2 years. He had not worked for the last 4 years since his alcohol consumption escalated. Within 2 months of his hospital discharge he relapsed and was again drinking alcohol heavily. He did not approach his GP, but took an overdose of paracetamol and benzodiazepines, and despite calling an ambulance died on arrival at the hospital.

This example illustrates several of the risk factors: previous deliberate self-harm, recent discharge from a psychiatric inpatient stay, alcohol dependence, and social isolation following marital breakdown.

Deliberate self-harm

Deliberate self-harm (DSH) refers to intentional poisoning or self-injury, whatever the motivation of the act. This is preferred to the terms 'attempted suicide' and 'parasuicide' in the UK, and as there is no clear categorical distinction between those who are and those who are not intending to die.

DSH is a behaviour and not a diagnosis. It is a heterogeneous phenomenon. The term DSH includes a poorly planned impulsive attempt in the setting of interpersonal distress, through repeated self-injury in an attempt to relieve unbearable inner tension, to an act that has been carefully planned and disguised to avoid discovery in someone with a severe depressive illness.

There are many contrasts between suicide and DSH. The majority of patients who present following DSH do not have severe mental illness. Females are at higher risk and the incidence of DSH reduces sharply with increasing age. Nevertheless, there are important overlaps; those who present to general hospitals following DSH form one of the highest risk groups for future suicide and account for 50% of those individuals who die by suicide.

Epidemiology

Variations in rates of DSH across countries may reflect differences in access to services, rather than true differences in prevalence as most recording systems rely on data obtained from general hospitals (Schmidtke *et al.* 1996). In England and Wales at the end of the 1990s there were an estimated 140 000 presentations to general hospitals annually following DSH, making it one of the most common reasons for an admission to a general hospital bed. It is unknown how many episodes are treated solely in primary care, but follow-up studies have found that the vast majority of repeat episodes involve a hospital attendance. DSH is often repetitive and of those presenting 50% have a previous history and up to 30% repeat within 1 year (Krietman and Foster 1991). A minority of individuals will repeat many times. Although rates of severe mental illness are low in this group, rates of personality disorder are high, in one study reported to be as high as 65% (Casey 1989). DSH is particularly common amongst those who have a borderline personality disorder and use self-injury as a means of regulating their emotions.

Management following DSH

There is no single intervention that has been shown to be effective following DSH in preventing either repetition or suicide (see Chapter 9). Some studies have evaluated the effect of social work interventions to tackle interpersonal, financial, and housing problems (Gibbons *et al.* 1978). It is known that those who deliberately self-harm have poor problem solving skills and cognitive behavioural approaches designed to improve these skills have been evaluated (Salkovskis *et al.* 1990). As DSH is often an impulsive act at a time of crisis, another approach aims to provide an alternative to DSH for the individual in crisis by offering an emergency card allowing crisis telephone consultation with mental health services (Evans *et al.* 1999). A Cochrane Review concluded that there was no evidence to suggest that any particular intervention was effective in reducing repeated DSH. Most studies were of insufficient sample size to detect clinically important effects, but there were trends favouring cognitive behavioural problem solving interventions and the provision of an emergency card (Hawton *et al.* 2000)

In practice, interventions offered to those presenting following DSH in the UK vary widely (Slinn *et al.* 2001). A psychosocial assessment will be offered to many, although not all, before discharge from hospital. This involves screening for major mental illness, and examining the interpersonal and social context of the episode of DSH. Only 10% are offered admission to a psychiatric inpatient unit, some who are already under mental health teams will be referred for urgent appointments and around a quarter will be referred back to their GP without follow-up. A variety of non-statutory agencies will be recommended, such as those addressing housing, marital, financial, and alcohol or substance abuse problems.

The role of the GP

It is most likely that the general practitioner will be involved with those who have been discharged from hospital following DSH. Although the role of the GP following DSH has not been formally evaluated it is important to assess the risk of suicide and, in particular, the strength of the wish to die. The GP needs to ask directly about symptoms and signs of depression, as well as signs of alcohol and drug abuse. There may be marked differences in mental state within hours or days of DSH. Frequently, patients will minimize the act of DSH and may feel ashamed. They may become cut off from the intense emotions experienced at the time of DSH. In this situation, it is important to spend some time encouraging the patient to name their feelings. Others may be hostile and demanding of care; in this situation empathic acknowledgement of feelings should be quickly followed by a more practical approach, focusing on strategies to cope with suicidal urges and intense emotions.

Case example

A 28-year-old man presented to his GP. He had left the general hospital 2 days earlier following an overdose of paracetamol. He was reluctant to attend the surgery, but had been persuaded to do so by his wife. At first he seemed hostile and unforthcoming about the episode of DSH. On careful questioning he had symptoms of depression including irritability, weight loss, and loss of interest. He admitted that he had argued with his wife and the overdose was an attempt to escape, rather than a wish to die. There were considerable stresses in his relationship and his wife has threatened to leave on a number of occasions. He was binge drinking and this had contributed to the financial hardship that the couple faced. After first acknowledging his distress, and then carefully explaining that both alcohol abuse and DSH are attempts to cope with the problems, but only reinforce them, his GP suggested that he attend an alcohol counselling service and also provided some information on a local debt advice agency. A review appointment in 1 week was arranged to establish whether symptoms of depression persisted.

At this appointment, should there have been continuing evidence of depression it would have been important to challenge the stigma, explaining that it is a treatable medical condition and providing any well-written patient information leaflets that are available. Treatment may consist of supportive therapy, cognitive behavioural therapy, and/or antidepressant medication and, if the latter, a selective serotonin reuptake that is safer in overdose would have been prescribed with advice about how long it would take to be effective and the common side effects.

Severe depressive illness

There is no categorical distinction between severe, moderate, and mild depressive illness. Different studies of treatment often use different cut off scores on continuous measures of depression to define severe depression. Although mild depressive disorder in primary care may be seen to be medicalizing social distress (see Chapter 4), the place of severe depression within the medical paradigm is less contentious. Although it is easier to recognize than milder forms of the illness, major depression is still not recognized in nearly a half of all those presenting to general practitioners, particularly if there is also a co-existing physical illness (Tylee *et al.* 1995).

Epidemiology

Lifetime risk of major depressive disorder is 10–25% for women and 5–12% for men. At any one time 5–9% of women and 2–3% of men are suffering from major depression. Epidemiological studies using well-standardized instruments indicate that severe depression is becoming more common particularly in the young (Bland 1997). Average age of onset is in the mid-twenties, although it can occur at any age. One year after the diagnosis, 40% still have symptoms sufficient for a current diagnosis of major depressive disorder, 20% some symptoms, although less severe, and 40% no mood disorder. About half of those who have a major depressive episode will experience a relapse at some time. The course of severe depression is variable, some individuals have clusters of episodes and others isolated ones separated by many years. In about two-thirds of cases there will be complete recovery from an episode.

Aetiology

Psychosocial stressors such as losses are important precipitants of a severe depressive illness particularly during early episodes; thereafter, there may be no discernible life event precipitating an episode. Early childhood experiences of loss and deprivation, such as unstable marital relationships and poor parenting all predispose to major depression in later life (Sadowki *et al.* 1999). Depression clearly runs in families and particular genes are likely to predispose to the development of severe depressive illness, although no genes have yet been identified that are definitely associated. Severe depression may be the first presentation of a bipolar illness in which previous hypomanic episodes have not come to medical attention. Careful history taking asking about protracted periods of elevated mood, excessive energy, and sleeplessness, including any family psychiatric history of bipolar illness, will help in establishing this. Physiological changes during a severe depressive episode such as alterations in REM sleep, raised cortisol, and impaired cellular immunity, are the same as those of an exaggerated and sustained stress response.

Clinical characteristics

Severe depression usually includes the three core symptoms of pervasive depressed mood, marked decreased in energy, and loss of interest or enjoyment. Some features of the so-called somatic syndrome will almost invariably be present namely:

* lack of emotional reactivity to events;
* waking much earlier than usual;
* depressed mood worse in the morning;
* psychomotor retardation (slowing in movement and thinking) or agitation;
* loss of weight, appetite, and libido.

Worthlessness or self-blame are very common, and may lead to suicidal ideas and suicidal acts. In addition, there may be psychotic symptoms and if so then the depressive illness is by definition severe. Delusions may follow from the sense of worthlessness and self-blame, and lead the individual to believe they are responsible for awful atrocities, that they have been financially ruined or have an incurable physical illness. Hallucinatory experiences include auditory hallucinations, often of a derogatory accusatory nature, and olfactory hallucinations, often of putrifaction or death.

Management

Severe depression can often be treated effectively with antidepressants given at a sufficient dose for a sufficient period of time. There is no evidence to suggest that one group of antidepressants is more effective than any other for first line treatment. Most patients will begin to respond after 3 weeks, but a therapeutic trial should last between 6 and 8 weeks. Although particular forms of psychotherapy such as problem solving treatment (Mynors-Wallis *et al.* 2000) may be just as effective as antidepressants alone in major depression, there is little evidence that generic counselling on it's own confers benefit for patients in primary care (Churchill *et al.* 1999; but see Chapters 10 and 18). There is a preference for psychotherapeutic approaches to the treatment of depression by the lay public; therefore, it is important to consider the availability of suitably trained therapists, given the lack of evidence to support the effectiveness of generic counselling. When a major depressive episode is particularly severe with marked suicidal ideas or profound retardation or agitation, then anti-depressant treatment will be essential, particularly medication with low toxicity in overdose such as selective serotonin reuptake inhibitors, or newer mixed serotonin and noradrenaline reuptake inhibitors (see Chapter 16). If psychotic symptoms develop then additional neuroleptic medication may be necessary for a short period. Electroconvulsive therapy, usually given as an in-patient, is particularly effective if there are psychotic features, and may be life-saving for an individual who is severely suicidal or suffering from profound self neglect. Other strategies used to treat severe depression in specialist settings include augmentation of antidepressants with lithium, thyroxine, or pindolol.

Apart from individual psychological and pharmacological treatments, attention should also be paid to the wider context in which depression is experienced, including the relationship with any partner. There is evidence that couple therapy, in which the relationship is seen to be both influencing and be influenced by the depression, may be just as effective in treating major depression as antidepressants alone (Leff *et al.* 2000). In practice, particularly for those with severe depression, combined treatment approaches are most often used.

Case example

A 40-year-old woman developed depression 3 months after she was attacked and robbed in the street. She had failed to be promoted in her work as an administrator within the local council. Her mother had suffered from depression and received inpatient treatment. She was divorced, but had recently started a new relationship. She presented to her GP tearful and lacking in energy requesting a sick note. Despite counselling that concentrated on a failed marriage, the attack in the street, and reactions to work problems, she continued to be depressed and attempted unsuccessfully to return to work. Several antidepressants at maximum dose were tried without success and she began to loose hope of ever getting better, her self care deteriorated, and she spent most of the day in bed. Following a referral to mental health services she started to attend a psychiatric day hospital and lithium was added to her antidepressant. Gradually, as her energy levels increased, she began to feel a sense of achievement through the tasks carried out in the day hospital and her mood improved. She felt more hopeful about the new relationship when after several joint sessions her partner understood more about her depression and became more supportive. She negotiated a gradual return to work through the occupational health service after a period of 18 months absence.

To conclude, depression, self-harm, and suicide are among the commonest and most significant of the many problems with which GPs are presented daily. Taking difficulties seriously, common sense, and recourse to antidepressants and various forms of psychotherapy can all have a significant impact on the course of this disabling and potentially lethal illness.

15 Substance misuse

Ilana Crome and Ed Day

General practitioners and their teams are in an excellent position to intervene in drug and alcohol problems. Treatment in the primary care setting can avoid the stigma that many people feel about attending a specialist addiction service and the teams may have the advantage of a long-term perspective on the patient's problems, as well as contacts with potential co-therapists such as family and friends. Furthermore, some of the developing evidence for the effectiveness of both pharmacological and psychological interventions in addictive behaviour has been derived from work in primary care settings.

Models of service delivery

The Department of Health 'Guidelines on management of drug misuse and dependence' acknowledges the importance of primary care in managing the problem, and specifically promote the 'shared care' model (Department of Health 1999c). In reality, general practitioners vary in their enthusiasm for managing substance misuse problems (Abed *et al.* 1990), but without a basic knowledge of the range of possible interventions it will be difficult to access the alternative available resources effectively. A variety of strategies have evolved to increase the effectiveness of the treatment of alcohol and drug misusers in primary care. In some areas a few GPs have become highly trained and special ized in management of these problems, whereas in others specialist drug services have taken the lead in developing 'shared care' schemes with GPs.

The term 'shared care' is widely used in medical practice, where primary care and specialist services work together in managing particular problems. The complex problems presented by drug misusers require effective collaboration between a number of different agencies, including GPs, drug misuse services, social and educational services, as well as the criminal justice system. All parties may benefit by developing a model that allows supported management of more straightforward cases in primary care, with more complex cases having specialist involvement. The GP feels less isolated, and can be reassured that more specialized counselling and monitoring are occurring. The specialist drug service can increase its access to information and links with the patients' own communities. Finally, the drug misuser may benefit from having appointments at home or in the GP's surgery, but with a specialized approach.

Different approaches to shared care

A variety of models have developed under the overall umbrella of shared care. One of the earliest schemes in Edinburgh developed in response to the spread of HIV among drug misusers (Greenwood 1992; Watson 2000). The central specialist service provides assessment and treatment recommendations to primary health care teams. This has met with a degree of success in that 70% of general practitioners participate in the scheme. A similar service is provided in Manchester, except that treatment is initiated by general practitioners with the support of a liaison team, with all general practitioners encouraged to prescribe (Carnwath *et al.* 2000). In Leeds, drug misuse is managed almost entirely within the resources of a general practice, with an addiction counsellor providing a secondary specialist level of care (Lawrence 2000). Gerada outlines a different type of intermediate service, where training and treatment is undertaken by a liaison service which focuses efforts on interested general practitioners who could become expert 'specialized generalists' and further encourage their peer group (Gerada *et al.* 2000). The Wirral has a specialist drug service led by a general practitioner that encompasses prescribing, outreach, GP liaison, general medical and mental health care, and young people's and pregnant drug users services. Here, however, attempts at re-integration with the patient's own general practitioner has not been as successful (Speed *et al.* 2000).

These differing models of care highlight the ways in which committed psychiatrists and primary care teams have found strategies to work together to meet the complex needs of drug misusers as effectively and efficiently as possible. Whatever the arrangement there will always be certain cases that require the input of specialist services (see Box 15.1). The type of service that

---

Box 15.1 **Categories requiring specialist services**

- Patients with co-morbid severe mental illness, such as schizophrenia or bipolar affective disorder
- Patients with severe physical illness, such as liver problems
- Patients who abuse multiple substances
- Patients who have frequent relapses of drug or alcohol use
- Patients who are very chaotic or who have unstable social circumstances
- Patients who require injectable substitute prescribing
- Patients requiring inpatient admission

emerges in a particular area will depend on a variety of factors, including existing service provision and personnel, prevalence and type of drug misuse, and geographical factors. They all aim to deliver a flexible service utilizing differing skills in the most effective manner, giving GPs the confidence and support to take on some responsibility for drug misuse problems themselves. However, although the exact arrangements may differ from area to area, it is important that all stakeholders are involved in their initial development. In addition to close contact between GPs and specialists, other important factors may be integrated: training, audit, locally agreed management guidelines and clearly defined responsibilities (Gerada 2000).

However, strategies for managing substance misuse problems must include more than simply offering treatment. Despite the fact that drugs are so commonly used and available, with devastating effects for some individuals and families, substance use remains one of the most highly stigmatized of behavioural problems and mental illnesses. The primary care team increasingly has a role in the prevention of the problem (Cryer 1999), and is at the heart of local policy responses in the substance misuse field, such as health education, public awareness campaigns, and community support. Interested general practitioners also have the capacity to train professionals and develop educational materials for clients, the general public, and other professionals. A few have become involved in seminal research and the dissemination of findings in the substance misuse field.

How common is substance use, misuse, and dependence?

Since the 1960s, increased availability of drugs and alcohol has led to an escalation in the use of a variety of both legal and illegal substances. Evidence gathered from many different sources (information on drug seizures, quantities of alcohol sold, offences, surveys of drug use, and notifications of drugs to agencies) indicates that substance use has increased in the last 30 years. It is now thought that over 60% of the population regularly use alcohol (with 5% dependent on it), 35% smoke cigarettes, 15% use cannabis, 5% use amphetamines, and possibly as many as 1–2% are using opiate drugs in a seriously problematic manner. Young people are being initiated into substance use at an earlier age (about 11–12 years old), and the association between smoking cigarettes, and drinking or drug taking means that polydrug use has now become an acceptable part of youth culture. There is also evidence to suggest that older people experience considerable drug- and alcohol-related morbidity as well. Thus, there is a high likelihood that individuals with both overt and covert substance misuse problems will present to primary care services on a regular basis.

What leads people into substance misuse?

Multiple factors are usually involved in the development of a substance misuse problem. These may include genetic predisposition, family factors, adverse life events, psychological symptoms, availability, social acceptability of the substance, peer pressure, and impoverished educational or work opportunities. Causation is seldom straightforward and it is usually possible to identify a combination of significant factors in any one person. However, it is well documented that depression, anxiety, and psychotic conditions are related to drug and alcohol problems, and substance misuse, in turn, may cause, complicate, or be a consequence of other mental health problems. American, European, and British research all suggests that about a third to half of people who are misusing substances have a mental health problem, and a similar proportion of those with a mental health problem are misusing substances.

The diagnosis and classification of substance misuse problems

The description and definition of terms are important. Successive editions of the *International Classification of Diseases* (8, 9 and 10) have produced specific symptom constellations for intoxication and withdrawal for all substances, as well as defining other terminology (WHO 1992). The term 'substance' means any medication or drug that alters the mind, while substance 'use' indicates that a substance is taken in a medically or socially acceptable manner, and that it is legal. 'Misuse' indicates that the substance is either not legal or else is used in a way that does not comply with medical recommendations, and 'harmful use' is defined as a pattern of substance use that is causing damage to health, but does not meet the criteria for dependence.

The term 'dependence' has a clear set of diagnostic criteria and has replaced the broader term 'addiction'. The ICD-10 states that three or more of the following must be experienced at some time during the previous year for a diagnosis of dependence:

1. A strong desire to take the substance.

2. Difficulties in controlling the use of the substance.

3. A withdrawal syndrome when substance use has ceased or been reduced. The physical symptoms of withdrawal vary across drugs, but psychological symptoms include anxiety, depression, and sleep disturbance. The individual may also report the use of substances to relieve the withdrawal symptoms.

4. Evidence of tolerance such that higher doses are required to achieve the same effect.

5. Neglect of interests and an increased amount of time taken to obtain the substance or recover from its effects

6. Persistent substance use despite evidence of its harmful consequences.

Table 15.1 The harmful physical effects of alcohol

System	Effects
Central and peripheral nervous system	Wernicke's encephalopathy—confusional state, nystagmus,ophthalmoplegia, and ataxia Korsakoff's syndrome—profound impairment of recent memory, relative preservation of remote memory and disorientation in time Mild-to-moderate cognitive impairment in long-term heavy drinkers Peripheral neuropathy—subjective paraesthesia to severe distal sensory and motor neuropathy Proximal myopathy
Hepatobiliary system	Liver damage—fatty change (usually asymptomatic) ˮ→ alcoholic hepatitis (pain in right hypochondrium, jaundice, or fever) ˮ → cirrhosis Complications of cirrhosis—portal hypertension, ascites, hepatic encephalopathy, primary liver cancer Chronic pancreatitis—severe pain, nausea, and vomiting Complications of chronic pancreatitis—pseudocysts, bile duct stenosis, portal vein thrombosis
Gastrointestinal system	Gastro-oesophageal reflux Oesophagitis Mallory–Weiss syndrome Alcoholic gastritis Carcinoma of the oesophagus is associated with alcohol and heavy smoking Poor small bowel functioning, diarrhoea, and malabsorption
Cardiovascular system	'Low risk' alcohol consumption (up to 3 units per day) protects middle-aged men against coronary heart disease 'High risk' alcohol consumption (more than 5 units per day in women and 7 units per day in men) increases the risk of stroke, hypertension, cardiomyopathy, and cardiac dysrhythmia
Endocrine system	Testicular atrophy and impotence in men Amenorrhoea, subfertility, and recurrent abortion in women Alcoholic pseudo-Cushing's syndrome—bloated facial appearance, obesity and hypertension
Skin	Palmar erythema Facial flushing Alcohol-related psoriasis

Almost every organ or system in the body may be affected by drugs and alcohol (see Table 15.1), and harmful physical effects may include cardiovascular, endocrine, respiratory, gastrointestinal, or neurological symptoms, as well as overdose, infections, or effects on the foetus. Some drugs have greater potential to cause harm than others, and alcohol, tobacco, heroin, methadone, amphetamine, and cocaine are highly likely to induce dependence. Cannabis, too is a dependence-inducing drug. LSD, ecstasy, and solvents also produce problems, but appear less likely to lead to the development of dependence.

Assessing the problem

Patients with a range of substance misuse problems may present to the general practitioner and other staff, and often the substance misuse problem is not the primary reason for consultation. Therefore, the primary health care team needs specific screening and assessment tools, as well as an awareness of the scope of the problem in order to be able to offer effective interventions. Many standardized assessment tools have been validated for use in the primary health care setting. The Alcohol Use Disorders Identification Test (AUDIT) is a 10-item screening instrument designed to screen for a range of drinking problems and in particular for hazardous use and harmful consumption. Scores for each item range from 0 to 4. A score of 8 or more is associated with harmful or hazardous drinking, while a score of 13 or more in women, and 15 or more in men, is likely to indicate alcohol dependence. CAGE (see Box 15.2) and MAST (Michigan Alcohol Screening Test) are also screening tools for the assessment of presence of alcohol problems. The Opiate Treatment Index (OTI) is a structured instrument that assesses six domains (drug use, HIV risk-taking behaviour, social functioning, criminality, health status, and psychological adjustment). Standardized instruments are also available for the assessment of severity of dependence, including the Severity of Alcohol Withdrawal Questionnaire (SADQ), Severity of Opiate Dependence Questionnaire (SODQ), and the Severity of Dependence Scale (SDS), but these are of more relevance to specialist services.

Box 15.2   **The CAGE questions**

- Have you ever felt you ought to **C**ut down on your drinking?
- Have people **A**nnoyed you by criticizing your drinking?
- Have you ever felt **G**uilty about your drinking?
- Have you ever had a drink first thing in the morning to steady your nerves (an **E**ye opener)?

Once a problem has been detected, the general practitioner can develop the assessment further. A non-judgemental approach is essential in constructing a picture of the nature and extent of the individual's problems, and particular attention should be paid to any risk-taking behaviour. Probing about the average daily use can be a useful method to establish severity, but corroboration may need to be sought from the individual's family, friends and colleagues. It is important to consider the range of potential co-morbid physical and psychological conditions, as well as any associated social problems. Further information should enable the practitioner to distinguish substance use, harmful use, and dependence, and to determine when psychological problems are due to substance use or other psychiatric illness. A proper initial assessment will ensure adequate estimation of risk, the safe initiation of effective therapies, appropriate referral to other specialist medical or voluntary services, and provide a baseline against which future strategies and outcomes may be measured.

Specialist substance misuse treatment services are likely to seek even more information, including a detailed assessment of both past, recent past (last 6 months to year) and present (last month) substance use (Glass *et al.* 1991). The age of initiation into smoking, alcohol and cannabis may provide some indication of the length of use. Each substance must be discussed in turn, including nicotine, alcohol, cannabis, amphetamine, cocaine, LSD, ecstasy, heroin, street methadone, benzodiazepines, and over-the-counter or prescribed medications. The quantity used, as well as route, length, pattern and context of substance use, and the development and severity of withdrawal symptoms are useful in the identification of the degree of problematic use. This will assist decisions about the administration of the extensive range of detoxification regimes, as well as substitute and maintenance prescribing. The previous treatment history, including self-detoxification, attempts at harm reduction, and any periods of abstinence are further pointers to the readiness or motivation of the client for change.

There are some investigations that may substantiate the individual's history. In the case of the alcohol misuser, biochemical tests of liver function (ALT and/or AST and GGT), and a haematological screen (including full blood count, serum folate, and B12) may be useful to gauge the extent of physical damage (Drummond and Ghodse 1999). Serum or breath alcohol levels, and CDT (carbohydrate deficient transferrin) may help to confirm a history of increasing or decreasing use from the patient. In some cases, clinical assessment of cognitive damage may be further substantiated by neuro-imaging or psychometric testing, but this is usually preceded by specialist assessment. For drug misusers, urine may be screened for a variety of misused substances (Wolff *et al.* 1999), both legal and illegal, and other investigations to consider are HIV, Hepatitis B and Hepatitis C testing. However, despite this large range of potential tests, the consensus is that the biochemical tests have limited usefulness without a comprehensive history. The more information a member of the primary health care team can elicit in order to understand the extent of the problems, the easier it will be to make decisions about appropriate management, including the provision of adjunctive medication or referral to specialist services.

The role of the primary care team in the identification of complications

There is a range of physical and psychological illnesses associated with the use, intoxication, withdrawal from or dependence on substances. All drugs have a particular intoxication syndrome, and many have a specific withdrawal syndrome or set of withdrawal symptoms (Table 15.2).

Table 15.2 Common signs and symptoms associated with intoxication and withdrawal

	Common signs and symptoms associated with intoxication	Common signs and symptoms associated with withdrawal
Alcohol	Facial flushing Ataxia Slurred speech Impaired attention	Sweating Insomnia Weakness Faintness Hyperthermia Fine to coarse tremor Seizures Tachycardia Hypertension Cardiac dysrhythmias Nausea and vomiting
Opiates	Nausea and vomiting Constipation Constricted pupils Dry mouth Sweating Drowsiness Respiratory depression Hypotension	Sweating Insomnia Gooseflesh Flushing Low-grade fever Running eyes and nose Sneezing Yawning Dilated pupils Shivering Psychomotor agitation Pains in muscles and joints Tachycardia Hypertension Nausea and vomiting Abdominal discomfort Diarrhoea
Stimulants	Dilated pupils Dry mouth Tachycardia Palpitations	Early-psychomotor agitation; Later-fatigue Weight gain

	Arrhythmias	
	Hypertension	
	Psychomotor agitation	
	Muscle twitching	
	Nausea and vomiting	
	Irregular respiration	
	Ataxia	
	Insomnia	
	Hyperthermia	
	Weight loss	
Benzodiazepines	Light-headedness	Sweating
	Drowsiness	Insomnia
	Confusion	Weakness
	Ataxia	Muscle twitching
	Muscle weakness	Psychomotor agitation
		Headache
		Tremor
		Tachycardia
		Palpitations
		Postural hypotension
		Anorexia
		Nausea
		Abdominal discomfort
		Diarrhoea

The role of the primary health care team in treatment of substance misuse

Interventions in drug and alcohol problems have a range of objectives, and it is important to try to tailor the approach to the individual. In some cases the objective will be to achieve and maintain abstinence from the substance of abuse. For example, patients with a long history of alcohol dependence, medical or psychiatric problems, or poor social support achieve better long-term outcomes if the goal is abstinence. However, this approach may not always be acceptable to the patient, and the GP may miss opportunities to bring about improvements in physical, psychological or social conditions by adhering rigidly to a policy that views abstinence as the only treatment goal. Setting more limited treatment targets can be effective at both an individual and population level, and the 'harm reduction' model has gained prominence in the last twenty years. The spread of the HIV virus in the early to mid-1980s and the associated risk of blood-borne infection via sharing needles led to the development of a 'hierarchical health message'. People were discouraged from taking drugs, but if they did so, it was suggested that they avoid injecting them. If they did inject, then it was suggested that they use sterile equipment and to avoid sharing with other drug users.

Alcohol

Psychosocial interventions

General practitioners can intervene across the whole spectrum of alcohol-related problems. Patients may present with a variety of alcohol-related problems (see Table 15.2), and adopting a harm reduction perspective can have wide-ranging effects. A number of randomized controlled trials have shown 'brief interventions' by GPs to be effective (Fleming *et al.* 1997). The simplest of these involves the use of a screening tool to identify harmful patterns of alcohol use, followed by brief advice (see Box 15.3).

However, other strategies suitable for use in primary care use a more extensive type of brief intervention consisting of screening and advice followed by three-five further sessions with a counsellor or suitably trained practice nurse. This allows a more detailed assessment of the pattern of alcohol consumption, the range of alcohol-related problems, and the degree of alcohol dependence. The use of a drinking diary may help increase motivation for change and allow the therapist to compare the patient's drinking level with the rest of the population. Feedback of blood test results may be helpful to stimulate discussion and increase knowledge of alcohol-related physical problems, and information booklets may be used.

Such opportunistic interventions are based on a public health model of care in which clinicians actively seek health risk factors among their patients. Their potential effectiveness has been demonstrated in a large number of clinical trials, including a large, multi-centre clinical trial by WHO, where 5 minutes of advice from a primary care physician about the importance of sensible drinking reduced consumption in hazardous and harmful drinkers by 30–40%.

The 'stages of change' model developed by Prochaska and DiClemente has become very influential in the conceptualization and subsequent management of

---

Box 15.3 **Brief advice following use of the screening tool**

Brief intervention

♦ 5–10 minutes in duration
♦ Personalized feedback about results of screening/blood tests
♦ Offering a 'menu' of alternative coping strategies
♦ Information about safe levels of drinking
♦ Provision of self-help materials
♦ Advice on reducing drinking
♦ Ventilation of anxieties and other problems
♦ Motivational interviewing techniques

Box 15.4   **The stages of change model**

- Precontemplation
- Contemplation
- Determination
- Action
- Maintenance
- Relapse

substance misuse problems. Prior to its inception there was a tendency to view motivation to change behaviour as a personal trait or an all-or-nothing phenomenon. Those that refused help, or who failed to benefit from it, were considered to have been 'lacking motivation'. Prochaska and DiClemente studied people who had managed to change their smoking behaviour without formal help. This led to the realization that change is rarely a sudden event, but instead occurs in steps or stages (see Box 15.4). Furthermore, motivation can be seen as the result of an interaction between the drinker and his or her environment, with the implication that it can facilitate and increase motivation for change.

This research has led to the development of a style of interviewing particularly suited to helping change problematic behaviour patterns. Motivational interviewing involves discussion about the personal costs and benefits of continued drinking when balanced against the health and social benefits that would follow a reduction in levels of consumption or abstinence.

Professionals in primary care may utilize knowledge of the stages of change model to employ a range of different cognitive-behavioural strategies at different stages of the problem. Motivational interviewing is well suited to moving patients towards a firm decision to stop drinking. Once they have accepted the need to change, it is important to work with the patient to generate realistic goals and to offer a menu of strategies to help reach these (see Box 15.5). Depending on available skills and resources, such interventions may be offered on an individual or group basis. Large scale studies such as Project MATCH have demonstrated the effectiveness of such interventions, with both cognitive-behavioural and motivational enhancement strategies producing major improvements not only on drinking measures but also in many other areas of life functioning (Project MATCH Research Group 1998).

Once withdrawal from alcohol is complete, 'relapse prevention' strategies can help support the patient in the goal of abstinence. The most common treatment outcome for addicts is relapse, with approximately 66% of all research participants returning to drinking by the 90-day follow-up assessment. Relapse prevention aims to offer alternative strategies to the 'revolving door' phenomenon

> Box 15.5   **Cognitive-behavioural strategies**
>
> ◆ Self-monitoring
> ◆ Setting drinking limits
> ◆ Controlling the rate of drinking
> ◆ Drink refusal skills
> ◆ Assertiveness training
> ◆ Relaxation training
> ◆ Development of alternative coping skills and rewards
> ◆ Identifying and challenging negative automatic thoughts

of relapse and withdrawal. The strategy aims to anticipate and prevent relapses from occurring, but if they do, to minimize the negative consequences and maximize learning from the experience. Rather than blaming a patient for difficulties that arise during the course of treatment, emphasis is placed on the specific context and situational factors in which the slip or relapse occurs.

Alcoholics Anonymous may also have much to offer the problem drinker and this approach can be easily integrated into a treatment programme involving other agencies. Self-referral to AA is simple and the only requirement for membership is a desire to stop drinking. The primary care team should be aware of the full range of local support services, including AA, and should be able to provide practical details to facilitate contact.

Pharmacological interventions

Once the individual has moved along the spectrum of alcohol problems towards dependence, it becomes more likely that pharmacological help may be needed to provide an effective intervention. In 'medicated' detoxification the severity of withdrawal symptoms is minimized (or completely suppressed) by the administration of a drug, with gradual reduction of the substitute medication after the peak of the withdrawal syndrome has passed (Mayo-Smith 1997). Detoxification is best seen as the start of the therapeutic process, rather than a treatment on its own, but in the case of severe alcohol dependence the process is also a harm-reduction measure as it may prevent other potentially life-threatening complications such as delirium tremens. The principles of home detoxification are presented in Box 15.6.

Most patients do not experience serious complications during alcohol withdrawal, and detoxification can usually be done safely, successfully, and cost-effectively at home (Finney *et al.* 1996). The GP will therefore often have a role in prescribing for these patients, sometimes in conjunction with a community alcohol team. However, patients with a history of withdrawal fits or

---

Box 15.6   **Principles of home detoxification**

- Daily or twice daily supervision to allow monitoring of withdrawal symptoms and the detection of complications, e.g. hallucinations
- Medication to prevent a withdrawal syndrome (chlormethiazole is no longer recommended due to the high risk of dependence and the dangers associated when it is consumed along with alcohol), e.g. chlordiazepoxide tablets 20–30 mg 4–6-hourly, titrating the dose against withdrawal symptoms. The dose is then gradually reduced over 10 days
- Carbamazepine has been shown to be effective in preventing withdrawal-related seizures (600–800 mg for the first 48–72 hours, then reduced by 200 mg per day)
- Multivitamin preparations are important to prevent the onset of the Wernicke–Korsakoff syndrome. An oral preparation containing at least 200 mg thiamine should be given for 1 month to all patients undergoing withdrawal

---

delirium tremens, severe medical or psychiatric problems, or little social support are likely to require inpatient admission.

Although psychosocial methods are the most commonly used treatment modalities for alcohol problems, there is a growing body of evidence for new forms of medication to reduce drinking in the rehabilitation phase of management (see Box 15.7). The general practitioner may have a role in prescribing these medications, usually after initiation by specialist services.

Box 15.7   **Medication to reduce drinking**

- Disulfiram inhibits aldehyde dehydrogenase, leading to potentially toxic blood levels of acetaldehyde if alcohol is consumed. It is most effective when used in a clinical setting that emphasizes abstinence and ensures that the medication is taken
- Acamprosate is believed to act as a GABA-receptor agonist. Acamprosate taken for 1 year by alcohol dependent patients who have undergone detoxification increases the number of days on which no alcohol is drunk during the treatment period (when combined with psychosocial therapy such as counselling). Benefits may continue for up to 1 year after stopping treatment
- Naltrexone is an opioid receptor antagonist and its use was prompted by animal studies that showed that alcohol consumption is reinforced by an interaction with the endogenous opioid system. Like Acamprosate, it appears to reduce relapse rate after abstinence

---

Even in specialist services these agents are not routinely administered (Drummond and Moncrieff 1997). Decisions depend on the history and severity of dependence, personality profile, psychological symptomatology, support network, and additional interventions. It should be noted that these medications are likely to be enhanced in combination with psychosocial interventions, and they should not be viewed as a simple answer to a complicated problem.

Drugs

General practitioners do not yet seem to be involved in managing drug misusers to the extent recommended by advisory bodies. This may be for a variety of reasons, including personal beliefs about the condition, a lack of knowledge as a result of inadequate training, anxieties about prescribing for drug users, fear of violence or disruption in the surgery, or disillusionment at the high rates of relapse. GPs perceive that drug misusers take up more consultation time than others (Deehan et al. 1997), and that the primary care setting is not suited to managing treatment contracts and the disagreements that sometimes ensue. In any one locality only a few general practitioners will generally be willing to treat drug misusers for fear of an uncontrollable demand for the service. Some studies have shown that GPs are seen as unsympathetic and lacking in knowledge about drug misuse (Telfer et al. 1990).

However, there are a number of potentially positive aspects to treating drug misuse problems in primary care. Surveys reveal that drug users perceive primary care services to be more accessible and responsive to their needs than hospital based services, with many expressing an overwhelming preference for detoxification or maintenance prescribing in general practice (Hindler 1995). GPs have contact with family and friends, and so may be alerted to an individual's drug use at an early stage. This may provide opportunities for education, harm minimization strategies or brief interventions. The facilities available in primary care enable a broad approach to the problem, including health checks, contraceptive advice and hepatitis screening. Furthermore, evidence is starting to show that satisfactory treatment outcomes can be obtained (Gossop et al. 1999).

Therefore, although GPs may not want to take on the full responsibility for prescribing, they should not overlook the other potentially useful work that can be done at an earlier stage of an individual drug-using career. The GP may have many roles:

- *Preventing misuse by careful prescribing of potential drugs of misuse*: the GP is usually the core prescriber of medications and so can do much to prevent dependence on drugs such as benzodiazepines or analgesics, as well as being suspicious of the possibility of misuse of medications such as codeine based analgesics or antihistamines bought 'over-the-counter'

(OTC). Any drug that alters a person's perception of their environment is particularly prone to abuse, and unless specific enquiries are made about OTC medications their use and abuse is likely to go unnoticed. Like any doctor working in a pressurized health service environment, the GP must be wary of the use of the prescription pad to end consultations with difficult or demanding patients.

+ *Reduction of harm associated with drug misuse*: injecting drug misuse carries a significant risk of infection, particularly when equipment is shared or poorly cleaned. Advice about improved injection technique and cleaning of equipment can be effective in reducing this risk, particularly when combined with the provision of clean needles and syringes via local needle exchange schemes. It is important to remember that this advice is equally applicable to injectors of drugs other than heroin (e.g. amphetamines, cocaine).

+ *Treatment of physical complications of drug misuse in general medical care*, such as cervical screening and hepatitis immunization.

+ *Assistance in withdrawal from opioids or other drugs of abuse*.

Opioids

An opiate-dependent drug user who wishes to stop using opiates abruptly or who is in the middle of a withdrawal syndrome may present as an emergency to the GP. Referral to drug services often takes some time and the GP may feel compelled to try to help. Furthermore, as heroin has become readily available in most areas of the UK, young people with short drug misuse histories increasingly present to primary care services. Long-term methadone maintenance is almost always inappropriate in these cases and detoxification may be the logical first treatment step. Although prescribing may be delayed for a few days, *it is vitally important that the general practitioner tests the patient's urine for evidence of opiate drugs if methadone is to be prescribed*. Laboratory tests are detailed and reliable, but slow, and 'dipstick' screening tests may be useful if an instant result is needed.

Patients using small amounts of heroin may be able to stop abruptly with purely symptomatic support. The first phase of therapy should include an assessment of the level of dependence (as described above), as well as any drug-related medical, psychological, and social problems. This should be accompanied by an attempt to develop a therapeutic alliance. An explanation of the likely withdrawal side effects and their time course can help to clarify any misunderstandings, and the GP may decide to prescribe the medications in Box 15.8 below for symptomatic relief.

Those with dependence who are also on higher doses of heroin or with longer histories of drug use may not be able to tolerate such a simple detoxification process, and will require assessment and management by a specialist

Box 15.8 **Symptomatic medications to be taken only if required**

Diazepam: up to 30 mg/day to reduce anxiety, muscle cramps and craving
Nitrazepam: 10 mg at night to aid sleep
Buscopan: 10 mg up to 6-hourly to reduce abdominal smooth muscle spasm
Lomotil: 10 mg initially, then 5 mg 6-hourly to reduce diarrhoea

drug treatment agency. However, the GP may be called upon to prescribe medication for a home detoxification under the supervision of a community drug worker, and this may take one of three forms:

- *Lofexidine plus symptomatic medication*: lofexidine is a non-opioid method of reducing opiate withdrawal symptoms. It is an analogue of clonidine, but despite its reduced hypotensive effect the dose should be built up gradually, and regular monitoring of blood pressure and pulse is important (see Box 15.9).

- *Dihydrocodeine plus symptomatic medication*: dihydrocodeine tablets or syrup can be used to substitute for the heroin and then gradually reduced over approximately 2 weeks. The major disadvantage of this method is the large number of 30 mg tablets needed each day (30 mg of dihydrocodeine is equivalent to 3 mg of methadone).

Box 15.9 **Monitoring of blood pressure and pulse**

Day 1	Blood pressure and pulse to be taken before first dose of lofexidine 0.2 mg in the morning. If blood pressure and pulse are stable, give second dose of lofexidine 0.2 mg in the evening. If diastolic blood pressure falls by over 30% from baseline or pulse falls below 55/minute, then omit second dose
Day 2	Check blood pressure and pulse. If satisfactory then lofexidine 0.2 mg four times daily
Day 3	Lofexidine 0.4 mg three times daily (depending on blood pressure and pulse)
Day 4	Stop the heroin. Lofexidine 0.4 mg four times daily (depending on blood pressure and pulse)
Day 5–14	Continue as above (outpatient clients being seen daily, except at weekends)
Day 15	Reduce dose of lofexidine to 0.4 mg three times daily
Day 16	Reduce dose of lofexidine to 0.2 mg three times daily
Day 17	Discontinue the lofexidine

* *Initiation and stabilization on methadone, followed by a slow reduction over a number of weeks*: methadone used in this way has become the mainstay treatment for opiate detoxification in the UK, but the evidence for its effectiveness is limited. It is also important to recognize the potential for overdose and death if methadone is not initiated at low doses (20–25mg) and slowly titrated against its effect.

Prescription of substitute medication such as methadone

'Substitute' prescribing implies the use of a legally prescribed drug instead of an illegal drug of unknown purity and quality. Methadone maintenance therapy (MMT) has been used for over 30 years in the management of opiate dependence, and research has demonstrated clear benefits in reducing illicit opioid use, HIV infection, and criminal activity (Marsch 1998). Its effectiveness appears to be dependent on a range of factors including dose, retention in treatment and psychosocial support. There is evidence to suggest that the regimes most successful at reducing illicit drug intake are those involving higher daily doses of the substitute drug (approximately 60–80 mg methadone), but that the prescription of high doses of drugs should only occur in conjunction with daily supervision and psychosocial interventions. Not surprisingly, the high-dose strategy is not often used in primary care in the UK. The provision of a limited period of methadone maintenance, but with the ultimate aim of reduction and detoxification, is the favoured approach. Indeed, many GPs are involved in the prescription and monitoring of methadone treatment under shared care schemes at different stages of the treatment plan. One situation in which it may be particularly feasible for general practitioners to be involved in prescribing is when long-standing methadone maintenance patients are stable.

Alternatives to methadone such as buprenorphine show considerable potential, but as yet are not widely used in the UK: Buprenorphine is a partial opiate agonist, and so produces less euphoria, sedation or respiratory depression than heroin. It also has a longer half-life, and discontinuation leads to less severe withdrawal symptoms. The evidence for its effectiveness is beginning to develop (Ling *et al.* 1998; Fischer *et al.* 1999).

Other drugs of abuse

The use of amphetamines is widespread in the UK, and there is extensive experience of treating cocaine and 'crack' cocaine users in the United States. However, the problem of stimulant abuse has tended to receive less attention than heroin abuse and there is little firm evidence on the best management strategy. Antidepressants, such as desipramine or fluoxetine, have been advocated to manage the craving and depressive symptoms of stimulant withdrawal, but with limited success. The relapse prevention strategies outlined above may offer the most promising treatment strategy, with referral to specialist services likely to be needed for the more complicated cases. Stimulant use may also carry a risk of precipitating psychiatric symptoms such as psychotic phenomena or depression (leading to suicide), and these will also need assessment and treatment.

The use of methylenedioxymethamphetamine (MDMA or 'ecstasy') by young people has increased dramatically in the last 15 years, mainly due to its association with a growing 'club culture' in the UK. It has stimulant effects similar to amphetamine combined with hallucinogenic properties, but users rarely present to medical services other than with complications such as depressive or anxiety symptoms. These are often brief and self-limiting, and should be treated in the usual manner.

Dependence on benzodiazepines is seen in a substantial number of people treated by primary care services. A useful treatment strategy may be to prescribe an initial maintenance period whilst other factors are stabilized, followed by a planned slow reduction of the benzodiazepine. The initial aim of such a programme is to convert the total benzodiazepine load to a single drug with a long half-life, such as diazepam. The starting dose and reducing regime are then negotiated between doctor and patient, aiming to minimize withdrawal symptoms. Clear criteria for review and goals of progress are also established before starting, and the frequency of reduction and stringency of required adherence to the regime vary with levels of motivation and co-morbid medical or psychosocial problems. Complicated cases with extensive co-morbidity may require a referral to specialist services and a period of inpatient treatment.

The use of substitute prescribing for heavy amphetamine users is a much-debated area that awaits further research clarification. However, although many specialist services advocate prescribing dexamphetamine sulphate in a similar manner to methadone, this treatment should never be instigated by a GP without specialist support.

Policy issues

Costs to the community

Substance misuse problems are estimated to cost the USA and Canada $250 billion and $20 billion, respectively, each year. In the UK, comprehensive figures are not available, but at a conservative estimate, £1.4 billion is spent on drugs and £2 billion on alcohol each year. Alcoholics cost the health services about two or three times more than the non-alcoholic general population. The cost of treatment for substance users in the UK is about £2000 per annum for inpatient treatment and £400 per annum for outpatient treatment. The average heroin user requires about £200 per week to maintain their habit. It has also been estimated that for every pound spent on treatment for drug misuse, £3 is saved (Healey *et al.* 1998). With these figures in mind, it is important to develop effective strategies for delivering the increasing range of effective treatments for substance misuse problems to as many people as possible.

General practitioners are frequently unsure of their competence in dealing with this group of patients. There are also doubts as to whether primary care is the most appropriate setting for the treatment of substance misusers. Furthermore, one cannot shy away from some of the unresolved and controversial issues that beset the treatment of substance misusers in general practice. These include equivocal evidence for the effectiveness of brief interventions delivered in primary care, the cost effectiveness of the range of treatment interventions in primary care, and also the unwillingness of drug misusers to register with and present to general practitioners (Merrill and Ruben 2000). There is also the gap between national policy which is strongly supportive of treatment at primary care level and, until very recently, the resources available to drive this forward. This new and much needed investment in training primary care practitioners and drugs workers will also need to be sustained over the longer term.

Special groups

The particular needs of women, e.g. pregnant users (Dawe *et al.* 1992), children and adolescents (Crome 1999a), older people (Crome and Day 2000), the homeless, the mentally disordered (Crome 1999b), and ethnic minorities, all of whom already access general practitioner services, need to be highlighted. The special factors affecting risk, accessibility to treatment, acceptability of treatment, and appropriateness of service provision, should not be overlooked in these groups, since they may be amongst the most in need, and their problems can not be addressed by any one practitioner or agency.

Many of the critical issues described earlier are epitomized by findings in the study of young people carried out in the first designated young people's (under 18-year-olds) drug service, which began in Stoke-on-Trent in 1995 (Crome *et al.* 2000). Of those that required a methadone reduction regime, 70% were injecting heroin, 70% were using more than one drug, and 70% were involved in criminal activities. In only 30% of cases were the parents together and in only 15% were both parents employed. Eighty per cent had taken no examinations and had left school prior to age 16. There was evidence of substance misuse in 40% of the families and chronic physical illness in 20% of the fathers. However, despite great social deprivation and multiple disadvantages, 80% were engaged and retained in treatment for at least 1 year. 'Treatment' included pharmacological and psychosocial interventions, as well as the collaboration of agencies, i.e. health, education, and social services. It is important to recognize that 40% of these young people had attended their GPs, and had been prescribed psychotropics for anxiety and depression, as well as analgesics for withdrawal symptoms, but for the variety of patient- and practitioner-orientated reasons described above, few of the GPs had learnt that their young patients were on heroin. Early intervention with this vulnerable group is far easier than attempted cure—10 years later.

Current scientific developments of direct relevance to primary care in the UK

The United Kingdom has historically played a seminal role in the development and evaluation of brief interventions by generalists in the addiction field. This legacy continues in the shape of two current large-scale substance misuse treatment trials in the UK that have direct relevance to general practitioners. Both are analysing outcome after relatively brief interventions of a type suitable for use in the primary care setting.

The United Kingdom Alcohol Treatment Trial (UKATT) is the largest of its kind ever undertaken in this country. Seven-hundred alcohol dependent patients in three sites in England and Wales are being randomized to two types of treatment intervention: MET (motivational enhancement therapy) and SNBT (social network behaviour therapy).

The National Treatment Outcome Study (NTORS) is evaluating the effectiveness of drug services in the UK. Twelve-hundred drug users are being followed up for 5 years. Initial indications are that treatment does influence substance use, injecting and sharing behaviour, and criminality, but has less impact on psychological symptoms and social adjustment.

There are many scientific developments that could lead to beneficial results. New techniques in the fields of brain imaging and neurochemistry may be relevant to the development and treatment of substance problems. The human genome project is likely to yield information regarding the origin of the predisposition to addiction and may produce results in terms of prevention and treatment. Many countries are gradually recognizing the problems addiction brings, and are prepared to invest in the treatment and prevention of addiction problems. The social, psychological and biochemical impairments that cause and contribute to substance problems need to be tackled simultaneously if any lasting change is to be made. The clinical key is the identification and management in the primary care setting.

16 Psychopharmacology

Adrian Feeney and David Nutt

Drug treatments form an important part of the general practitioner's repertoire of responses to mental health problems. In cases of anxiety disorders or depression, drugs are often initiated in primary care, while antipsychotics more often in the hospital setting. In recent years there has been a dramatic increase in the number of new drugs available to treat both depression and psychosis. Effective prescribing in primary care is based on correct diagnosis, and thorough knowledge of the efficacy and side effects of a few well-chosen agents. In the age of ever more limited drug budgets the selection of a newer and often markedly more expensive drug must be carefully justified. However, drug cost may not be the only factor, which dictates cost-effectiveness of prescribing. This chapter will consider the treatments of depression, anxiety disorders, insomnia, and psychosis in turn.

The placebo effect

The placebo effect is an improvement in symptoms associated with the administration of a tablet, which contains no active ingredient. It is related to the individual's expectation of symptom improvement, and may be enhanced by personal contact and empathy from health professionals and carers. Since placebo response rates for depression and psychosis vary between 20 and 60% this effect is an important consideration when interpreting the response to a drug in both the individual and drug trial samples. The ethics of the use of placebos for conditions for which there are effective drugs available has been questioned. It is impossible to establish whether the response to a drug in a trial is a true drug effect unless there is a placebo control arm. Trials lacking a placebo arm may yield misleading results and lead to the use of ineffective drugs. An intriguing question is whether the improvement seen with clinically effective drugs comprises both drug and placebo effects. For instance in depression trials improvement that is both delayed and sustained is suggestive of a true antidepressant drug effect (Quitkin 2000).

Depressive disorder (ICD-10 criteria)

Diagnosis of a depressive episode is based on the presence for at least 2 weeks of two of three core features (low mood, reduced energy, or loss of interest or enjoyment). There are some associated features (Box 16.1) and some physiological disturbances (biological features, Box 16.2) that, if present, also help to make the diagnosis. Untreated, a depressive episode lasts on average between three and six months and occasionally as long as a year (Angst 1992), the aim of an antidepressant is to shorten these illness episodes.

Choosing an antidepressant

As yet there is no firm evidence that in primary care any specific antidepressant has greater efficacy than the others. The task of the prescriber is to select the antidepressant with the side-effect profile, which is most suitable for each patient. However, the response of an individual patient's depressive symptoms is difficult to predict. While a particular antidepressant may prove to be extremely effective in one patient it may be ineffective in another. If an antidepressant has been given at

---

Box 16.1 **Associated features of a depressive episode**

- Reduced concentration and attention
- Reduced self-esteem and self-confidence
- Ideas of guilt and unworthiness
- Pessimistic views of the future
- Ideas of deliberate self-harm or suicide
- Disturbed sleep
- Reduced appetite

Box 16.2 **Biological symptoms**

- Weight loss
- Early morning wakening (2 hours earlier than usual)
- Libido reduced
- Diurnal mood variation (mood worst in the morning)
- Motor retardation or agitation
- Appetite worse
- Emotional reactivity lost (inability to respond to happy events)
- Interest and pleasure lost

an adequate dose for a sufficient trial period (generally 6 weeks) the next step is to prescribe an antidepressant with a different mechanism of action. Changing from one antidepressant to another requires careful planning and adequate interval between agents (Bazire 2000). The concomitant administration of two antidepressants that both alter serotonin can cause a rare, but serious syndrome of serotonin excess, the serotinergic syndrome. This syndrome is characterized by agitation, restlessness, sweating, diarrhoea, fever, hyperpyrexia, lack of co-ordination, confusion, myoclonus, and tremor. Treatment is cessation of the offending drugs and supportive measures (Gillman 1999).

If a patient has failed two courses of antidepressants and remains depressed it would be reasonable to refer them for a psychiatric opinion (Anderson *et al.* 2000). This would provide a review of the diagnosis. The Maudsley protocol for the treatment of depression suggests at this point that the second antidepressant should be augmented with lithium and if that is ineffective a course of electroconvulsant therapy (ECT) should be considered (Taylor *et al.* 1999).

A universal feature of drug treatment of depression is the delay (lasting between 1 and 3 weeks) after starting the antidepressant before the mood begins to lift. Unfortunately, the side effects are often evident before the therapeutic benefit is apparent and this may lead to poor compliance. Such side effects can be minimized by introducing the antidepressant at sub-therapeutic doses and gradually increasing to the therapeutic dose. Compliance can be improved by warning patients of the side effects, reassuring them that they are likely to be transient and matching the drugs side-effect profile to the patient.

In general, an adequate course of antidepressant should be at least 6 months in duration, the depressive symptoms should have resolved at least 4 months before stopping, and the patient should be without undue external stress (Prien and Kupfer 1986). An inadequate duration of treatment leads to relapse (Figure 16.1). In those patients who have already suffered three previous depressive episodes, and the likelihood of further relapse is as high as 90%, there is a case for continuation therapy as a prophylactic measure (Forshall and Nutt 1999). If there is a psychotic component to the depressive episode then an antipsychotic drug should be used in combination with an antidepressant (Spiker *et al.* 1985).

Antidepressant discontinuation reactions

Discontinuation reactions can be seen on abrupt withdrawal or dose reduction of any of the antidepressants. Common symptoms include disturbance of the gastrointestinal system, sleep disturbance, associated affective symptoms (low mood, anxiety, and irritability) and somatic symptoms (sweating, headaches, and lethargy; Haddad *et al.* 1998). Discontinuation of the SSRIs can be associated with dizziness, numbness, and paraesthesia (Coupland *et al.* 1996). Features that help to differentiate between discontinuation reactions and relapse of depression are listed in Table 16.1.

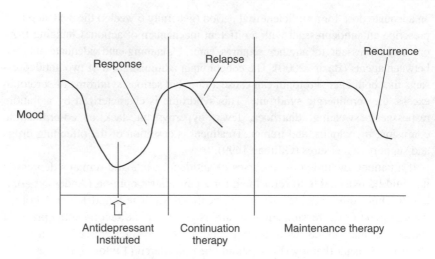

Fig 16.1 Possible responses to antidepressant therapy

Table 16.1 Features that help to differentiate between discontinuation reactions and relapse of depression

	Discontinuation reaction	Depressive relapse
Speed of onset	Abrupt	Gradual
Duration	Short-lived (<21 days)	May be chronic
Effect of reintroducing antidepressant	Resolves quickly	No effect in short-term

Tricyclic antidepressants (TCAs)

These are among the older agents, and as such are off patent and available in cheaper generic preparations. They work by blocking the re-uptake of serotonin and noradrenaline to a greater or lesser extent. The side effects of promoting serotonin and noradrenaline are listed in Boxes 16.3 and 16.4, respectively. They also act as antagonists at the muscarinic, histaminergic and alpha-1 adrenoceptors (Table 16.2). Thus the side effect profile of any given TCA can be deduced with knowledge of its effects on neurochemistry. Dothiepin has been commonly chosen for those depressed patients with concomitant insomnia since its anti-histaminergic action is sedating. However, like all the other TCAs with

> Box 16.3 **Serotonin side effects**
>
> - Nausea
> - Headache
> - Diarrhoea
> - Insomnia
> - Discontinuation syndrome
> - Agitation
> - Akathisia
> - Reduced libido
> - Lack of orgasm or ejaculation

> Box 16.4 **Noradrenaline side effects**
>
> - Agitation
> - Insomnia
> - Sweating

the exception of lofepramine, it is cardio-toxic in overdose. The therapeutic dose of a tricyclic is that which is equivalent to 150 mg of amitriptyline. TCAs therapeutic ranges are listed in Table 16.3.

The selective serotonin re-uptake inhibitors (SSRIs)

These are newer antidepressants and throughout the 1990s have only been available as patented drugs. These patents are about to start lapsing and, consequently, competitively priced generic versions will soon be available. This class includes fluvoxamine, fluoxetine, sertraline, paroxetine, and citalopram.

Table 16.2 Antagonists at the muscarinic, histaminergic, and alpha-1 adrenoceptors

Anti-muscarinic	Anti-histaminergic	Anti-α1
Constipation	Weight gain	Hypotension
Dry mouth	Drowsiness	Dizziness
Constipation		Drowsiness
Drowsiness		
Urinary hesitancy		

Table 16.3 The tricyclics

Drug	Therapeutic dose range/day
Amitriptyline	125–150 mg
Clomipramine*	125–150 mg
Imipramine	150–200 mg
Lofepramine[†]	140–210 mg
Nortriptyline[†]	75–100 mg
Dothiepin	125–150 mg

*Predominantly blocks serotonin re-uptake.
[†] Predominantly blocks noradrenaline re-uptake.

Their mechanism of action is, as their name suggests selective inhibition of the re-uptake of serotonin and this is also responsible for their side effects (Box 16.3). Fluoxetine has a long half-life (6 weeks) and, thus, a long washout period. It is also more alerting than the other SSRIs and this can be usefully exploited in depressed patients with retardation.

They all inhibit to some extent the cytochrome p450 system and consequently have interactions with drugs metabolized by this system. Of the SSRIs, sertraline inhibits this system the least and may therefore be suitable for patients on complex treatment regimes.

The monoamine oxidase inhibitors (MAOIs)

These were the first antidepressant drugs to be discovered. They irreversibly and non-selectively inhibit both monoamine oxidase A and B enzymes. These enzymes are responsible for metabolizing serotonin, noradrenaline, dopamine, and tyramine. It is thought that by preventing the metabolism of these amines the MAOIs promote the activity of the monoamine system.

The major problem with the MAOIs is that they prevent the metabolism of tyramine by the MAO in the intestine. This amine is found in a variety of foods including cheese, pickled herrings, Bovril, and alcohol. If tyramine-containing food is eaten, then significant quantities of tyramine can enter the brain and displace the large intracellular stores of catecholamines, which have accumulated as a result of the MAO inhibition. This can lead to catastrophically raised blood pressure. This dietary restriction has made the MAOIs less popular and psychiatrists now generally only initiate them when other less problematic drugs have failed. MAOI side effects are shown in Box 16.5. MAOIs may cause toxicity when given in combination with other drugs, which promote increased concentrations of neurotransmitters (antidepressants, sympathomimetics, and

Box 16.5 **Side effects of MAOIs**

- ◆ Orthostatic hypotension
- ◆ Sexual dysfunction
- ◆ Dietary restrictions
- ◆ Insomnia

opioids). MAOIs therefore complicate the choice of additional medication for patients taking them.

A new variant of this class, moclobemide, is a selective reversible inhibitor of monoamine oxidase A (RIMA). This drug does not have the same dietary restrictions and can be used as an adjunct to other antidepressants.

Newer antidepressants

The side effect profile of the following newer agents can be deduced with knowledge of their receptor activity (see Boxes 16.3 and 16.4, and Table 16.2).

- ◆ Venlafaxine is an example of a serotonin and noradrenaline re-uptake inhibitor (SNRI). It has been likened to clomipramine but without the troublesome tricyclic activity at other receptors (Table 16.2). It may cause either hypotension or hypertension, and thus blood pressure should be checked before starting and after dose increases. It has two pharmacological profiles; at doses less than 150 mg it acts as an SSRI and at higher doses it also blocks the re-uptake of noradrenaline.
- ◆ Reboxetine is a noradrenaline re-uptake inhibitor (NARI). It has an alerting effect by enhancing noradrenaline and the second of its twice-daily doses should not be given after mid-afternoon in order to avoid sleep disruption. It may be particularly useful in those patients who are suffering motor retardation or lethargy.
- ◆ Mirtazepine is an antagonist at $5HT_2$ and $5HT_3$ post-synaptic receptors (which reduces some serotonergic side effects; Box 16.3) and histaminergic receptors at doses of 30 mg/day or less. At higher doses it also acts as an α_2 adrenoceptor antagonist action pre-synaptically (causing increased synaptic noradrenaline). Thus, lower doses are sedating due to the anti-histaminergic activity and higher doses are alerting due to the raised noradrenaline levels. A significant side effect is weight gain due to appetite stimulation.
- ◆ Nefazodone acts as a $5\,HT_2$, histamine and α_1 adrenoceptor antagonist, and also weakly inhibits the release of both serotonin and noradrenaline.

Trazodone is similar to nefazodone, but lacks the noradrenaline re-uptake inhibition and is more sedating. Both drugs are appropriate treatments of depression in which insomnia is a significant component.

Anxiety and the anxiety disorders

When the demands of life outstrip an individual's resources that individual is under stress, and one response to this is a sense of unease and threat, which is manifest as anxiety. It is important to distinguish between this sub-syndromal anxiety and the specific anxiety disorders. Sub-threshold anxiety is extremely common in primary care. When faced with a patient complaining of such anxiety it is worth considering the following:

◆ Is the anxiety disabling?

◆ How long is it likely to last?

◆ Is this patient likely to develop dependence to or abuse benzodiazepines?

◆ Is there a non-pharmacological approach (Box 16.6), which would be effective?

Treatment may be indicated if level of functioning is reduced. A benzodiazepine such as diazepam carefully policed as a limited course of less than 2 weeks would be appropriate for short-lived anxiety, for instance, after an acute stressor. Benzodiazepines would be unsuitable for more chronic forms of low-grade anxiety since the risk to benefit ratio of dependence versus relief of symptoms would be unfavourable. In these cases non-pharmacological approaches would be more appropriate.

The treatment of the anxiety disorders is based on accurate diagnosis. The sub-classification of the anxiety disorders with their distinguishing features is displayed in Table 16.4 (Feeney and Nutt 1999). There is good evidence that psychological therapies (particularly Cognitive Behavioural Therapy) are effective in treating the anxiety disorders; however, their availability is limited. Drug treatments are much more readily available and are also effective in the anxiety disorders with the exception of specific phobias.

Box 16.6   **Measures to reduce sub threshold anxiety**

◆ Reduce stressors
◆ Regular exercise
◆ Relaxation techniques, meditation/yoga
◆ Fewer than six cups of tea or coffee per day

Table 16.4 Sub-classification of anxiety disorders and their distinguishing features (adapted from Feeney and Nutt 1999)

Anxiety disorder	Core feature of anxiety	Prescribing options
Generalized anxiety disorder	Persistent worries	Buspirone then SSRI or TCA or Venlafaxine then benzodiazepine*
Panic disorder	Spontaneous and triggered panic attacks Fear of dying during attack	Paroxetine or citalopram or tricyclic then MAOI (phenelzine) benzo-diazepine*
Social phobia	Under social scrutiny fear of making a fool of oneself	(CBT) or SSRI then MAOI or RIMA then benzodiazepine*
Post-traumatic stress disorder	Precipitated by severe stress or manifest by: reliving the event dissociation hyper-vigilance	MAOI or SSRI or nefazodone
Specific phobia	Fear and avoidance of a specific object	Cognitive-behavioural therapy
Obsessive-compulsive disorder	Intrusive thoughts (obsessions) and actions (compulsions)	SSRI or clomipramine

*Avoid use of benzodiazepines in patients with a history of substance dependence (APA guidelines).

There are two broad classes of anxiolytics, the antidepressant agents and the benzodiazepines. The former take weeks to relieve anxiety and doses at least as large if not larger than those required to treat depression are needed. There is a time lag between instituting the antidepressant drug and the relief of the symptoms, which can vary between 4 and 8 weeks. If there has been no improvement in symptoms within three months of treatment then an agent from a different class should be selected (Nutt and Bell 1997). Some authors suggest treating for about 6 months at first presentation and up to 2 years in patients suffering from recurrent illness.

Benzodiazepines give relief from anxiety symptoms more immediately. Courses of benzodiazepines that last longer than 3 weeks are associated with the withdrawal symptoms on cessation in up to one third of patients (Hallstrom 1993). As already mentioned, such withdrawal symptoms can commonly include anxiety, insomnia, irritability, and nausea. The American Psychiatric Association (Salzman 1991) has made recommendations that benzodiazepines should be carefully targeted, and the prescriber be aware that the risk of dependence is increased with increase dose and duration of treatment. However, there are patients whose anxiety disorder does not respond to any other medication and in this select group with adequate supervision benzodiazepines have been proposed as a relatively safe and effective treatment (Nutt 1996). Benzodiazepines should not be given to patients with a history of substance abuse.

Hypnotics

Insomnia (difficulty going to sleep, staying asleep, or waking up early) is a common problem. Sleep disturbance may be secondary to physical illness and mood disorders (depressive or hypomanic episode). It is therefore important to consider this possibility and to treat the underlying cause if present.

Non-drug interventions are indicated initially for primary insomnia. These include reassurance (so as to alleviate worry about not sleeping, which then perpetuates the insomnia), identification of any precipitants, and practical steps to promote a regular sleep routine (Box 16.7) (Wilson and Nutt 1999). Some prescribed medication can also cause insomnia: antidepressants (the SSRIs fluvoxamine and fluoxetine, and MAOIs), B agonists (salbutamol) and B blockers.

If these measures have proved unsuccessful over several weeks then there is a case for offering hypnotic medication for 1 or 2 weeks in order to try to re-establish a normal pattern of sleep. For those patients who are unable to re-establish a normal sleep pattern intermittent use of a hypnotic (once or twice a week) may be helpful. By giving hypnotics in this fashion the patient can feel reassured that they can be guaranteed a good night's sleep at least on those occasions. This also avoids continuous use of such sedatives, which may be associated with problems of tolerance and withdrawal.

The choice of hypnotic

The first hypnotics available were chloral hydrate and the barbiturates. These, in common with chlormethiazole, can be fatal at doses only a few times greater than therapeutic levels. The advent of the benzodiazepines was hailed as a major

---

Box 16.7 **Practical steps to promote sleep**

- ◆ No day time napping
- ◆ Regular hours of rising and retiring
- ◆ Daytime exercise and exposure to daylight
- ◆ Establish a relaxing bedtime routine
- ◆ Avoid stimulants, alcohol, and cigarettes in the evening

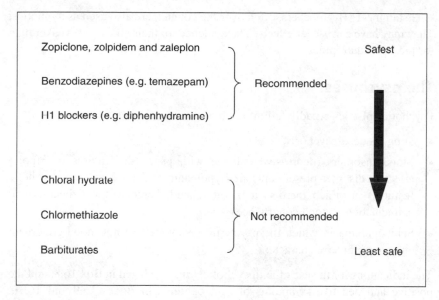

Fig 16.2   Relative safeties of sedative drugs.

step forward as they were relatively safe in overdose and made the older agents obsolete (Figure 16.2). Benzodiazepines are still used as hypnotics. Short half-life drugs like temazepam ($t_{1/2}$ = 8 hours) are suitable for patients who need to be alert the following morning. Longer half-life drugs (nitrazepam, $t_{1/2}$ = 25 hours) have a carry-over effect, which can usefully be exploited in those patients who suffer daytime anxiety.

More recently the newer non-benzodiazepine drugs, which are also agonists at the benzodiazepine receptor, have been introduced. This group comprises zopiclone, zolpidem, and zaleplon. It has been suggested that dependency is less of a problem with these drugs than with the benzodiazepines (Lader 1997). Zaleplon has an extremely short half-life (3 hours). The patient is encouraged to use it 1 hour after retiring only on those nights when they have failed to fall asleep naturally, thus theoretically reducing the risk of dependence. It also has the advantage of having less potential for hangover drowsiness the next morning.

In the wake of concerns regarding the benzodiazepines causing a withdrawal syndrome thioridazine, an antipsychotic, became a popular alternative sedative and anxiolytic drug. However, thioridazine causes cardiotoxicity (QTc interval prolongation and ventricular arrhythmias). In December 2000, the Committee on Safety of Medicines decided to restrict its use to second-line treatment of schizophrenia only, on the basis that the balance of risks benefits was unfavourable in all other conditions.

Histamine-1 (H_1) blockers, often over the counter, are also used as hypnotics. They may have carry-over effects. The evidence for their efficacy is weaker than for the benzodiazepines.

The psychoses

Psychotic episodes broadly fall into one of three categories:

* Drug-induced psychosis.
* Mood disorders (depressive episode with psychotic features or bipolar affective disorder present episode hypomanic or depressive with psychotic features) in which there is a mood related theme to the delusions and hallucinations (mood congruence).
* Schizophrenia in which the psychotic symptoms are not mood congruent and have a bizarre character.

The indications for the use of antipsychotic drugs are listed in Box 16.8, and the positive and negative symptoms of schizophrenia in Boxes 16.9 and 16.10, respectively.

Box 16.8   Indications for antipsychotics

* Positive symptoms of schizophrenia (Figure 16.2)
* Negative symptoms of schizophrenia (Box 16.8)
* Agitation associated with psychosis
* (Hypo)manic episode
* Acute confusional state (including delirium tremens)
* Depressive episode with psychotic symptoms

Box 16.9   Positive symptoms of schizophrenia

* Delusions
* Hallucinations
* Disorganized speech
* Disorganized behaviour
* Catatonia
* Agitation
* Language abnormalities

Box 16.10 **Negative symptoms of schizophrenia**

- ◆ Blunted affect
- ◆ Poverty of speech
- ◆ Poor rapport
- ◆ Passivity
- ◆ Social withdrawal
- ◆ Lack of spontaneity
- ◆ Poor attention
- ◆ Anhedonia
- ◆ Stereotyped thinking
- ◆ Lack of motivation
- ◆ Emotional withdrawal

Extra-pyramidal side effects (EPSEs)

All drugs with antipsychotic properties share the common feature of dopamine-2 (D_2) receptor blockade. D_2 receptor blockade is probably responsible for the reduction in delusions and hallucinations. However, D_2 receptor blockade in the basal ganglia is responsible for EPSEs. The EPSEs are listed as the mnemonic ADAPT (Figure 16.3).

Acute dystonia is an early side effect of such blockade, which is manifest by spasm of the neck, tongue, jaw, and eye muscles. Other manifestations seen in the first weeks and months of treatment are akathisia (motor restlessness especially in the limbs which may be accompanied by subjective tension) and Parkinsonism (slowness of movement, muscle rigidity, abnormal gait, and more rarely tremor). Acute dystonia, akathisia, and Parkinsonism all respond to anti-cholinergics (e.g. procyclidine).

Tardive dyskinesia is a late onset EPSE that is the most problematic manifestation of these side effects and may be irreversible. It is characterized by abnormal movements (protrusion of the tongue and chewing, sucking and pouting movements of the mouth, and writhing movements of the head neck and trunk).

Extrapyramidal side effects	Time course
Acute	early
Dystonia	
Akathisia	↓
Parkinsonism	
Tardive dyskinesia	late

Fig 16.3 Extra-pyramidal side effects.

Long-term use of procyclidine may contribute to the development of tardive dyskinesia. Established tardive dyskinesia may respond to clozapine (Lieberman *et al.* 1991). To avoid EPSEs the smallest effective dose of an antipsychotic must be given.

Conventional antipsychotic or atypical?

The simplest definition of an atypical antipsychotic is one, which at therapeutic doses does not cause EPSEs. The prototypical agent for atypicals is clozapine and this is the only antipsychotic to have proven efficacy in treatment resistant psychosis (Kane *et al.* 1988). Clozapine has a complex receptor binding profile and it is not yet clear as to the mechanism for its enhanced efficacy. However, clozapine can cause fatal agranulocytosis. This limits its use to those who have failed to respond to an adequate dose of two other antipsychotics and necessitates regular full blood count monitoring.

The pharmaceutical industry has created a new generation of antipsychotic drugs over the last decade in an attempt to mimic the efficacy of clozapine without neutropenia: the atypicals risperidone, olanzapine, quetiapine, and amisulpiride. A recent meta-analysis concluded that atypicals were of similar efficacy to conventional antipsychotics at a dose equivalent to 12 mg or less of haloperidol, and did, indeed, cause fewer EPSEs, but had similar overall tolerability to the established antipsychotics (Geddes *et al.* 2000). No consensus has yet been reached about the place of the atypicals in the treatment of non-treatment resistant schizophrenia. While on the one hand Geddes and his colleagues suggest that atypicals are appropriate for those patients who do not respond to a standard dose of conventional antipsychotic or experience severe EPSEs, on the other, the Maudsley Guidelines propose that atypicals should be used as a first line treatment (Taylor *et al.* 1999). At present, it appears that the prescriber must weigh up the increased risk of EPSEs associated with conventional antipsychotics against the considerable extra cost of atypicals.

The choice of an antipsychotic drug should be made so as to match the side-effect profile to the patient. Young men with first presentation of psychosis are at high risk of EPSEs and it would be appropriate to consider an atypical. The elderly are vulnerable to antipsychotics with a marked anti-muscarinic component, and thus thioridazine and olanzapine are better avoided. The more sedative antipsychotics (chlorpromazine, olanzapine, and quetiapine) are useful in the agitation of acute psychosis.

The atypicals are markedly more expensive than the older antipsychotics. However, the prescribing expenses represent only a fraction of the total costs of care of a patient with schizophrenia. In one American study, it was shown that for patients classified as 'high hospital users' those treated with clozapine incurred significantly less health care expense when compared to those treated with

Table 16.5 Commonly used antipsychotics

Drug	Dose range	Indications	Side effects
Chlorpro-mazine	25–250 mg TDS	Use only in acutely psychotic agitated patients	Sedation[†] EPSEs common Hyperprolactinaemia Hypotension* Cardiotoxicity**
Haloperidol	2–4 mg TDS	Delirium tremens, as unlike chlorpromazine, does not reduce the seizure threshold	EPSEs doses > 12 mg Hyperprolactinaemia
Sulpiride	200–1200 mg BD	Psychosis without agitation	EPSEs rarely Hyperprolactinaemia
Thioridazine	50–200 mg TDS	Restricted to 2nd line treatment of schizophrenia due to cardiotoxicity	Sedation[†] Hypotension* EPSEs rarely Cardiotoxicity**
Risperidone	1–3 mg BD adult 0.25–1 mg BD elderly	Liquid and depot preparations available	EPSEs doses>6 mg Anxiety
Olanzapine	10–20 mg OD	Especially if sedation required for Anti-muscarinic, less suitable for the elderly	Sedation[†] EPSEs doses>15 mg Weight gain
Quetiapine	75–400 mg BD adult 25–75 mg BD elderly	Especially if sedation required If co-morbid Parkinson's disease	Sedation[†] Hypotension* Weight gain
Amisulpiride	200–800 mg BD	In the obese, less weight gain than other atypicals	Hyperprolactinaemia
Clozapine	25–900 mg OD	Proven efficacy in treatment resistant Schizophrenia (21) Established tardive dyskinesia (20)	Agranulocytosis Sedation[†] Hypotension* Hypersalivation Weight gain

*Hypotension due to anti-α_1;
[†]sedation due to anti-H_1;
**cardiotoxicity due to anti-muscarinic activity (Table 16.2).

haloperidol due to less inpatient time (Rosenbeck *et al.* 1999). However, for the GP, whose individual prescribing is subject to scrutiny, reduction in total health care costs at the expense of their own prescribing budget is of little comfort.

The antipsychotics presently available are listed in Table 16.5 with their dose ranges and indications.

The management of acute psychotic episode (schizophrenic or affective)

For the general practitioner faced with a new presentation of psychotic symptoms the first task is to manage the acute distress of patient and family sensitively (see Chapter 13). Explanation of the role neurochemicals play and reassurance that prognosis is improved with the correct treatment will help to form the basis of a working alliance with the patient. Ideally, the next step is a drug-free assessment by a psychiatrist. At this stage, the possibility of a drug-induced psychosis is considered and urine tests performed. If symptoms prove too difficult to contain then the first choice sedative should be a benzodiazepine such as diazepam. If a benzodiazepine is inadequate to sedate an acutely disturbed patient in the community then it is reasonable to give an antipsychotic drug. Using the principles described above one of the more sedative antipsychotics (chlorpromazine, olanzapine, and quetiapine) would be a reasonable first choice in the agitation of acute psychosis.

Benzodiazepines and neuroleptics act synergistically, and combining these two classes of drug in the most agitated patients may provide good sedation with less risk of side effects.

Maintenance treatment for schizophrenia

About 80% of those diagnosed with schizophrenia will go on to have two or more episodes. It is at present impossible to identify those who would not go on to have a recurrence without medication, thus necessitating long-term treatment for all. Risk of relapse is increased five-fold on cessation of antipsychotic medication (Robinson *et al.* 1999). The key element to successful long-term drug treatment of psychosis is compliance.

Whichever antipsychotic has been chosen an adequate trial is 6 weeks at a dose equivalent to between 250–750 mg chlorpromazine. If this proves ineffective then a second drug from a different group should be tried for a further 6-week trial. At this stage, compliance should be investigated and if in doubt an alternative strategy would be a depot.

Bipolar affective disorder

Bipolar affective disorder is characterized by episodes of hypomania or mania with or without depressive episode. The short-term management of a hypomanic phase is a sedative antipsychotic and for a depressive phase an antidepressant.

Once the diagnosis has been established patients suffering bipolar affective disorder are often started on a mood stabilizer by their psychiatrist in order to reduce the frequency of episodes. The most commonly used mood stabilizer is lithium. The kidneys eliminate this drug and therefore the relationship between the oral dose and plasma concentration is dependent upon renal function. Before starting lithium the urea and electrolytes, ECG and thyroid function need to be checked. Patients are usually started on 400 mg/day and the dose titrated upward until the plasma concentration (twelve hours post dose) is between 0.6 and 1.0 mmol/l. There is a risk of toxicity with plasma concentrations of greater than 1.0 mmol/l. Toxicity is characterized by tremor, ataxia, dysarthria, nystagmus, and convulsions. It is important to consider the possibility of lithium toxicity when patients on this drug present even with non-specific symptoms. The monitoring of lithium levels (3-monthly) and thyroid function (6-monthly) may either be dealt with by a lithium clinic organized by the local psychiatry service or by the GP and practice nurse. The anticonvulsants carbamazepine and sodium valproate are also used as mood stabilizers.

Conclusion

Non-pharmacological interventions are often more appropriate first choice for presentations of insomnia, and mild anxiety and depression. Psychotropic medication commonly prescribed in general practice can be broadly divided into treatments for depression, anxiety, insomnia, and psychosis. These conditions may be difficult to diagnose. However, a clear diagnosis is an important platform upon which to institute treatment. A thorough knowledge of a core of psychotropic drugs, their indications, their use, and their side effects will equip the GP to deal with these conditions. A good rule of thumb when prescribing any psychotropic is that it is always best, where possible to start and stop these drugs gradually. While drug therapy is by no means the sole treatment response to psychiatric illness its careful use can relieve suffering and be cost-effective.

17 Trauma and post-traumatic stress disorder

Gwen Adshead

For part of the week, I work in a clinic in the middle of London that offers a service for survivors and victims of trauma, and we try to work closely with GPs and other members of primary care teams who 'carry' our patients between appointments. From this perspective, I want to explore the impact of traumatic events on individuals and on communities as a whole, and look at what this may mean for providers of primary care. Traumatic stress experiences are common in 'everyday' life and mental health professionals need to think about the impact of trauma on mental health in order to understand their patients' complaints. It may also be useful to draw on disability, rather than disease models in order to appreciate some of the difficulties of survival after trauma.

The word trauma comes from the Greek 'to pierce'; and in everyday speech, 'trauma' refers to those events that are unexpected, sudden, shocking, and associated with life-threat. We tend to think of trauma or traumatic events as being unusual when compared to the events of everyday life. However, it may be that this view is rather narrow and somewhat optimistic. After all, it is only in the developed world that sudden threat to life is unusual; even in the West, rates of interpersonal violence can be so high as to be an every day occurrence for some groups of people.

An early classification system defined a traumatic stressor as 'outside the range of usual human experience' (American Psychiatric Association 1994). However, this definition was modified as it became clear that there are many experiences that are 'usual', but still traumatic, such as being a victim of crime. Perhaps the real point here is that there is no such thing as a 'usual' human experience.

The definition of trauma

Most accounts of trauma have focused on events that are dramatic, shocking, and unexpected. Threat to human life and helplessness in the face of life-threatening events are key features of traumatic stressors, as described in the Diagnostic and Statistical Manual criteria for Post-Traumatic Stress Disorder (Box 17.1; PTSD, APA 1994).

> **Box 17.1   DSM-IV criteria for Post-traumatic Stress Disorder (PTSD) (abbreviated)**
>
> ---
>
> Criterion A: the person has been exposed or witnessed an event involving death or threatened death. The person's response involved intense fear, helplessness, or horror
>
> Criterion B: the traumatic event is re-experienced in one of five ways, e.g. dreams, flashbacks, distress at reminders
>
> Criterion C: persistent avoidance of stimuli associated with the event (three of seven), e.g. diminished interest, detachment, avoidance of reminders
>
> Criterion D: symptoms of hyperarousal, e.g. insomnia, irritability, hyper-vigilance
>
> Criterion E: duration of disturbance over 1 month
>
> Criterion F: the disturbance causes impairment or distress

As suggested, the definition of trauma has moved away from something apparently objective: 'usual human experience', 'events which would distress almost everyone', to something more subjective: 'intense fear and helplessness'. The objective-subjective distinction is important and, in some respects, is political in nature, insofar as identifying objective criteria for disorders can lead to the diagnostic process becoming the province of 'experts'. The more the criteria resemble scientific data the more they can be described and codified by experts; these 'expert' generalizations are being made by those who remain external to the experience.

Emphasis on subjective criteria, in contrast, places the ownership of the labelling process with the one who has the experiences. There is no 'usual human' or 'everyone' who would feel the same in the same setting; there is the individual's story of their experience, which is constructed by them and has a validity that cannot be deconstructed by an outside 'expert'. Only someone who has actually had the experience can say whether they felt 'intense fear and helplessness'.

For mental health sciences, this tension poses a difficulty in relation to post-traumatic psychological morbidity. If the criterion for trauma is too subjective, then post-traumatic stress will be difficult to study using traditional scientific paradigms. If it is too 'objective', it risks defining social reality in a way that is essentially normative, i.e. how we think it should be, not how it is. This process may stimulate the criticism that psychiatric practice is often about imposing social norms and not about diagnosis of disease.

Trauma in different communities

There is data available about the prevalence of traumatic events in the community. However, we have to consider which community? Not all communities are the same in the extent of their exposure to violence or its place in the life of the community. There are many communities in the world where civil strife and violence are relatively common, such as Algeria, Somalia, or the former Yugoslavia at the present time. However, exposure to violence can still cause traumatic stress reactions, even though the violence is frequent and predictable.

There are communities where there is a long history of violence and bad feeling, but where traumatic events may be uncommon; for example, the annual number of deaths from road traffic accidents in Northern Ireland exceeds the number of deaths annually from terrorism. Both causes of death may be understood as traumatic, but death or injury by terrorism is scrupulously noted, examined, and discussed as evidence of community discord. This anxious attention may be compared with the relative lack of attention given to family homicide in England and Wales, even though the number of deaths by family homicide annually exceed the number of deaths by terrorism. The point here is that the community 'decides' what is or is not 'traumatic' in relation to its own values and priorities.

It is important to consider that reporting bias may influence our ideas about the prevalence of fearful events and, therefore, what constitutes trauma. In many cultures, some types of life-threatening events are never reported to anyone and can therefore erroneously be thought uncommon. In England and Wales, there is evidence that physical and sexual violence in the home is significantly under-reported. A recent study of rape suggests that only a third of rapes are reported (Home Office 2000) and the latest data on domestic violence suggests that this is also under-reported. Reporting is less likely if the victim thinks they will not be believed, so that the question of what is or is not 'believable' becomes important for the patient and the primary care provider. Who can decide whether something is 'believable'? Experts' perceptions of the believability of traumatic events are likely to affect the readiness with which they make such diagnoses.

Trauma in Western communities: 'ordinary trauma'

What types of trauma can the GP or primary care worker expect to have to deal with in practice? Estimates of lifetime prevalence of traumatic events range from 40 to 69% and one study (using a broad definition of trauma) found a prevalence of 89% (Breslau 1998). These data suggest that far from being unusual, traumatic events actually are likely to affect *most* people at some time in their lives and that only a minority will never experience any traumatic stressor. The commonest type of trauma is the sudden unexpected death of a close friend or relative. Many GPs will already offer post-bereavement visits, but some practices do not; it may sometimes be difficult for the practice to know when a bereavement has occurred. It may also not be appreciated how many people can be involved in the response to a bereavement. Hearing about trauma to others is also common and, although frequently missed, is a cause of traumatic stress itself. The most frequent types of trauma are not gender specific, but rape and sexual assault are more common in women, while physical assault, accidents, and witnessing violence are more common in men. One problem with this data is that victims who experience assaults that run contrary to gender stereotype (such as male victims of sexual assault) may face scepticism and disbelief, leading to isolation and under-reporting.

Vulnerable populations

Children and the elderly are also at risk of exposure to traumatic stressors. Children most obviously may be at risk of violence within the home, either by witnessing violence or experiencing it at the hands of their caretakers. Data indicates that the prevalence of physical abuse of children is between 20 and 30%, a substantial minority. Urban adolescents may be at particular risk of exposure to violence (Berton and Stabb 1996).

Elderly people with a history of exposure to trauma may commonly present first to their GPs and primary care teams, often through the context of other medical problems. Their history of trauma may be compounded by the loss-events that are commoner with advancing age. Combinations of previous trauma and new stressors may result in the development of delayed stress reactions. This is particularly true of elderly men who survived military service; of the four million veterans who returned from Vietnam, 30–40% had symptoms of PTSD, and even higher proportions developed substance abuse and mood disorders. Some 30 years on, these problems may be exacerbated by physical frailty and loss of contact with other survivors. The elderly are actually less at risk of becoming a victim of violence, but are more fearful of it, probably because they are aware of their frailty.

In addition to the native communities at risk of exposure to traumatic stress, there are immigrant populations who arrive after escaping from traumatic experiences in other countries. Primary care workers, especially those in urban areas, can expect to meet people who have survived persecution, torture, war, and sometimes mass homicide of whole social or family groups. Their experiences may be comparatively unusual, but their mental health needs both resemble and differ from others exposed to violence and fear. Similar problems include poor housing and lack of employment; different ones entail difficulties with language, literacy, and cultural alienation. Cultural beliefs and attitudes are likely to affect how male and female refugees understand and present their problems.

The key point for GP management is the recognition of significant cultural differences. For example, a torture survivor from Iran may develop depression that needs to be understood in terms of his cultural and religious experiences, and perhaps his political identity as a dissident and immigrant. However, he may still benefit from the usual treatments for depression, such as medication.

The impact of crime

Interpersonal criminal violence is one of the commoner causes of traumatic stress. One community study of crime (Mayhew *et al.* 1993) reported over a million physical assaults that had taken place over the previous year; half of which had taken place within the home between partners (see Chapter 4). There is evidence that criminal victimization unfairly affects the poor and disadvantaged, who are at twice the risk of assault than educated or more affluent populations. This means that people who already have an increased risk of physical and psychological morbidity because of social inequalities are then exposed to an even greater risk arising through violence.

GPs are likely to see victims of street violence and victims of domestic violence (male and female, adult and child). Such people may not automatically be thought of as victims of crime, so it may be helpful to recall that exposure to *any* interpersonal violence is a potent risk factor for PTSD and other post-traumatic conditions. In this context, the increase in violence to GPs, and to other staff in surgeries, means that GPs themselves and their colleagues may be at risk of developing such disorders. A colleague who has been assaulted, while at work may well develop symptoms that need to be understood as post-traumatic in origin, and which are likely to have a profound effect on work performance.

Perhaps one of the most potent stressors faced by people is sudden unexpected death caused by homicide. The term 'homicide' includes all violent deaths perpetrated by others, which may result in later legal convictions for murder or manslaughter. In this situation, an individual is faced not only with a sudden unexpected death, but also with the aftermath of violent crime. It is important to appreciate that the response to this goes far beyond 'ordinary' bereavement. There is good evidence that bereavement by homicide causes clinical distress beyond normal grief and increases the risk of developing disorders such as pathological bereavement reactions, and PTSD (Thompson *et al.* 1998). There are between 5–600 homicides annually in England and Wales, and the distress from these affects multiple members of families across generations, so that every year at least 2000 people will be dealing with the aftermath of homicide. It should also be remembered that homicide perpetrators may be members of the same family and may also be bereaved.

Accidents and illness

Accidents, especially car accidents, are a common cause of traumatic stress. A significant minority of individuals will develop post-traumatic stress reactions after car accidents, regardless of the severity of injury. Car accidents are also the cause of sudden unexpected death in at least 4000 cases annually in the UK.

The sudden threat of loss of health and well being caused by illness could also be considered a traumatic stressor, and a number of reports describe post-traumatic stress reactions in patients after strokes or other types of unexpected illness (Kutz *et al.* 1994; Sembi *et al.* 1998). Surgical procedures, especially those performed as emergencies, can be traumatic. This is particularly the case with obstetric surgery, where not only the mother's health, but also a baby's life may be at risk. Menage (1993) found a high incidence of PTSD in a sample of women undergoing obstetric or gynaecological procedures.

Thus, in general practice, members of primary care teams can expect to see many people with histories of exposure to traumatic events. In one study, 38% of primary care patients referred for anxiety or depression had been exposed to 'intense fear and helplessness' (Samson *et al.* 1999). Any ordinary person may be exposed to criminal violence, either directly or indirectly, or be bereaved suddenly by illness, accident, or homicide. It is not the rarity of events that makes them traumatic, but rather their association with intense feelings of fear and helplessness, and the sudden and unexpected loss of (or threat of loss to) safety and security.

What happens after trauma: PTSD and other experiences

The conscious experience of intense fear and helplessness reflects the neurophysiology of acute fear reactions in the frontal cortex and other areas of the brain responsible for processing fear and threat (LeDoux 1998; Bremner 1999). There is evidence that central cortisol release is neurotoxic if it becomes chronic, with subsequent impact on adrenergic stress responses (Yehuda and McFarlane 1995). This neural 'toxicity' has an existential equivalence in terms of the individual's sense of self and identity, which may equally be injured or damaged, both consciously and unconsciously. In this respect, there may be a link with accounts of stress from evolutionary biology; just like other mammals, in ordinary life, we are faced with regular threats to life (Sapolsky 1994). It seems that the perception of impending death, combined with the apparent (or real) inability to protect oneself, causes not only an intense neurophysiological response, but also has a profound effect on the individual's sense of themselves, their world, and their relationships.

A number of diagnostic labels have been applied to psychological morbidity after trauma. PTSD is a diagnosis that has attracted considerable debate. The present consensus is that PTSD is not an expectable reaction to extreme stress, but a specific pathological reaction (Yehuda 1997). It has a particular neuroendocrinological profile, distinct from the other disorders it resembles, such as anxiety and depression. PTSD itself is the psychological expression of the failure of the sympathetic nervous system to 'switch off' after the individual has been exposed to fear-inducing stimuli. This failure itself is caused by a dysregulation of cortisol secretion (Yehuda 1997).

It is, in fact, comparatively unusual for people to develop PTSD after trauma. PTSD occurs in only 25–30% of cases of exposure to trauma, although the risk is increased after some types of trauma such as interpersonal victimization. Depression is the commonest pathological reaction to loss and traumatic events; this is unsurprising given the association of traumatic events and sudden loss events. Substance abuse is also common, and may represent attempts by the individual to self-medicate for symptoms of anxiety and persistent arousal. Other types of distress include anxiety disorders, and other types of mood disorder characterized by the experience of persistent guilt or shame (Box 17.2).

Acute fear and loss

What is the connection between trauma and the development of these disorders? In what sense are they 'caused' by trauma? Some of the debates about PTSD mirror earlier discussions about pathological bereavement reactions (Bowlby 1980). Clearly, nearly everyone will be distressed after the death of a loved person, but only a small proportion of people will go on to develop pathological bereavement reactions, which are more likely when the bereavement is sudden or premature (Parkes 1972). The debate about bereavement is relevant to debates about the nature of trauma, because of the common theme of loss. Loss events are common in every culture. However, when losses are unexpected, unpredictable, and associated with fear and helplessness, they may be traumatic. Traumatic bereavement is one example; but loss of home or community may also be traumatic losses, even if there has been no loss of life. This is the common experience of many refugees. Survivors of interpersonal violence often describe the loss of a sense of safety or trust in others. People who have suffered these experiences are also at an increased risk of losing their jobs, their partners and even their mental health as result of developing post-traumatic stress reactions (Davidson *et al* 1991).

If loss and the meaning of loss are part of the explanation for the psychologically harmful effects of traumatic events, then fear reactions are another. Fear is associated with perceptions of and reactions to threat: flight or fight may follow fear. In healthy individuals, fear is managed using cognitive

---

Box 2   **Other post-traumatic mental disorders**

- ◆ Depression
- ◆ Substance misuse (especially alcohol)
- ◆ Panic disorder and phobic avoidance
- ◆ Dissociative experiences

models of safety and security—what Bowlby called 'internal working models' (Bowlby 1982). These models are both intrapersonal and interpersonal; they are models (or schemata) of the self at times of threat, and the self-and-other at times of threat. Exposure to traumatic experiences causes feelings of fear and helplessness. At these times, individuals will both consciously and unconsciously seek out safety, and internal working models of secure states will be evoked. If the stressor evokes overwhelming feelings of fear, the psychological mechanisms may not be able to 'hold' the feelings of physiological arousal. The individual feels out of control, both physically and psychologically, which in turn increases the feelings of fear and helplessness. If the fear experience is comparatively short-lived (minutes, rather than hours), then the individual will start to regain control once safety is established and anxiety begins to reduce. After such brief fear experiences, most people will experience acute stress symptoms over the next 2–3 months. These will gradually reduce in frequency and intensity until the individual reaches homeostasis again (Horowitz 1978). Memories of the fearful event become incorporated into the individual's narrative history; it is not forgotten, but it no longer evokes such overwhelming feelings of fear.

Chronic fear and shame

The model described above presupposes two things: first, that the fear experience stops completely, and, secondly, that the individual has internal working models of safety to access at times of fear. If the fearful experience continues for a long period, or the individual cannot bring to mind any secure sense of self, or model of help, then the psychological and physiological systems for the management of fear will become dysregulated. The long-term affects of chronic fear are not well understood. The best available data comes from studies of adults and children who have been exposed to fear for long lengths of time. Data about adults comes from studies of POW and Holocaust survivors, and from studies of battered women. From these studies, chronic fear and helplessness seems to be associated with depressive symptoms, disorders of bodily experience, and disorders of the experience of self; what has been called 'complex PTSD' (Herman 1992; Roth *et al.* 1997; Ford and Kidd 1998). Data about the affects of chronic fear in children also come from the Holocaust literature, but also from follow-up studies of children into adulthood. Exposure to repeated physical violence in childhood is associated with an increased perception of threat, a decreased capacity to make friendships, increased aggression and decreased empathy with others. It is likely that these affects are mediated by both psychological and physiological accommodation to fear (Bremner 1999).

Several authors have noted the similarities between accounts of complex PTSD and the diagnostic features of Borderline Personality Disorder (BPD). There is some evidence to suggest that complex PTSD is common in primary care settings (Dickinson *et al.* 1998). These authors studied the prevalence of symptoms associated with complex PTSD in women who attended GP practices with unexplained physical symptoms and a history of childhood trauma. All had symptoms of psychiatric distress, and a subset was highly symptomatic in four domains: depression, PTSD, dissociative symptoms, and somatization symptoms (see Chapter 5). This highly symptomatic profile was associated with all types of family violence, especially a history of combined physical and sexual abuse in childhood. There is an increasing understanding that personality disorder in adulthood is associated with early childhood trauma and adversity, and that many of the negative manifestations of personality disorder may reflect chronic maladaptive responses to fear and loss, especially in relation to carers (Herman 1992).

Perhaps the crucial effect of chronic fear reactions is the impact on the narrative that the fearful individual builds up about the world and her place in it. Specifically, this narrative will not only offer an account of fear and helplessness, it will also provide an account of the availability and usefulness of helpers and caregivers. The relevance of this for primary care is that children and adults who have been exposed to fearful experiences may find it hard to trust others, even those who offer help. These patients may be very demanding of help, but unable to make good use of it—sometimes because they fear that help will suddenly vanish, or the helper will become an attacker, or that the help is not enough for their need. Given the limit to resources in the NHS, this fear is sometimes justified; people who are chronically fearful may need reassurance that limits to care are not indicative of personal threat.

Survival and disability

PTSD and other diagnostic labels tend to construe the psychological sequelae of trauma as 'disease' and for some people this may be helpful. A rather different approach to working with survivors is to think about the process of living with past trauma events, and to consider the importance of each person's vulnerability and resilience. The shift of language from 'victim' to 'survivor' is not just a matter of political correctness, but also a statement about agency. The term 'victim' implies powerlessness and helplessness, and emphasizes vulnerability. The term 'survivor' emphasizes resilience, the capacity for endurance and perseverance in the face of traumatic challenge. These two terms do not represent a dichotomy. People who experience trauma are neither victims nor survivors; they are both and both states of mind need to be borne in mind.

A disability perspective assumes that people will cope well generally, but accepts that they will have intermittent crises, especially at times of new stress. This implies the need to take a long-term view in planning support and care, and a focus on using specialist services as a source of help from time to time, but not as a solution. This is an approach that will be familiar to primary care workers, but less so to those who work in specialist services.

If chronic stress reactions are regarded as types of disability, it has the advantage of lessening the sense of alienation described earlier. Survivors of traumatic events often describe feeling cut off from the 'normal' world they used to inhabit. Like those who are disabled physically, they see the 'normal' world as favouring those who apparently feel no fear or vulnerability. They may feel anger, and a sense of grievance that further disables them because it fosters resentment, rather than action. Finding meaning in suffering becomes a crucial existential task, which includes trying to reconnect to the world; what Frankl called a 'lesson in living' (Frankl 1959).

This discussion does not mean that the disease model of PTSD has no validity. For many individuals, especially those who have experienced a short-lived episode of trauma and were previously in good health, the disease model with its implication of a return to normality, will be appropriate. PTSD does exist and can be treated. As a diagnostic model it applies less well to those who have experienced repeated and/or extremes of traumatic events, such as those who have become refugees or prisoners of war. It may be that 'complex PTSD' is a better term for the constellation of psychological problems faced by such people, because it includes the impact of chronic trauma on the sense of self and on interpersonal relating.

Assessment

Many trauma survivors will present first to their GPs or other members of the primary care team. However, they may not complain directly of their history of trauma, since they are likely to find it difficult to trust another person, no matter how well intentioned. They may feel intense shame or guilt about their experience, which makes disclosure difficult. Talking about the trauma often results initially in an exacerbation of symptoms and active avoidance of reminders of the trauma is a diagnostic phenomenon. It is therefore more common for people to present with either unexplained somatic complaints, symptoms of hyperarousal (especially insomnia), and new or worsened substance misuse.

Key points include finding out when the trauma took place and what has prompted presentation now. This has implications for treatment; stress responses as a result of recent trauma require different interventions to those that took place many years earlier. Previous physical and mental health may be indicators of prognosis; generally, the better a person's pre-traumatic health, the more likely they are to make a good recovery from a new stressor. Here, the GP's experience of the patient and information from the GP records are invaluable; often the most obvious sign that a person is suffering a traumatic stress reaction is an increase in illness behaviour as recorded in the notes.

Assessment of individuals with a history of traumatic stress needs to include attention to pre-traumatic patterns; especially previous experience of trauma or fear, and the individual's usual style of coping. Continuing flashbacks or nightmares may indicate that the individual is still dealing with fearful affects, whereas withdrawal, depression, and mood swings may indicate that the individual is struggling with sad, guilty, or shameful feelings. A substance abuse history is essential, partly because many people manage their feelings with alcohol or drugs, and partly because, if they do this, it may interfere with effective treatment. Irritability, combined with substance misuse may result in violence, which is most often expressed towards partners.

Treatment: words and memories

Experientially, there are two difficulties that survivors describe most often: the first is in connection with memory and the second with language. Survivors of trauma report different types of memory disturbance; repetitive, intrusive, or fragmented memories of the trauma, cut off from normal autobiographical memory, are a problem for some, and are characteristic of PTSD (Brewin *et al.* 1996), whilst others report an experience of 'blankness' or amnesia around the time of traumatic events.

Survivors often find it hard to speak about their experiences, as though language fails in the face of recalled fear and other intolerable affects. What they then have to wrestle with is, literally, 'unspeakable'. The language difficulty may be related to the memory difficulty and both may combine in a way that makes any type of thinking about the traumatic experience hard. The sense of a memory that cannot be incorporated into the person's past, and an experience which cannot be put into speech, increases the sense of alienation and fragmentation that many survivors of traumatic events describe. Their disorders of memory and language distort their conscious experience of themselves by disrupting their sense of autobiography (Holmes 1996; Damasio 1999). Experience and emotion may be expressed somatically if narrative is not available; several of the early studies noted the frequency of psychosomatic complaints in trauma survivors.

Case

A woman presented to her doctor with a 'burning' sensation on micturition, and frequency. All routine investigations were normal, as were the more specialist examinations. A psychological cause was sought. It transpired that she was a survivor of a fire in a nightclub several years before. She had gone to the club with a good friend, and had left her for a moment when she went to the washroom to urinate. The fire broke out minutes later, and the alarm was raised. She found herself unable to get out the way she had come, but she managed to escape through a window. Her friend died in the fire.

An ordinary desire to urinate became a potent somatic memory that triggered unconscious grief and unexpressed guilt; the 'burning' she described was a poignant example of her attempt to express the memory in verbal fragments. Expression of grief and guilt in words lead to a marked reduction in her urinary symptoms.

Perhaps the greatest difficulty for survivors of trauma is that life does not stand still for them while they recover. Survivors of accidents, assaults, and bereavements are not immune from the ordinary stresses of Western life: redundancy, poor housing, and further trauma, such as crime or bereavement. Another case example may illustrate this:

An elderly man presented in the clinic with symptoms of increasing anxiety, panic attacks, and nightmares. These nightmares related to his experiences as a Japanese prisoner of war some 50 years earlier. He had never had symptoms before; in fact, he had prided himself on his post-war fitness and engagement with life. He had taken up motorbike racing, and been a DIY enthusiast, even doing his own roof repairs until well into his late sixties. Chronic osteoarthritis in both hips was now decreasing his mobility. He feared having an operation, but could no longer ride his motorbike or climb on the roof. His awareness of his physical frailty and his loss of health was an unconscious reminder of a time when to be immobile or vulnerable at all, significantly increased the likelihood of death. In his nightmares, he was in the camp again, but now as an old man: he knew what lay ahead. He knew he would never be able to survive without the physical health, luck, and determination that had saved him half a century ago. Recent deaths of fellow POWs may also have been a trigger for his new anxiety.

There is some reason to think that traumatic victimization actually increases the risk of further trauma (Breslau 1998). However, this may apply more to victims of criminal violence than to other types of survivor who may be more resilient. Many asylum seekers and refugees are individuals who have found courage and psychological stamina to face escaping from persecution and enduring the hardships of flight. Once safe, however, they face continuing problems of loneliness, isolation, and sometimes further victimization in the form of racism and rejection by the immigration services. All this must be managed, while still struggling to come to terms with experiences of abrupt flight and loss.

Treatment: specific interventions

Treatment interventions may be psychological and pharmacological; they may also involve the social world and community of the trauma survivor. The community aspect is most relevant to the issue of safety; treatment efficacy is likely to be reduced if the patient is still not safe. This is often an issue for victims of family or street violence, and for refugees who lack housing or income.

Once safety is established, the therapeutic intervention indicated depends on the symptom profile. Patients who present with largely fear-based symptoms, such as nightmares and intrusive memories, will benefit from fear-based paradigms, such as exposure therapy (Tarrier *et al.* 2000). This involves asking patients to go over their experience in detail: in speech, on tape, and sometimes in writing. Gradually, the fear reduces and patients have less inclination to avoid thinking about or feeling their experience. Exposure therapy is an effective treatment for simple PTSD where the traumatic experience has been time-limited or unrepeated.

Shame and depression are commoner after chronic trauma or after interpersonal violence. For patients with these symptoms, anti-depressants combined with cognitive therapy may be effective. There is evidence that serotonergic medication is a good first line treatment, especially for chronic stress reactions (Turner 1999). Pharmacological treatment needs to be vigorous, using higher dosages than for depression alone (see Chapter 16). For many patients, seeing their GP for their medication is a vital part of the treatment programme. In our clinic we prefer our GP colleagues to hold the responsibility for prescribing, so that there is some joint 'ownership' of the treatment between the patient, the specialist, and the GP.

Both cognitive and exposure therapies can be carried out via an interpreter for those patients who do not speak English: the essential aspect is the patient has an alliance with the therapist and understands why they are being asked to do certain tasks. Interestingly, some patients will say that they prefer to carry out their therapy in English, even if a native speaking therapist can be found for them. Such patients often say that this is because English is associated with safety in a way their own language is not.

Although most of the empirical evidence comes from individual treatment approaches, group therapies have also been used to good effect. Group treatments were first described for soldiers suffering from war trauma in the 1940s. Later, group therapy was used for Vietnam veterans, in both inpatient and outpatient settings. There is evidence to suggest that group therapy can be effective for trauma reactions, especially chronic stress reactions. Most group therapy has used an homogenous group model, putting survivors of similar traumatic experiences together. The strength of the group approach is that it addresses the experience of isolation and dissociation that trauma survivors often feel. This may be of especial relevance for those who have been disconnected from their home communities. However, there are situations where a heterogenous group reduces a sense of isolation by the discovery of similarity in apparently different experiences. We have also found that it is not unusual for refugees from one country to be very resistant to being in groups with their countrymen, especially in those places where they have fled civil war. We do not always know the full story of peoples' lives before a war, or their flight from home—sometimes the identity of perpetrator and victim becomes confused when there is civil strife. In a group we ran for refugees from the former Yugoslavia, the members had nothing in common except that they were refugees. Their profound differences of money, class, and religious belief were sad reminders of the strife that had made them flee for their lives.

All psychotherapies deal with narrative. There has been considerable interest in the relevance of narrative in relation to traumatic memories and fear experience, where the fearful experience is disconnected from the life story. Most therapies for traumatic stress reactions involve the patient in telling their story in some form or other. This may take the form of a spoken narrative which is taped, and to which they listen. There has been some interest in the use of *written narratives* as part of therapy for PTSD (Resick and Schnicke 1993). For those who have suffered torture or political violence, narratives in the form of a written or witnessed testimony may be valuable as a way of affirming the value of individual survival, and reassurance that individual experience matters. Such work is a good example of trauma therapy that can be carried out in primary care by the GP.

Conclusion

I hope that I have been able to demonstrate that primary care workers are likely to meet many people who are trauma survivors, and who may be experiencing chronic or acute fear reactions. The people who attend the GP most often are also most at risk: children, the elderly, women, and people who lack emotional language to deal with stressors. Traumatic stress reactions may be caused by *any* life-threatening experience, which includes serious medical illness, emergency operations, and accidents, even those that do not cause much physical injury. The *perception* of life-threatening events or hostility, and the experience of fear or helplessness, and its meaning in terms of their own life-story, may be more psychologically damaging than any actual injury.

Finally, let me think about the primary care worker as a *potential victim* of traumatic stress: first, as a possible member of a traumatized community and, secondly, by virtue of what has been called '*vicarious traumatization*'. After any community trauma, it is the primary care services that may notice the impact on the community first, but the effects may last many years after the original event. In the UK we may think about the primary care professionals in the towns of Lockerbie, Hungerford, or Dunblane. Professionals may have the difficulty of being both members of a traumatized community, but also those expected to help the community recover. This situation can be an argument for contact with 'outsiders' to support primary care teams, rather than bringing in outside specialists to deal with the community directly. The best evidence to date suggests that where an event has affected a whole community, it is helpful for the community to be and work together.

Vicarious traumatization is a different problem, and one that afflicts all health care professionals. Arguably the most difficult part of health care is supportive work for those long-term problems that may never resolve or fully recover. It can be hard to sit and listen to someone else's account of feeling helpless and horrified; normal human empathy means that, at least briefly, we share some of the horror and the helplessness. If there is little the primary carer can do to make things better, this can add to the helplessness a sense of frustration and anxiety. Thus the carers become at risk of vicarious trauma reactions; depression and anxiety; and adoption of maladaptive strategies to cope with these feelings, such as substance misuse, or hostility and rejection of patients. Training and education about such feelings can help carers to manage and digest them (see Chapters 6, 7, and 10).

Finally, as noted earlier, GPs and primary health care workers, like anyone else, may be exposed to traumatic events at work and in their private lives. As health care professionals we may have to ask ourselves searching questions about how we look after ourselves and our colleagues, and especially about our unconscious investment in never being a patient, but always a carer. What we must not do is to assume that traumatic experiences always happen to someone else. Extraordinary trauma happens to ordinary people.

N.B.: The cases are clinically accurate but fictitious.

18 Psychological therapies

Glenys Parry and John Cape

All mental health practitioners and GPs use psychotherapeutic skills in the course of their routine care of patients. Our focus in this chapter is on psychotherapy undertaken as a specialist treatment by trained practitioners for whom the provision of psychological therapy is their dedicated role. We concentrate on NHS-provided psychological therapy and on treatment provided in secondary care, and the indications for referral thereto from primary care. Counselling and psychological treatments in primary care have been discussed in Chapter 10.

There are many types of psychotherapy. The most common approaches in the NHS are cognitive-behaviour therapy, psychoanalytic (also called psycho-dynamic) psychotherapy, and systemic therapy, although cognitive-analytic therapy and interpersonal psychotherapy are also increasingly used.

Cognitive behaviour therapy is a pragmatic combination of concepts and techniques from cognitive and behaviour therapies, common in clinical practice. *Behavioural therapy* is a structured therapy originally derived from learning theory, which seeks to solve problems, and relieve symptoms by changing behaviour and the environmental factors that control behaviour. Graded exposure to feared situations is one of the commonest behavioural treatment methods and is used in a range of anxiety disorders. *Cognitive therapy* is a struc-tured treatment approach derived from cognitive theories. Cognitive techniques (such as challenging negative automatic thoughts) and behavioural techniques (such as activity scheduling and behavioural experiments) are used with the main aim of relieving symptoms by changing maladaptive thoughts and beliefs.

A number of different therapies draw on psychoanalytic theories, although they differ in terms of technique. *Focal psychodynamic therapy* identifies a central conflict arising from early experience that is being re-enacted in adult life, producing mental health problems. It aims to resolve this by the relation-ship with the therapist giving new opportunities for emotional assimilation and insight. This form of therapy is sometimes time-limited, with anxiety aroused by the ending of therapy being used to illustrate how re-awakened feelings about earlier losses, separations, and disappointments may be experienced dif-ferently. *Psychoanalytic psychotherapy* is a longer-term process (usually lasting for at least a year or more) in which there is a combination of support and the re-enactment of unconscious conflicts in the relationship with the therapist, which are worked through with interpretation in a developmental process.

Systemic and family therapists understand individual problems by considering the relevance of family relationships, and the impact of the wider social and economic context on people's lives, their well being and their mental health. Therapeutic work is undertaken with individuals, couples, or families, and may include consultation to wider networks, such as other professionals working with the individual or the family. Therapy aims to identify and explore patterns of belief and behaviour in roles and relationships, and therapists actively intervene to change family structure and enable people to decide where change would be desirable, and to facilitate the process of establishing new, more fulfilling, and useful patterns (see Chapters 5 and 9).

Some practitioners, especially psychologists and counsellors, will use a number of different approaches to psychotherapy, either with different patients or mixing approaches with the same patient. Other practitioners specialize and only provide one kind of psychotherapy.

Counselling is a broad term, used in mental health services to mean therapeutic counselling and as such it overlaps with psychotherapy. Therapeutic counselling commonly describes approaches that are shorter-term and with patients who have less severe problems. This arises from its historic focus on maximizing psychological health, rather than treating psychopathology and dysfunction. Therapeutic counselling historically was most commonly person-centred (humanistic) counselling, but increasingly forms of counselling are provided matching each of the psychotherapies—psychodynamic counselling, cognitive behavioural counselling, etc. (East 1995). A further source of confusion in the UK is that a dedicated mental health professional providing psychological treatments in primary care is commonly called a counsellor, whatever their training and type of psychological therapy provided.

Organization of psychotherapy services

The Department of Health Review of NHS Psychotherapy Services in England (Department of Health 1996) found wide variation in the availability and organization of psychotherapy services in the NHS. The extent to which specific types of psychotherapy (e.g. cognitive-behavioural, psychodynamic, systemic) are available, and how they are accessed, organized and co-ordinated varies widely across the country. In most areas there is more than one service within a Trust providing dedicated psychological therapy services. The independent types of psychotherapy service may be characterized by:

+ Type of therapy provided (e.g. psychodynamic, cognitive-behavioural, systemic).

- Professional group leading on organization and provision of the service (e.g. psychiatry/consultant psychotherapist, clinical psychology).
- Service for specific patient groups (e.g. eating disorders, personality disorders).

Thus, in a particular geographical area, there may be a predominantly psychoanalytic psychotherapy service organized by a consultant psychotherapist, a service providing cognitive-behavioural and other psychological therapies organized by a psychology department, and a specialist eating disorder service that includes provision of a range of individual and group psychotherapies to patients with eating disorders.

Poor co-ordination between the different psychological therapy services within a Trust was often noted by respondents to the Department of Health (1996) survey. Different services within a locality or even within one Trust may have no commonly agreed criteria for referral, separate information systems, poor communication between services, and inadequate cross-referral arrangements. It is likely that from the perspective of primary care it is frequently difficult to know what services are available or most appropriate for specific patients.

The history of development of psychotherapy provision within the NHS helps explain this lack of integration between local psychotherapy services. Psychotherapy departments led by consultant psychiatrists trained in psychoanalytic psychotherapy began to be established prior to establishment of the NHS in the 1930s and 1940s (Pedder 1989). Independent of these psychotherapy departments, clinical psychologists began to provide behavioural and then cognitive-behavioural therapy services to both secondary and primary care in the late 1960s and early 1970s (Hackman 1993). Although psychotherapy departments are no longer usually exclusively psychoanalytic (Royal College of Psychiatrists 1991) or psychology services exclusively cognitive-behavioural, the organizational independence of these services frequently remains.

The independent development of counselling in primary care has been a further factor adding to the complexity. This began in the 1970s, funded initially through Family Practitioner Committees, then Family Health Services Authorities. The growth in the number of counsellors employed in General Practice in the early 1980s (Abel-Smith *et al.* 1989) was sustained by flexible use of funding following the 1987 White Paper *Promoting Better Health* and then taken further by some fund-holding practices.

A move to integrated provision of psychotherapy services has taken place over the past six years in line with the recommendations of a joint working party of the British Psychological Society and Royal College of Psychiatrists (Binns *et al.* 1994). This was further spurred by the Department of Health (1996) Psychotherapy Review. Proposals for and reports on integrated psychotherapy services are increasingly being published (Holmes and Mitchison 1995; Knowles 1997). There have also been developments in the integration of services with primary care, with psychological therapy departments managing counsellors working in primary care (see description in Chapter 10).

A further development has been consideration of how to map psychological therapy service provision onto the needs of a population. The level of psychological morbidity presenting in primary care (Goldberg and Huxley 1992) far outstrips the availability of psychotherapy services. A tension exists between providing services to patients with more severe and complex disorders who need longer-term psychotherapy, and to patients with less severe problems who can be effectively treated in shorter-term therapies. Models describing integrated tiers of services are beginning to appear (Paxton et al. 2000). These provide brief and short-term psychological therapies at or close to primary care by generalist psychotherapy practitioners trained to provide more than one type of psychotherapy (e.g. cognitive-behavioural and systemic). The generalists are backed up by specialist provision for more complex cases requiring longer-term psychotherapy. The tiers of psychotherapy provision need to be integrated with other mental health provision (Holmes 1996; Paxton et al. 2000).

Significant psychotherapy provision also exists outside the NHS in most of the UK, through both voluntary organizations and independent practitioners. Voluntary organizations providing psychotherapy services are at times funded by the NHS or Local Authority Social Services Departments. In considering referral to voluntary and independent practitioners, GPs and other referrers in discharging their duty of care, need to be satisfied about the competence in psychotherapy of the practitioners to which patients are being referred. This should at minimum involve establishing that the psychotherapy practitioner is accredited through one of the two national accreditation bodies—British Confederation of Psychotherapists, UK Council of Psychotherapy—or through the British Psychological Society or Royal College of Psychiatrists. Each of these keeps registers of practitioners in psychological therapy and has formal procedures to investigate complaints of malpractice against practitioners.

This raises the complex issue of the training required to practice psychotherapy. There are many different routes to psychotherapeutic competence. In the NHS psychotherapy is most commonly practised by clinical psychologists, psychiatrists with specialist training, and an increasing number of other mental health professionals, particularly mental health nurses and occupational therapists who undertake post-qualification training in one or other form of psychotherapy. Clinical psychologists tend to have the broadest grounding in different models of psychological therapy, but do not necessarily train to specialist level in any one, although some do. As such, they are often called on at the secondary care level to help those patients within Community Mental Health Teams who are not easily suited to straightforward support or to offer assessment. Psychiatrists qualifying in psychotherapy 'major' as Specialist Registrars in Psychotherapy in one of the three main modalities of therapy, with the other two taken as 'minors' and tend to work in specialist tertiary psychotherapy units.

There are a number of trainings available that lead to registration as a psychotherapist with the UK Council for Psychotherapy or the British Confederation of Psychotherapists. These are usually of at least 4 years' duration. Most people who train as adult psychotherapists without a prior mental health qualification work in the private sector, although the number employed in the NHS is increasing. Child psychotherapists, on the other hand, have long been employed in the NHS. The sheer variety of trainings can be confusing to the GP and even more so to the patient. The issue is of great importance because of the immense trust engendered in the psychotherapeutic relationship, the harm that is done by betrayal of that trust and the power of incompetence to cause deterioration. For these reasons, competence to practice, adherence to an ethical code, and professional accountability are essential. GPs or patients should never be afraid to ask frankly about any practitioner's training and qualifications to practice.

Effectiveness and outcomes of psychotherapy

Evidence for the effectiveness of psychological therapies has existed since the first meta-analytic reviews two decades ago (Smith and Glass 1977; Shapiro and Shapiro 1982). Influential reviews for the Department of Health by Roth and Fonagy (1996), and for the American Psychological Association Task Force on empirically validated psychological therapies (DeRubeis and Crits-Christoph 1998; Nathan and Gorman 1998) have summarized evidence for the efficacy of psychological therapies for specific conditions (depression, personality disorders, etc). Mackay and Barkham (1998) provide an overview of good quality reviews of the evidence for psychological therapies in specific conditions, commissioned for the Department of Health guideline on treatment choice in psychological therapies (Department of Health 2001).

There are, however, significant gaps in the evidence. The empirical research on psychotherapy has concentrated on brief and structured forms of psychotherapy with fewer studies on longer-term psychotherapies. Studies of the effectiveness of psychotherapy in patients with complex and co-morbid problems are lacking as controlled trials have focused on establishing efficacy in patients with discrete conditions (Aveline *et al.* 1995; Clarke 1995; Barkham and Mellor-Clark 2000). Pragmatically, within the NHS where most patients are seen by GPs and there is evidence that GPs can be effective in managing psychological problems (Cape *et al.* 2000), a key under-researched question is the circumstances under which psychotherapy is more effective and cost effective than good quality GP psychological management. This is a different research question from whether primary care counselling is cost effective compared with 'usual GP treatment', which has been addressed albeit with mixed results (King *et al.* 2000; Rowland *et al.* 2000; Simpson *et al.* 2000).

Patients wanting help for psychological problems may have acute symptoms of distress, chronic distress symptoms, and/or characterological or interpersonal symptoms, even if presenting with a single diagnosable condition such as major depressive disorder. There is evidence that these different kinds of symptom require increasing lengths of psychotherapy for resolution (Barkham *et al.* 1996; Kopta *et al.* 1994). Acute distress symptoms, such as crying and pessimism, resolve most quickly, followed by chronic distress symptoms, such as self-blame, with characteristic and interpersonal problems, such as frequent arguing and difficulties with intimacy, needing more lengthy treatment. Based on the evidence of differential responsiveness of different kinds of symptoms, Howard *et al.* (1993) suggested that psychotherapy follows three phases. In this model, therapy begins with reversal of demoralization (remoralization), continues with remediation of long-standing symptoms, and concludes with rehabilitation where maladaptive patterns of dealing with life are unlearned and better patterns established. Attention to the dose–response relationship in psychotherapy also gave rise to a reanalysis of the data that led Eysenck in 1952 to claim that psychotherapy was no more effective than spontaneous remission. The re-analysis showed that the impact of a few months of psychotherapy was equivalent to the impact of 2 years of other forms of help (McNeilly and Howard 1991).

Guidance on psychotherapy for primary care practitioners

With the increasing range of psychological therapies available in the NHS, together with the independent development of primary care counselling over the past three decades, there has been a need for guidance for GPs on psychotherapy and, in particular, on referrals to psychological therapies including counselling.

Much useful guidance is available, particularly on which cases are considered appropriate to be referred by GPs for brief counselling in primary care and which to secondary care psychotherapy and mental health services (Bond 1995; Friedli and King 1996; Parker *et al.* 1997). However, this guidance has generally not been developed systematically and recommendations are not specifically related to the evidence on which they are based (Cape and Parry 2000). Such evidence-based guidance for primary care on referrals for psychotherapy was first developed as part of the US Agency for Health Care Policy and Research (AHCPR) depression guidelines for primary care (AHCPR 1993). In the UK, a local evidence-based guideline for counselling and psychological therapies (Cape *et al.* 1998) received some attention in part through being summarized in a *British Medical Journal* ABC Guide to psychological therapies publication (Richardson 1997). The development of the Department of Health funded national treatment choice in psychological therapies and counselling guideline (2001) has been described by Parry (2000a).

The evidence-based guidance from these sources focuses on general principles regarding appropriateness of referrals for psychological therapies and on choice of psychological therapy, rather than on choice of counselling or psychotherapy service (e.g. a primary versus a secondary care-based service). As indicated above, organization of psychotherapy services varies widely and the boundaries between what is provided in primary care and in secondary care are likely to continue to change with the development of Primary Care Trusts in the UK. Choice of an appropriate service also depends on local variable factors, such as waiting times and accessibility, and on idiosyncratic factors such as a given GP's personal knowledge of the therapist or service being referred to. The implication of this variation is that any evidence-based guidance on choice of psychological therapies needs to be adapted to local circumstances. GPs need the evidence base for referral to different types of therapy, but to be optimally useful this needs to be supplemented by details of specific services that provide the recommended treatments and practitioners who have the appropriate skills. Inevitably, in many localities there will be a gap between best referral practice based on research evidence and the constraints of local provision.

General recommendations on appropriateness of referrals for psychological therapies from evidence-based guidelines can be summarized as covering areas of *general appropriateness for psychotherapy*, the importance of the *therapeutic relationship, patient variables, therapist variables*, and the importance of *case complexity*. Recommendations on the choice of specific psychological therapies relate to *condition*. Each of these is summarized below. The Department of Health Guideline (2001) gives details of the evidence on which these are based.

Appropriateness for psychotherapy

Patients with a wide variety of mental health problems are suitable for psychotherapy. The Department of Health Guideline (2001) focuses on common mental health problems, such as depression, anxiety, eating disorders, personality disorders, and some common somatic problems with psychological features. For patients with more severe problems (schizophrenia, severe depression) psychological therapies have been shown to be a useful adjunct to pharmacological treatments.

Therapeutic relationship

A good working relationship between psychotherapist and patient is important for all psychological therapies. Adequacy of working relationship depends on both the skills of the psychotherapist, the personality of the patient, and on the interaction between these two. Perhaps one implication of this for the GP is to prepare a patient referred for psychotherapy for their part in this relationship, and explain the need to give the therapy and therapist a 'fair trial'. Another implication is that a patient who is hostile to or suspicious of the idea of a psychological therapy is much less likely to benefit, however impressive the research evidence for the effectiveness of a particular approach for a particular condition.

Patient variables

Patient motivation for psychotherapy and preference for a specific type of psychotherapy should be considered. Interest in self-exploration and capacity to tolerate frustration in relationships may be particularly important for success in psychoanalytic and psychodynamic therapies.

Therapist variables

As in other areas of medicine, extensive training, and experience in a specific form of psychotherapy and in specific types of patient problems are likely to be beneficial for treatment. The skill and experience of the therapist should therefore be taken into account. More complex problems and those where patients are poorly motivated require more skilful therapists (see Chapters 8 and 10). In practice, inexperienced therapists under supervision often see patients with complex and longstanding difficulties, but the GP should reserve the right to specify that a senior practitioner sees such a patient.

Treatment length

Therapies of fewer than eight sessions are unlikely to be optimally effective for most moderate to severe mental health problems. Often 16 sessions are required for symptomatic relief and more for lasting change.

Case complexity

As well as requiring more skilled and experienced psychotherapists, complex cases benefit from longer treatments. Complexity can be assessed in terms of multiple presenting psychological problems (co-morbid conditions), co-existing personality disorders, and prior unsuccessful episodes of psychotherapy treatment.

Choice of specific psychological therapies

Patients who are *adjusting to life events*, *illnesses*, *disabilities*, or *losses* may benefit from brief therapies such as counselling. However, counselling is not recommended as the main intervention for severe and complex mental health problems or personality disorders.

Where *post-traumatic stress disorder* (PTSD) is present, psychological therapy is indicated, with best evidence for cognitive behavioural methods (see Chapter 17). Patients with PTSD can expect to receive substantial help from psychological therapy even in the absence of a complete cure. The differential effectiveness of different types of treatment has not been established, with best evidence for the benefit of systematic desensitization (graded exposure) and related approaches (stress inoculation therapy and eye movement desensitization). Prolonged re-exposure (flooding) may exacerbate some symptoms (depression, anger, alcohol use) and graded re-exposure is generally more acceptable to patients. Psychodynamic therapy and hypnotherapy have also shown benefit. However, single-session routine debriefing following traumatic events does not prevent PTSD and is not recommended.

Depression may be treated effectively with a number of therapies, with best evidence for cognitive therapy or interpersonal therapy (see Chapter 14). Other brief structured therapies for depression may be of benefit, such as psychodynamic therapy and counselling.

Anxiety disorders with marked symptomatic anxiety (panic disorder, agoraphobia, social phobia, obsessive-compulsive disorders, generalized anxiety disorders) are likely to benefit from cognitive behaviour therapy.

Psychological intervention should be considered for *somatic complaints* with a *psychological component*, with most evidence for CBT in the treatment of chronic pain and chronic fatigue. For irritable bowel syndrome, promising results have been obtained with psychodynamic-interpersonal therapy, cognitive behaviour therapy, psychodynamic psychotherapy, and hypnosis (see the story of May and her GP, Chapter 4).

A co-existing diagnosis of *personality disorder* may make treatment of the presenting mental health problem more difficult and possibly less effective; indications of personality disorder include forensic history, severe relationship difficulties, repeated self-harm, and recurrent complex problems. However, structured psychological therapies delivered by skilled practitioners can contribute to the longer-term treatment of personality disorders (see Chapter 5). Available therapies include dialectical behaviour therapy, psychoanalytic day hospital programmes, therapeutic communities, cognitive analytic therapy, schema-focused cognitive therapy, and psychoanalytic therapy.

Eating disorders can be treated with psychological therapy. Best evidence in bulimia nervosa is for CBT, IPT and family therapy for teenagers. Treatment usually includes psycho-educational methods. There is little strong evidence on the best therapy type for anorexia (see Chapter 12).

Future developments

Predicting the future is perilous, but instructive, helping to trace a direction of travel, to make some links between aspirations and achievable realities. With the development of national guidelines and the inclusion of psychological therapies into the National Service Framework for Mental Health (Department of Health

1999a), the NHS is at last beginning to take psychotherapy seriously. These therapies are moving from the margins of the NHS, where fragmented, patchy services were inaccessible to many people, into the mainstream of mental health care. We predict that those referring patients and the patients themselves will increasingly expect minimum acceptable standards of provision, greater availability of safe and effective therapies, and more reliable service delivery systems. There is a greater awareness of the right of the public in general and patients in particular to have good information about psychological therapies, and to make informed choices in relation to referral. The principle that psychotherapy practice should be informed by research seems irreversibly established (Parry 2000b). The infrastructure for commissioning such research is also being established through the implementation of NHS Priorities and Needs R&D Funding. Finally, practitioners of these therapies working in the NHS will increasingly be required to demonstrate their competence, both through initial qualification and in the routine evaluation of therapy outcomes.

References

Abed, R.T. and Neira-Munoz, E. (1990) A survey of general practitioners' opinion and attitude to drug addicts and addiction. *British Journal of Addiction* **85**, 131–6.

Abel-Smith, A., Irving, J. and Brown, P. (1989) Counselling in the medical context. In: W. Dryden, D. Charles-Edwards and R. Woolfe (eds) *Handbook of Counselling in Great Britain*. London: Tavistock/Routledge.

Agency for Health Care Policy and Research (1993) *Depression in Primary Care*. London: HMSO.

Ainsworth, M.D.S., Blehar, M., Waters, E. and Wall, S. (1978) *Patterns of Attachment*. Hillsdale: Erlbaum.

Alderson, P. (1998) The importance of theories in health care. *British Medical Journal* **317**, 1007–10.

Allebeck, P. (1989) Schizophrenia: a life-shortening disease, *Schizophrenia Bulletin* **15**, pp. 81–9.

Alpern, L. and Lyons Ruth, K. (1993) Preschool-children at social risk—chronicity and timing of maternal depressive symptoms and child-behavior problems at school and at home. *Development and Psychopathology* **5**, 371–87.

American Psychiatric Association (1994) *Diagnostic and Statistical Manual*, Version 4. Washington: American Psychiatric Press.

Amis, M. (1991) *Time's Arrow*. London: Penguin.

Anderson, I.M., Nutt, D.J. and Deakin, J.F. (2000) Evidence-based guidelines for treating depressive disorders with antidepressants: a revision of the 1993 British Association for Psychopharmacology guidelines. *Journal of Psychopharmacology* **14**, 3–20.

Andrews, G. and Jenkins, R. (1999) Substance Use Disorders. In: *Management of Mental Disorders*, Vol. 2, pp. 477–515. London: WHO Collaborating Centres in Mental Health.

Angst, J. (1992) The epidemiology of depressive disorder. *European Neuro-psychopharmacology* Suppl. 95–8.

Apley, J. (1974) *The Child with Abdominal Pain*, 2nd edn. Oxford: Blackwell Scientific Publications.

Appleby, L., Warner, R., Whitton, A. and Faragher, B. (1997) A controlled study of fluoxetine and cognitive-behavioural counselling in the treatment of postnatal depression. *British Medical Journal* **314(7085)**, 932–6.

Appleby, L., Koren, G. and Sharp, D. (1999) Depression in pregnant and postnatal women: an evidence-based approach to treatment in primary care. *British Journal of General Practice* **49(447)**, 780–2.

Aristotle (2000) *Physics* IV II 219 b1. Quoted in U. Eco Time. In: K Lippincott and U. Eco (eds) *The Story of Time*, pp. 10–15. London: Merrell Holberton.

Armstrong, D. (2000) The temporal body. In: R. Cooter and J. Pickstone (eds) *Medicine in the 20th Century*, pp. 247–59. Amsterdam: Harwood Academic Publishers.

Armstrong, K.L., Fraser, J.A., Dadds, M.R. and Morris, J. (1999) A randomized, controlled trial of nurse home visiting to vulnerable families with newborns. *Journal of Paediatrics and Child Health* **35**(3), 237–44.

Asberg, M., Traskman, L. and Thoren, P. (1976) 5-HIAA in cerebral spinal fluid: a biochemical suicide predictor? *Archives of General Psychiatry* **33**, 1193–7.

Asen, K.E. and Tomson, P. (1992) *Family Solutions in Family Practice*. Lancaster: Quay Books.

Asen, E. and Tomson, P. (1997) Getting into family systems medicine. *Thinking Families* **7**, 4–5.

Aveline, M., Shapiro, D.A., Parry, G. and Freeman, C.P.L. (1995) Building research foundations for psychotherapy practice. In: M. Aveline and D. A. Shapiro (eds) *Research Foundations for Psychotherapy Practice*. Chichester: Wiley.

Bacaltchuk, J., Trefiglio, R.P., de Oliveira, I.R., Lima, M.S. and Mari, J.J. (1999) Antidepressants versus psychotherapy for bulimia nervosa: a systematic review. *Journal of Clinical Pharmacology and Therapy* **24**, 23–31.

Bachrach, L.L. (1988) Defining chronic mental illness: a concept paper, *Hospital and Community Psychiatry*, **39**, pp. 383–8.

Balint, M. (1957) *The Doctor, His Patient and the Illness*, Millennium edition, 2000. Edinburgh: Churchill Livingstone.

Balint, E., Courtenay, M., Elder, A., Hull, S. and Julian, P. (1993) *The Doctor, the Patient and the Group. Balint Revisited*. London: Routledge.

Bammer, *et al.* (2000) The impact of retention of expansion of an Australian public methadone programme. *Drug and Alcohol Dependence* **58**, 173–80.

Banasiak, S.J., Paxton, S.J. and Hay, P.J. (2000) Cognitive-behavioural guided self-help for bulimia nervosa in primary care. Paper presented at the Academy of Eating Disorders, 9th International Conference on Eating Disorders, New York, 4–7 of May.

Barbee, R. and Feldman S. (1970) A three year longitudinal study of the medical interview and its relationship to student performance in clinical medicine. *Journal of Medical Education* **45**, 770–6.

Barkham, M. and Mellor-Clark, J. (2000) Rigour and relevance: the role of practice-based evidence in the psychological therapies. In: N. Rowland and S. Goss (eds) *Evidence-based Counselling and Psychological Therapies*. London: Routledge.

Barkham, M., Rees, A., Stiles, W.B., Shapiro, D.A. and Hardy, G.E. (1996) Dose-effect relations in time-limited psychotherapy for depression. *Journal of Consulting and Clinical Psychology* **64**, 927–35.

Barraclough, B. M., Bunch, J., Nelson, B., *et al.* (1974) A hundred cases of suicide: clinical aspects. *British Journal of Psychiatry* **125**, 355–73.

Bashir, K., Blizard, B., Bosanquet, A., Bosanquet, N., Mann, A. and Jenkins, R. (2000) The evaluation of a mental health facilitator in general practice: effects on recognition, management, and outcome of mental illness. *British Journal of General Practice* **50**, 626–9.

Bateson, G. (1972) *Steps to an Ecology of Mind*. New York: Ballantine Books.

Bazire, S. *The Psychotropic Drug Directory, The Professionals' Pocket Handbook and Aide Memoire 2000*. Lancaster: Quay Books.

Beitchman, J.H., Zucker, K.J., Hood, J.E., DaCosta, G.A. and Akman, D. (1992) A review of the long-term effects of child sexual abuse. *Child Abuse and Neglect* **16**, 101–18.

Bell, D. (1996) A primitive mind of state. *Psychoanalytic Psychotherapy* **7**, 1–11.

Bell, M. (1994) How primordial is narrative? In: C. Nash (ed.) *Narrative in Culture*, pp. 172–98. London: Routledge.

Berger, J. and Mohr, J. (1967) *A Fortunate Man: the story of a country doctor*. Harmondsworth: Penguin Press.

Berton, M.W. and Stabb, S.D. (1996) Exposure to violence and PTSD in urban adolescents. *Adolescence* **31**, 488–98.

Bhugra, D. (ed.) (1996) *Homelessness and Mental Health*. Cambridge: Cambridge University Press.

Bifulco, A., Moran, P.M., Ball, C. and Bernazzani, O. (2002) Adult attachment style: its relationship to clinical depression. *Social Psychiatry and Psychiatric Epidemiology* **37(2)**, 50–59.

Bifulco, A., Moran, P., Ball, C. and Jacobs, C. (2000) Attachment Style Interview (ASI). Unpublished manuscript.

Binns, M., Hobbs, M., Kosviner, A., McClean, E. and Parry, G. (1994) *Psychological Therapies for Adults in the NHS*, a joint statement by the British Psychological Society and the Psychotherapy Section of the Royal College of Psychiatrists.

Bion, W. (1967) *Second Thoughts*. London: Heinemann.

Birchwood M., Todd, P. and Jackson, C. (1998) Early intervention in psychosis. *British Journal of Psychiatry* **172** (suppl. 33), 53–59.

Bisaga, A. and Popik, P. (2000) In search of a new pharmacological treatment for drug and alcohol addiction: N-methyl-D-aspartate (NMDA) antagonists. *Drug and Alcohol Dependence*.

Bland, R.C. (1997) Epidemiology of affective disorders: a review. *Canadian Journal of Psychiatry – Revue Canadienne de Psychiatrie* **42**, 367–77.

Bloch, D.A. and Doherty, W.J. (1998) The collaborative family healthcare coalition. *Families, Systems and Health* **16**, 3–5.

Blondal, T., Gudmondsonn, L. J., Olafsdottir, I., Gustavsson, G. and Westin, A. (1999) Nicotine nasal spray with nicotine patch for smoking cessation: randomised trial with six year follow up. *British Medical Journal* **318**, 285–9.

Blum, J.D. (1978) On changes in psychiatric diagnosis over time. *American Psychologist* **33**, 1017–31.

Bond, T. (1995) The nature and outcomes of counselling. In: J. Keithley and G. Marsh (eds) *Counselling in Primary Health Care*. Oxford: Oxford University Press.

Bourne, S. (1976) Second opinion: a study of medical referrals in a seminar for general practitioners at the Tavistock Clinic, London. *Journal Royal College of GPs* **26**, 487–95.

Bower, P., Byford, S., Sibbald, B., Ward, E., King, M., Lloyd, M. and Gabbay, M. (2000) Randomised controlled trial of non-directive counselling, cognitive-behaviour therapy, and usual general practitioner care for patients with depression. II: Cost effectiveness. *British Medical Journal* **321**, 1389–92.

Bowlby, J. (1980) *Attachment, Separation and Loss. Vol. 3. Loss.* London: Hogarth.

Bowlby, J. (1982) *Attachment and Loss: Vol. I. Attachment*, 2nd edn. New York: Basic Books.

Bradbury, M. (2000) *To the Hermitage*. London: Picador.

Brazelton, T.B. (1992) *Touchpoints. Your Child's Emotional and Behavioural Development*. Harmondsworth: Penguin Books Ltd.

Bremner, J. (1999) Does stress damage the brain? *Biological Psychiatry* **45**, 797–805.

Breslau, N. (1998) Epidemiology of trauma and post-traumatic stress disorder. In: R. Yehuda (ed.) *Psychological Trauma*. Washington: American Psychiatric Press.

Brewin, C., Dalgleish, T and Joseph, S. (1996) A dual representation theory of post-traumatic stress disorder. *Psychological Review* **103**, 670–86.

Bridges, K. and Goldberg, D. (1985) Somatic presentations of DSM-3 psychiatric disorders in primary care. *Journal of Psychosomatic Research* **29**, 563–9.

Briscoe, M. (1986) Identification of emotional problems in postpartum women by health visitors. *British Medical Journal* **292**, 1245–7.

British Medical Association (2000) *Eating Disorders, Body Image and the Media*. London: BMJ Publications.

Britten, N. (1998) Psychiatry, stigma and resistance: psychiatrists need to concentrate on understanding, not simply compliance. *British Medical Journal* **317**, 763–4.

Brook, A. (1995) The eye and I: psychological aspects of disorders of the eye. *Journal of the Balint Society* **23**, 13–16.

Brook, A. and Temperley, J. (1976) The contribution of a psychotherapist to general practice. *Journal of the Royal College of General Practitioners* **26**, No. 163, 86–95.

Brook, A., Elder, A. and Zalidis, S. (1998) Psychological aspects of eye disorders. Turning a blind eye: some reflections on a multi-disciplinary seminar. *Journal of the Royal Society of Medicine* **19**, 47–53.

Brookfield, S. (1986) *Understanding and Facilitating Adult Learning*. Buckingham: Open University Press.

Broom, B. (1997) *Somatic Illness and the Patient's Other Story*. London: Free Association Books.

Browne, K. and Freeling, P. (1967) *The Doctor–Patient Relationship*. Edinburgh: E. and S. Livingstone.

Brugha, T.S., Wheatley, S., Taub, N.A., Culverwell, A., Friedman, T., Kirwan, P., *et al.* (2000) Pragmatic randomized trial of antenatal intervention to prevent post-natal depression by reducing psychosocial risk factors. *Psychological Medicine* **30**, 1273–81.

Brugha, T.S., Wing, J.K. and Smith, B.L. (1989) Physical health of the long-term mentally ill in the community. Is there unmet need? *British Journal of Psychiatry* **155**, 777–81.

Bryant-Waugh, R. and Lask, B. (1999) *Eating Disorders—A Parents Guide*. Harmondsworth: Penguin Books.

Buist, A., Westley, D. and Hill, C. (1999) Antenatal prevention of postnatal depression. *Archives of Womens Mental Health* **1**, 167–73.

Burd, M. (1996) A Model of Teamwork in the Community. In: K. Abel, M. Buszewicz, S. Davison, S. Johnson and E. Staples (eds) *Planning Community Mental Health Services for Women*. London: Routledge.

Burd, M. and Donnison, J. (1994) Partnership in Clinical Practice. *Clinical Psychology Forum* **63**, 22–5.

Burns, T. and Bale, R. (1997) Establishing a mental health liaison attachment with primary care. *Advances in Psychiatric Treatment*, **3**, 219–24.

Burns, T. and Cohen, A. (1998) Item-of-service payments for general practitioner care of severely mentally ill persons: does the money matter? *British Journal of General Practice* **48**, 1415–16.

Burns, T. and Kendrick, T. (1997) Care of long-term mentally ill patients by British general practitioners. *Psychiatric Services* **48**, 1586–8.

Burns, T., Millar, E., Garland, C., Kendrick, T., Chisholm, B. and Ross, F. (1998) Randomized controlled trial of teaching practice nurses to carry out structured assessments of patients receiving depot antipsychotic injections. *British Journal of General Practice* **48**, 1845–8.

Burton, M. (1998) *Psychotherapy, Counselling and Primary Care Assessment for Brief and Longer-term Treatment*. London: John Wiley.

Byrne, P. and Long, B. (1976) *Doctors Talking to Patients*. London: HMSO.

Calasso, R. (1994) *The Marriage of Cadmus and Harmony*. London: Vintage.

Calvino, I. (2000) *Why Read the Classics?* London: Vintage

Canguilhem, G. (1978) *On the Normal and the Pathological*. Dortrecht: Reidel Publishing Co.

Cape, J. and Parry, G. (2000) Clinical practice guidelines development in evidence-based psychotherapy. In: N. Rowland and S. Goss (eds) *Evidence-based Counselling and Psychological Therapies*. London: Routledge.

Cape, J., Hartley, J., Durrant, K., Patrick, M. and Graham, J. (1998) Development of local clinical practice guideline to assist GPs, counsellors and psychological therapists in matching patients to the most appropriate psychological treatment. *Journal of Clinical Effectiveness* **3**, 97–140.

Cape, J., Barker, C., Buszewicz, M. and Pistrang, N. (2000) General practitioner psychological management of common emotional problems (I): definitions and literature review. *British Journal of General Practice* **50**, 313–18.

Carnwath, T., Gabbay, M. and Barnard, J. (2000) A share of the action: general practitioner involvement in drug misuse treatment in Greater Manchester. *Drugs: education, prevention and policy* **7**, 235–50.

Carpenter, J. and Treacher, A. (1993) *Using Family Therapy in the Nineties*. Oxford: Blackwell.

Carroll, K.M. *et al.* (1998) Treatment of cocaine and alcohol dependence with psychotherapy and disulfiram. *Addiction* **93**, 713–28.

Carter, J.C. and Fairburn, C.G. (1998) Cognitive behavioural self help for binge eating disorder: a controlled effectiveness study. *Journal of Consulting and Clinical Psychology* **66**, 616–23.

Casey, P.R. (1989) Personality disorder and suicide intent. *Acta Psychiatrica Scandinavica* **79**, 290–5.

Cassano, G.B. *et al.* (1996) A randomised, double-blind study of alpidem vs placebo in the prevention and treatment of benzodiazepine withdrawal syndrome. *European Psychiatry* **11**, 93–9.

Cecchin, G. (1987) Hypothesising, circularity and neutrality revisited: an invitation to curiosity. *Family Process* **26**, 405–13.

Cecchin, G., Lane, G. and Ray, W.A. (1992) *Irreverence; a strategy for therapists' survival*. London: Karnac.

Chambers, R. and Campbell, I. (1996) Anxiety and depression in general practitioners: associations with type of practice, fundholding, gender and other personal characteristics. *Family Practice* **13**, 170–3.

Chaplin, R., Gordon, J., and Burns, T. (1999) Early detection of antipsychotic side-effects, *Psychiatric Bulletin* **23**, 657–60.

Christie-Seely, J. (ed.) (1984) *Working with the Family in Primary Care*. New York: Praeger.

Churchill, R., Dewey M., Gretton, V., Chilvers, C. and Lee, A. (1999) Should general practitioners refer patients with major depression to counsellors? A review of current published evidence. *British Journal of General Practice* **49**, 738–43.

Clarke, G. (1995) Improving the transition from basic efficacy research to effectiveness studies: methodological issues and procedures. *Journal of Consulting and Clinical Psychology* **63**, 718–25.

Coccaro, E.F., Siever, L.J., Klar, H.M., Muarer, G., *et al*. (1989) Serotonergic studies in patients with affective and personality disorders: correlates with suicidal and impulsive aggressive behaviour. *Archives of General Psychiatry* **46**, 587–99.

Cogill, S.R., Caplan, H.L., Alexandra, H., Robson, K.M. and Kumar, R. (1986) Impact of maternal postnatal depression on cognitive- development of young-children. *British Medical Journal* **292(6529)**, 1165–7.

Cole-Kelly, K. (1992) Illness stories and patient care in the family practice context. *Family Medicine* **24**, 45–8.

Cooper, P. (1993) *Bulimia Nervosa*. London: Robinson.

Cooper, P.J. and Murray, L. (1997) Prediction, detection, and treatment of postnatal depression. *Archives of Disease in Childhood* **77(2)**, 97–9.

Cooper, P.J. and Murray, L. (2000a) A controlled trial of the long term effect of psychological treatment of postpartum depression: I impact on maternal mood. *British Journal of Psychiatry* **183**, 77–84.

Cooper, P.J. and Murray, L. Preventive intervention for postpartum depression: a controlled trial. *In preparation*.

Cooper, P.J., Coker, S. and Fleming, C. (1996a) An evaluation of the efficacy of supervised cognitive behavioural self-help for bulimia nervosa. *Journal of Psychosomatic Research* **40**, 281–7.

Cooper, P.J., Murray, L., Hooper, R. and West, A. (1996b) The development and validation of a predictive index for postpartum depression. *Psychological Medicine* **26**, 627–34.

Cooper, P.J., Tomlinson, M., Swartz, L., Woolgar, M., Murray, L. and Molteno, C. (1999) Post-partum depression and the mother-infant relationship in a South African peri-urban settlement. *British Journal of Psychiatry* **175**, 554–8.

Counsellors in Primary Care (2000) Professional Counselling and Primary care: guidelines and protocols.

Coupland, N.J., Bell, C.J. and Potokar, J.P. (1996) Serotonin reuptake inhibitor withdrawal. *Journal of Clinical Psychopharmacology* **16**, 356–62.

Courtenay, M.J.F. and Hare, M. (1978) Difficult doctors. *Journal of the Balint Society* **7**, 14–18.

Cox, J.L., Holden, J.M. and Sagovsky, R. (1987) Detection of postnatal depression—development of the 10-item Edinburgh Postnatal Depression Scale. *British Journal of Psychiatry* **150**, 782–6.

Cox, J.L., Murray, D. and Chapman, G. (1993) A controlled-study of the onset, duration and prevalence of postnatal depression. *British Journal of Psychiatry* **163**, 27–31.

Crisp, A.H., Joughin, N., Halek, C. and Bowyer, C. (1996) *Anorexia Nervosa. The Wish to Change.* Hove: Psychology Press.

Crome, I.B. (Guest ed.) (1999a) Special Issue Substance misuse and young people: substance misuse and young people. Treatment interventions: looking towards the millenium. *Drug and Alchol Dependence,* **55**, 247–63.

Crome, I.B. (Guest ed.) (1999b) Substance misuse and psychiatric comorbidity: towards improved service provision. *Drugs Education Prevention and Policy* **6**, 151–74.

Cromwell O. (1650) Letter to the General Assembly of the Church of Scotland, 3 Aug.

Cronen, V.E., Johnson, K.M. and Lannamann, J.W. (1982) Paradoxes, double binds, and reflexive loops: an alternative theoretical perspective. *Family Process* **21**, 91–112.

Cryer, C. P., Jenkins, L. M., Cook, A. C., Ditchburn, J. S., Harris, C. K., Davis, A. R. and Peters, T. J. (1999). The use of acute and preventative medical services, by a general population: relationship with alcohol consumption. *Addiction,* **94**, 1523–32.

Cutrona, C.E. and Troutman, B.R. (1986) Social support, infant temperament, and parenting self-efficacy—a mediational model of postpartum depression. *Child Development* **57**, 1507–18.

Damasio, A (2000) *The Feeling of What Happens.* New York: William Heinemann.

Dammers, J. and Wiener, J. (2001) Developing a role for counselling in the primary care team. In: J. Keithley and G. Marsh (eds) *Counselling in Primary Health Care,* 2nd edn. Oxford: Oxford University Press.

Dane, G. (1998) *Reading Ophelia's Madness.* London: Pegasus Press.

Davidson, J. *et al.* (1991) PTSD in the community. *Psychological Medicine* **21**, 713–21.

Davies, M.L. (1997) Shattered assumptions: time and the experience of long-term HIV positivity. *Social Science Medicine* **44**, 561–71.

Davies, P. (2000) General practitioners' main interest is people. *British Medical Journal* **321**, 173.

Davies, R., Olmsted, M.P. and Rockert, W. (1990) Brief group psychoeducation for bulimia nervosa: assessing the clinical significance of change. *Journal of Consulting and Clinical Psychology* **58**, 882–5.

Davis, J.M., Schaffer, C.B., Killian, G.A., Kinard, C. and Chan, C. (1980) Important issues in the drug treatment of schizophrenia, *Schizophrenia Bulletin,* **6**, 70–87.

Davis, M.D., Wagner, E.G. and Groves, T. (2000) Advances in managing chronic disease. *British Medical Journal* **320(7234)**, 525–6.

Dawe, S., Gerada, C. and Strang, J. (1992). Establishment of a laison service for pregnant opiate dependent women. *British Journal of Addiction,* **87**, 867–71.

Day, C. and Wren, B. (1994) Journey to the center of primary care: primary care psychology in perspective. *Clinical Psychology Forum* **63**, 3–6.

De Rubeis, R.J. and Crits-Christoph, P. (1998) Empirically supported individual and group treatments for adult mental disorders. *Journal of Consulting and Clinical Psychology* **66**, 37–52.

De Zwaan, M., Bailer, U., El-Giamal, N., Leenkh, C. and Strand, A. (2000) Guided self-help versus cognitive behavioural, group therapy in the treatment of bulimia nervosa. Paper presented at the World Psychiatric Congress, Paris France, 26–30 June, 2000.

Department of Health (1992) *Health and Personal Social Services statistics for England.* London, HMSO.

Department of Health (1995) *Sensible Drinking: the report of an interdepartmental working group.* London: Department of Health.

Department of Health (1998b) *A Contract for Health: Our Healthier Nation.* London, HMSO.

Department of Health (1996a) *A Review of Strategic Policy on NHS Psychotherapy Services in England.* London: NHS Executive.

Department of Health (1996b) *Task Force to Review Services for Drug Misusers. Report of an Independent Review of Drug Treatment Services in England.* London: HMSO.

Department of Health (1999) Research and Development in the NHS: A Srategic Review. London: HMSO.

Department of Health (1999a) *National Service Framework for Mental Health.* London: HMSO.

Department of Health (1999b) *Saving Lives: Our Healthier Nation.* London. HMSO.

Department of Health (1999c) *Drug Misuse and Dependence—Guidelines on Clinical Management.* London: HMSO.

Department of Health (2001) *Treatment Choice in Psychological Therapies and Counselling: an evidence-based clinical practice guideline.* London: HMSO.

Deys, C., Dowling, E. and Golding, V. (1989) Clinical psychology: a consultative approach in general practice. *Journal of the Royal College of General Practitioners* **39**, 342–4.

Dickinson, L.M., deGruy, F.V. Dickinson, P. and Candib, L (1998) Complex post-traumatic stress disorder: evidence from the primary care setting. *General Hospital Psychiatry* **20**, 214–24.

Diego, M. and Field, T. (2000) *Biochemical Profiles and Activity Levels of Fetuses of Depressed Mothers.* Paper presented at the International Conference on Infant Studies, Brighton, UK.

Dinan, T.G. (1999) The physical consequences of depressive illness. *British Medical Journal* **318**, 826.

Doll, R., Peto, R., Hall, E., Wheatley, K. and Gray, R. (1994) Mortality in relation to consumption of alcohol: 13 years' observations on male British doctors. *British Medical Journal* **309**, 911–18.

Doran, C.M. *et al.* (1998) General practitioners' role in preventive medicine: scenario analysis using smoking as a case study. *Addiction* **93**, 1013–22.

Douglas, J. (1992) *How to Treat your Doctor:* London: Bloomsbury.

Dowling, E. (1994) Closing the gap: consulting in a general practice. In: C. Huffington and H. Brunning (eds) *Internal Consultancy in the Public Sector: case studies,* pp. 75–86. London: Karnac.

Doyle, R. (1996) *The Woman Who Walked Into Doors.* London: Jonathan Cape.

Drake, R.E., Mercer-McFadden, C., Mueser, K.T., McHugo, G.J. and Bond, G.R. (1998) Review of integrated mental health and substance abuse treatment for patients with dual disorders. *Schizophrenia Bulletin* **24(4)**, 589–608.

Draper, J. and Weaver, S. (1999) Exploring blocks to effective communication in the medical interview. *Education for General Practice* **10**, 14–20.

Drummond, C.D., and Moncrieff, J. (1997). New drug treatments for alcohol problems: a critical appraisal, *Addiction*, **92(8)**, 939–49.

Drummond, C.D., and Ghodse, H. (1999) use of investigations in the diagnosis and management of alcohol use disorders. *Advances in Psychiatric Treatment,* **5**, 366–75.

Drummond, D.C., Thom, B., Brown, C., Edward, G. and Mullan, M. (1990) Specialist versus general practitioner treatment of alcohol drinkers. *Lancet* **336**, 915–18.

Dymond (in prep.) *Moderators of Outcome Following a Preventive Intervention for Postpartum Depression.* Reading: University of Reading.

East, P. (1995) *Counselling in Medical Settings.* Buckingham: Open University Press.

Eastaugh, A., Higginson, I. and Webb, D. (1998) Palliative care communication workshops for general practitioners and district nurses. *Education for General Practice* **9**, 331–6.

Eastman, N. (1999) Who should take responsibility for antisocial personality disorder? *British Medical Journal* **318**, 206–7.

Edwards, G., Marshall, E.J. and Cook, C.C.H. (1997) *The Treatment of Drinking Problems.* London: Gaskell.

Egeland, B. and Erickson, M.F. (1990) Rising above the past: strategies for helping new mothers break the cycle of abuse and neglect. *Zero to Three* **11**, 29–35.

Eisler, I., Dare, C., Hodes, M., Russell, G., Dodge, E. and Le Grange, D. (2000) *Family therapy for adolescent anorexia nervosa: the result of a controlled comparison of two family interventions.* Journal Child Psychol Psychiatry **41**, 727–36.

Elder, A. (1987) Moments of change. In: A. Elder and O. Samuel (eds) *While I'm Here, Doctor. A Study of the Doctor Patient Relationship.* London: Tavistock Press.

Elder, A. (1996) Primary care and psychotherapy. In: Conference Proceedings: Future directions of psychotherapy in the NHS: Adaptation or Extinction. *Psychoanalytic Psychotherapy* Suppl., **10**.

Elliot, S.A., Leverton, T.J., Sanjack, M., Turner, H., Cowmeadow, P., Hopkins, J. and Bushnell, D. (2000) Promoting mental health after childbirth: a controlled trial of primary prevention and postnatal depression. *British Journal of Clinical Psychology* **39(3)**, 223–41.

Engel, G.L. (1997) The need for a new medical model: a challenge to biomedicine. *Science* **196**, 129–36.

Evans, J., Reeves, B., Platt, H., Liebenau, A., Goldman, D., Jefferson, K. *et al.* (2000) Impulsiveness, serotonin genes and repetition of deliberate self harm (DSH). *Psychological Medicine* **30**, 1327–34.

Evans, M.O., Morgan, H.G., Hayward, A. and Gunnell, D.J. (1999) Crisis telephone consultation for deliberate self harm patients: effects on repetition. *British Journal of Psychiatry* **175**, 23–7.

Eysenck, H.J. (1952) The effects of psychotherapy: an evaluation. *Journal of Consulting Psychology* **16**, 319–24.

Fairburn, C.G. (1995) *Overcoming Binge Eating.* Guildford: New York.

Farrell, E. (1995) *Lost for Words.* London: Process Press Ltd.

Farthing, M.J.G. (1995) Irritable bowel, irritable body, or irritable brain? *British Medical Journal* **310**, 171–5.

Feeney, A.J. and Nutt, D.J. (1999) Current pharmacological approaches to anxiety. *Prescriber* **10(22)**, 69–80.

Feeney, J.A. and Noller, P. (1990) Attachment style as a predictor of adult romantic relationships. *Journal of Personality and Social Psychology* **58**, 281–91.

Ferriman, A. (2000) The stigma of schizophrenia. *British Medical Journal* **320**, 522.

Field, T. (1992) Infants of depressed mothers. *Development and Psychopathology* **4**, 49–66.

Field, T.M., Sandberg, D., Garcia, R., Vegalahr, N., Goldstein, S. and Guy, L. (1985) Pregnancy problems, postpartum depression, and early mother infant interactions. *Developmental Psychology* **21**, 1152–6.

Field, T.M., Healy, B., Goldstein, S. and Perry, S. (1988) Infants of depressed mothers show 'depressed' behaviour. *Child Development* **59**, 1569–79.

Field, T.M. (1984) Early interactions between infants and their postpartum depressed mums. *Infant Behaviour and Development* **7**, 517–22.

Finney, J.W., Hahn, A. and Moos, R.H. (1996) The effectiveness of inpatient and outpatient treatment for alcohol abuse: the need to focus on mediators and moderators of setting effects. *Addiction*, **91**, 1773–97.

Fonagy, P., Leigh, T., Steele, M., Steele, H., Kennedy, R., Mattoon, G. *et al.* (1996) The relation of attachment status, psychiatric classification, and response to psycho-therapy. *Journal of Consulting and Clinical Psychology* **64(1)**, 22–31.

Ford, J. and Kidd, P. (1998) Early childhood trauma and disorders of extreme stress as predictors of outcome with chronic PTSD. *Journal of Traumatic Stress* **11**, 743–63.

Forshall, S. and Nutt, D.J. (1999) Maintenance pharmacotherapy of unipolar depression. *Psychiatric Bulletin* **23(6)**, 370–3.

Foster, T., Gillespie, K. and McClelland, R. (1997) Mental disorders and suicide in Northern Ireland. *British Journal of Psychiatry* **170**, 447–52.

Fraise, P. (1963) *The Psychology of Time*. London: Eyre and Spottiswode.

Frankl, V (1959) *Man's Search for Meaning*, 3rd edn. New York: Simon and Schuster/Touchstone Books.

Freeling, P. and Barry, S. (1982) *In-service Training—a Study of the Nuffield Courses of the Royal College of General Practitioners*. Windsor: NFER-Nelson Publishing.

Friedli, K. and King, M. (1996) Counselling in general practice—a review. *Primary Care Psychiatry* **2**, 205–16.

Fugelli, P. (1999) *Rød resept. Essays om perfeksjon, prestasjon og helse*, p. 14. Oslo: TanoAschehoug.

Gadamer, H-G. (1996) *The Enigma of Health. The Art of Healing in a Scientific Age*.

Gannick, D. (1995) Situational disease. *Family Practice* **12**, 202–8.

Gask, L., Sibbald, B. and Creed, F. (1997) Evaluating models of working at the interface between mental health services and primary care. *British Journal of Psychiatry* **170**, 6–11.

Geddes, J., Freemantle, N., Harrison, P. and Bebbington, P. (2000) Atypical antipsy-chotics in the treatment of schizophrenia: systematic overview and meta-regression analysis. *British Medical Journal* **321**, 1371–6.

Geddes, M. and Medway, J. (1977) The symbolic drawing of the family life space. *Family Process* **16**, 219–28.

General Medical Council (1993) *Tomorrow's Doctors*. London: General Medical Council.

George, C. and West, M. (1999) Developmental vs. social personality models of adult attachment and mental ill health. *British Journal of Medical Psychology* **72**, 285–303.

George, C., Kaplan, N. and Main, M. (1985) Adult Attachment Interview. Unpublished manuscript.

Gerrard, J., Holden, J.M., Elliott, S.A., McKenzie, P., McKenzie, J. and Cox, J.L. (1993) A trainers perspective of an innovative program teaching health visitors about the detection, treatment and prevention of postnatal depression. *Journal of Advanced Nursing* **18**, 1825–32.

Ghodse, A.H. (1997) *Drugs and Addictive Behaviour A Guide to Treatment*, 2nd edn.

Gibbons, J.S., Butler, J., Urwin, P. *et al.* (1978) Evaluation of a social work service for self-poisoning patients. *British Journal of Psychiatry* **133**, 111–18.

Gillman, P.K. (1999) The serotonin syndrome and its treatment. *Journal of Psychopharmacology* **13**, 100–9.

Glover, V. and Gitau, R. (2000) *Fetal and Maternal Hormonal Stress Responses*. Paper presented at the International Conference on Infant Studies, Brighton, UK.

Goldberg, D. and Huxley, P. (1992) *Common Mental Disorders*. London: Routledge.

Goldberg, D. and Gourney, K. (1997) *The General Practitioner, the Psychiatrist and the Burden of Mental Health Care*, Maudsley Discussion Paper No. 1. London: Maudsley Hospital.

Good, B.J. (2000) Clinical narratives and the study of contemporary doctor–patient relationships. In: G. L. Albrecht, R. Fitzpatrick and S. C. Scrimshaw (eds) *Handbook of Social Studies in Health and Medicine*, p. 246. London: Sage.

Goodlad, S. (ed.) (1995) *Students as Tutors and Mentors*. London: Kogan Page.

Good, M.J.D. and Good, B.J. (2000) Clinical narratives and the study of contemporary doctor-patient relationships. In: G.L. Albrecht, R. Fitzpatrick and S.C. Scrimshaw (eds) *Handbook of Social Studies in Health and Medicine*. London: Sage.

Goody, J. (1968) Time; social organisation. In: D. L. Sills (ed.) *The International Encyclopaedia of the Social Sciences*. London: Macmillan Co.

Gordon, P. and Plamping, D. (1996) Primary health care: its characteristics and potential. In: P. Gordon and D. Plamping (ed.) *Extending Primary Care*. Oxford: Radcliffe.

Graham, H. and Sher, M. (1976) Social work and general medical practice: personal accounts of a three-year attachment. *British Journal of Social Work* **6**, 2–8.

Graham, H., Senior, R., Lazarus, M. and Mayer, R. (1992) Family therapy in general practice: views of referrers and clients. *Journal of the Royal College of General Practitioners* **45**, 25–8.

Gray, D.P. (1994) In: I. Pullen, G. Wilkinson, A. Wright and D. P. Gray (eds) *Psychiatry and General Practice Today*. London: Royal College of Psychiatrists/Royal College of General Practitioners.

Gray, R.P.A.P.S. *et al.* (1999) A national survey of practice nurse involvement in mental health interventions. *Journal of Advanced Nursing*, **30**, 901–6.

Greco, M., Buckley, J. and Francis, W. (1997) Triads: an effective method for learning the art of listening. *Education for General Practice* **8**, 329–34.

Greenhalgh, T. and Hurwitz, B. (1998) Why study narrative? In: T. Greenhalgh and B. Hurwitz (eds) *Narrative Based Medicine*, pp. 3–16. London: BMJ Books.

Grol, R. (1981) *To Heal or to Harm*. London: Royal College of General Practitioners.

Groves, J.E. (1978) Taking care of the hateful patient. *New England Journal of Medicine* **298**, 883–8.

Gunnell, D.J., Peters, T.J., Kammerling, R.M. and Brooks, J. (1995) Relation between parasuicide, suicide, psychiatric inpatient admission, and socioeconomic deprivation. *British Medical Journal* **311**, 226–30.

Hackman, A. (1993) Behavioural and cognitive psychotherapies: past history, current applications and future registration issues. *Behavioural and Cognitive Psychotherapy*, Suppl. 1, 16–21.

Haddad, P., Lejoyeux, M. and Young, A. (1998) Antidepressant discontinuation reactions. *British Medical Journal* **316**, 1105–6.

Haley, J. (1976) *Problem-solving Therapy*. San Francisco: Jossey-Bass.

Hallett, C. (1995) Child abuse: an academic overview. In: P. Kingston and B. Penhale (eds) *Family Violence and the Caring Professions*. London: Macmillan.

Hallstrom, C. (1993) *Benzodiazepine Dependence*. Oxford: Oxford University Press.

Hambling, S. (1998) In: A. Hibble (ed.) *Report on the Second Cambridge Conference on Higher Professional Education for General Practice*. Cambridge: Office of Postgraduate General Practice Education, Anglia Deanery.

Hardy, G.E., Aldridge, J., Davidson, C., Rowe, C., Reilly, S. and Shapiro, D.A. (1999) Therapist responsiveness to client attachment styles and issues observed in client-identified significant events in psychodynamic-interpersonal psychotherapy. *Psychotherapy Research* **9**, 36–53.

Harris, E.C. and Barraclough, B. (1997) Suicide as an outcome for mental disorders. A meta-analysis. *British Journal of Psychiatry* **170**, 205–28.

Haste, F., Charlton, J., and Jenkins, R. (1998) Potential for suicide prevention in Primary Care? An analysis of factors associated with suicide. *British Journal of General Practice* **48(436)**, 1759–63.

Hawton, K., Townsend, E., Arensman, E., Gunnell, D., Hazell, P., House, A. *et al.* (2000) Psychosocial versus pharmacological treatments for deliberate self harm (Cochrane review), In: *The Cochrane Library*, Issue 3. Oxford: Update Software.

Hay, P.J. and Bacaltchuk, J. (2000) Psychotherapy for bulimia nervosa and binging (Cochrane Review) In: *The Cochrane Library*, Issue 1. Oxford: Update Software.

Hazan, C. and Shaver, P. (1987) Romantic love conceptualized as an attachment process. *Journal of Personality and Social Psychology* **52**, 511–24.

Heaney, S. (1995) *Crediting Poetry: the Nobel Lecture 1995*. Oldcastle: Gallery Press.

Heath, I. (1995) *The Mystery of General Practice*. London: Nuffield Provincial Hospitals Trust.

Heath, I. (1998) Following the story. In: T. Greenhalgh and B. Hurwitz (eds) *Narrative Based Medicine*, pp. 93–102. London: BMJ Books.

Heath, I. (1999) There must be limits to the medicalisation of human distress. *British Medical Journal* **318**, 440.

Heath, I. (2000) Dereliction of duty in an ageist society. *British Medical Journal* **320**, 1422.

Heidegger, M. (2000) *Being and Time*. Oxford: Blackwell.

Heinicke, C.M., Fineman, N.R., Ruth, G., Recchia, S.L., Guthrie, D. and Rodning, C. (1999) Relationship-based intervention with at-risk mothers: outcome in the first year of life. *Infant Mental Health Journal* **20**, 349–74.

Herman, J. (1992) A syndrome in survivors of prolonged and repeated trauma. *Journal of Traumatic Stress* **5**, 377–91.

Herz, M.I. and Lamberti, J.S. (1995) Prodromal symptoms and relapse prevention in schizophrenia. *Schizophrenia Bulletin* **21**, 541–51.

Herz, M.I., Lamberti, J.S., Mintz, J., Scott, R., O'Dell, S.P., McCartan, L. *et al.* (2000) A program for relapse prevention in schizophrenia: a controlled study. *Archives of General Psychiatry* **57**, 277–83.

Herzog, W., Deter, H.C., Fiehn, W. and Petzold, E. (1997) Medical findings and predictors of long-term physical outcome in anorexia nervosa: a prospective, 12-year follow-up study. *Psychological Medicine* **27**, 269–79.

Hill, K. (1995) *The Long Sleep: young people and suicide*. London: Virago Press.

Hodgkin, P. (1996) Medicine, postmodernism, and the end of certainty. *British Medical Journal* **313**, 1568–9.

Holden, J.M., Sagovsky, R. and Cox, J.L. (1989) Counseling in a general-practice setting—controlled-study of health visitor intervention in treatment of postnatal depression. *British Medical Journal* **298(6668)**, 223–6.

Holland, J. (1995) *A Doctor's Dilemma: stress and the role of the carer*. London: Free Association Books.

Holloway, F. (1988) Prescribing for the long-term mentally ill. A study of treatment practices. *British Journal of Psychiatry* 152, pp. 511–15.

Holmes, J. (1993) *John Bowlby and Attachment Theory*. London: Routledge.

Holmes, J. (1996) *Attachment, Intimacy, Autonomy*. New York: Jason Aronson.

Holmes, J. (1998a) The changing aims of psychoanalytic psychotherapy: an integrative perspective. *International Journal of Psycho-Analysis* **79**, 227–41.

Holmes, J. (1998b) The psychotherapy department and the community mental health team: bridges and boundaries. *Psychiatric Bulletin* **22**, 729–32.

Holmes, J. and Mitchison, S. (1995) A model for an integrated psychotherapy service. *Psychiatric Bulletin* **19**, 209–13.

Holmes, R. (1998b) *Coleridge—Darker reflections*. London: Harper Collins.

Horowitz, M. (1978) *Stress Response Syndromes*, 2nd edn. New Jersey: Northvale.

Howard, K.I., Leuger, R., Maling, M. and Martinovich, Z. (1993) A phase model of psychotherapy: causal mediation of outcome. *Journal of Consulting and Clinical Psychology* **61**, 678–85.

Howie, J.G.R., Heaney D.J., Maxwell, M., Walker, J.J., Freeman, G.K. and Rai, H. (1999) Quality at general practice consultations: cross sectional survey. *British Medical Journal* **319**, 738–43.

Hunter, K.M. (1991) *Doctors' Stories*. Princeton: Princeton University Press.

Hurwitz, B. (2000) Narrative and the practice of medicine. *Lancet* **356**, 2086–9.

Huygen, F.J.A. (1978) *Family Medicine. The Medical Life History of Families*. London: Royal College of General Practitioners.

Irvine, H., Bradley, T., Cupples, M. and Boohan, M. (1997) The implications of teenage pregnancy and motherhood for primary health care: unresolved issues. *British Journal of General Practice* **47(418)**, 323–6.

Jacobson, A. and Richardson, B. (1987) Assault experiences of 100 psychiatric in-patients: evidence of the need for routine inquiry. *American Journal of Psychiatry* **144**, 908–13.

James, W. (1956) The dilemma of determinism. In: W. James (ed.) *The Will to Believe and Other Essays in Popular Philosophy*, pp. 145–83. Dover: New York.

Jaques, E. (1965) Death and the mid-life crisis. *International Journal of Psycho-Analysis* **46**, 502–14.

Jenkins, H. (1989) Family therapy with one person: a systemic framework for treating individuals. *Psihoterapija* **19**, 61–3.

Jenkins, H., and Asen, K.E. (1992) Family therapy without the family: a framework for systemic practice. *Journal of Family Therapy* **14**, 1–14.

Jenkins, R., Bebbington, P., Brugha, T.S., Farrell, M., Lewis, G. and Metzler, H. (1998) British psychiatric morbidity study. *British Journal of Psychiatry* **173**, 4–7.

Johnson, D.A. (1981) Studies of depressive symptoms in schizophrenia, *British Journal of Psychiatry* 139, 89–101.

Johnson, S. and Thornicroft, G. (1993) The sectorisation of psychiatric services in England and Wales. *Social Psychiatry and Psychiatric Epidemiology* 28, 45–7.

Johnstone, E.C., Frith, C.D., Leary, J., Owens, D.G., Wilkins, S. and Hershon, H.I. (1991) Background, method, and general description of the sample. *British Journal of Psychiatry* Suppl. **13**, 7–6.

Jones, B. (1990) Working together: a description of residential multidisciplinary workshops. *Postgraduate Education for General Practice* **1**, 154–9.

Kane, J.M., Honigfeld, G., Singer J. and Meltzer, H.Y. (1988) Clozapine and the treatment-resistant schizophrenic: double-blind comparison with chlorpromazine. *Archives of General Psychology* **45**, 789–96.

Keilen, M., Treasure, T., Schmidt, U. and Treasure, J. (1994) Quality of life measurements in eating disorders, angina, and transplant candidates: are they comparable? *Journal of the Royal Society of Medicine* **87**, 441–4.

Keithley, J., Bond, T. and March, G. (2002) Counselling in primary care, 2nd edn. Oxford: Oxford University Press.

Kendrick, T. (1996) Cardiovascular and respiratory risk factors and symptoms among general practice patients with long-term mental illness. *British Journal of Psychiatry* **169**, 733–9.

Kendrick, T. (2000) Why can't GPs follow guidelines on depression? *British Medical Journal* **320**, 200–1.

Kendrick, T., Sibbald, B., Burns, T. and Freeling, P. (1991) Role of general practitioners in care of long term mentally ill patients. *British Medical Journal* **302(6775)**, 508–10.

Kendrick, T., Burns, T., Freeling, P. and Sibbald, B. (1994) Provision of care to general practice patients with disabling long-term mental illness: a survey in 16 practices. *British Journal of General Practice* **44(384)**, 301–5.

Kendrick, T., Burns, T. and Freeling, P. (1995) Randomised controlled trial of teaching general practitioners to carry out structured assessments of their long term mentally ill patients. *British Medical Journal* **311(6997)**, 93–8.

Kendrick, T., Burns, T., Garland, C., Greenwood, N. and Smith, P. (1999) Are specialist mental health services being targeted on the most needy patients? The effects of setting up special services in general practice. *British Journal of General Practice* (In press).

Kermode, F. (1968) *The Sense of Ending*. Oxford: Oxford University Press.

Kernberg, O. (1999) Psychoanalysis, psychoanalytic psychotherapy and supportive psychotherapy: contemporary controversies. *International Journal of Psychoanalysis* **80**, 1075–91.

Kessler, D., Lloyd, K., Lewis, G. and Pereira Gray, D. (1999) Cross sectional study of symptom attribution and recognition of depression and anxiety in primary care *British Medical Journal* **318**, 436–40.

King, L.S. (1992a) *Medical Thinking*. Princeton: Princeton University Press.

King, M. and Nazareth, I. (1996) Community care of patients with schizophrenia: the role of the primary health care team. *British Journal of General Practice* **46(405)**, 231–7.

King, M., Sibbald, B., Ward, E., Bower, P., Lloyd, M., Gabbay, M. and Byford, S. (2000) Randomised controlled trial of non-directive counselling, cognitive-behaviour therapy and usual general practitioner care in the management of depression as well as mixed anxiety and depression in primary care. *National Coordinating Centre for Health Technology Assessment* **4**, 83–9.

King, M.B. (1989) Eating disorders in a general practice population. Prevalence, characteristics and follow-up at 12–18 months. *Psychological Medicine* Suppl. **14**, 16–22.

King, M.B. (1992) Management of patients with schizophrenia in general practice (Editorial). *British Journal of General Practice* **42(361)**, 310–11.

Kirwan, M. and Armstrong, D. (1995) Investigation of burnout in a sample of British general practitioners. *British Journal of General Practice* **45**, 259–60.

Kleinman, A. (1987) Anthropology and psychiatry: the role of culture in cross-cultural research on mental illness. *British Journal of Psychiatry* **151**, 447–54.

Knowles, J. (1997) 'The Reading model': an integrated psychotherapy service. *Psychiatric Bulletin* **21**, 84–7.

Kobak, R.R. and Hazan, C. (1991) Attachment in marriage—effects of security and accuracy of working models. *Journal of Personality and Social Psychology* **60**, 861–9.

Kopta, S.M., Howard K.I., Lowry, J.L. and Beutler, L.E. (1994) Patterns of symptomatic recovery in psychotherapy. *Journal of Consulting and Clinical Psychology* **62**, 1009–16.

Kreitman, N., and Foster, J., (1991) The construction and selection of predictive scales, with special reference to parasuicide. *British Journal of Psychiatry* **159**, 185–192.

Kuhn, T.S. (1967) *The Structure of Scientific Revolutions*. Chicago: University of Chicago Press.

Kuipers, L. and Bebbington, P. (1988) Expressed emotion research in schizophrenia: theoretical and clinical implications. *Psychological Medicine* **18**, 893–909.

Kutz, I. *et al.* (1994) PTSD in myocardial infarction patients: prevalence study. *Israel Journal of Psychiatry and related science*, **31**, 48–56.

Lamarque, P. (1994) Narrative and invention: the limits of fictionality. In: C. Nash (ed.) *Narrative in Culture*, pp. 131–55. London: Routledge.

Landabaso, M.A. *et al.* (1998) A randomised trial of adding fluoxetine to a naltrexone treatment programme for heroin addicts. *Addiction* **93**, 739–44.

Launer, J. (1994) Psychotherapy in the GP surgery: with and without a secure therapeutic frame. *British Journal of Psychotherapy* **11**, 120–6.

Launer, J. (1996) Towards Systemic General Practice. *Context* **26**, 42–5.

Launer, J. (1998a) Teaching systemic general practice: a guide to conducting group exercises. *Education for General Practice*, **9**, 344–347.

Launer, J. (1998b) Teaching systemic general practice: some basic exercises. *Education for General Practice* **9**, 441–3.

Launer, J. (1999a) Teaching systemic general practice: developing interview skills. *Education for General Practice* **10**, 72–5.

Launer, J. (1999b) Teaching systemic general practice: using supervisors and teams. *Education for General Practice* **10**, 176–9.

Launer, J. (1999c) Teaching systemic general practice: developing skills for complex problems. *Education for General Practice* **10**, 282–6.

Launer, J. and Lindsey C. (1997) Training for systemic general practice: a new approach from the Tavistock Clinic. *British Journal of General Practice* **47**, 453–456.

Leach, E.R. (1971) *Rethinking Anthropology*. London: LSE Monographs.

Le Doux, J.E. (1998) *The Emotional Brain: The Mysterious Underpinnings of Emotional Life*. London: Weidenfeld & Nicholson.

Leff, J. (1994) Working with the families of schizophrenic patients. *British Journal of Psychiatry* Suppl **23**, 73–6.

Leff, J., Vearnals, S., Wolff, G., Alexander, B., Chisholm, D., Everitt, B. *et al.* (2000) The London Depression Intervention Trial: randomised controlled trial of antidepressants *v.* couple therapy in the treatment and maintenance of people with depression living with a partner: clinical outcome and costs. *British Journal of Psychiatry* **177**, 95–100.

Lester, D. (1995) The concentration of neurotransmitter metabolites in the cerebrospinal fluid of suicidal individuals: a meta-analysis. *Pharmacopsychiatry* **28**, 45–50.

Levinas, E. (1969) *Totality and Infinity*. Pittsburgh: Dusquesne University Press.

Lewis, G. and Appleby, L. (1988) Personality disorder: the patients psychiatrists dislike. *British Journal of Psychiatry.*

Lieberman, J.A., Saltz, B.L., Johns, C.A. *et al.* (1991) The effects of clozapine on tardive dyskinesia. *British Journal of Psychiatry* **158**, 503–10.

Ling, W., Charuvastra C., Collius, J.F. *et al.* (1998) Buprenorphine maintenance treatment of opiate dependence: a multicenter randomised clinical trial. *Addiction*, **93**, 475–86.

Livesey, P.G. (1996) *The GP Consultation*. Oxford: Butterworth Heinemann.

Louden, P. and Graham, H. (1998) Working with an elderly couple: thinking families. *Context* **12**, 39–43.

MacIntyre, A. (1981) *After Virtue: a study in moral theory*. London: Duckworth.

Mackay, H., and Barkham, M. (1998) *Report to the National Counselling and Psychological Therapies Clinical Guidelines Development Group: evidence from published reviews and meta-analyses, 1990–98*. Leeds: Psychological Therapies Research Centre, University of Leeds.

Main, M. and Goldwyn, R. (1991) Adult attachment classification system, version 5. Unpublished manuscript.

Main, T. (1978) Some medical defences against involvement with patients. *Journal of the Balint Society* **7**, 3–11.

Mandl, K.D., Tronick, E.Z., Brennan, T.A., Alpert, H.R. and Homer, C.J. (1999) Infant health care use and maternal depression. *Archives of Pediatrics and Adolescent Medicine* **153**, 808–13.

Mann, D. (1999) The generalized transference in general practice. In: J. Lees (ed.) *Clinical Counselling in Primary Care*. London: Routledge.

Manning, C. (1999) Come back Balint—all is forgiven. *bmj.com*, accessed 14 February 1999.

Marinker, M. (1973) The doctor's role in prescribing. The medical use of psychotropic drugs. *Journal of the Royal College of General Practitioners* **23**, Suppl. 2.

Marinker, M. (1978) The chameleon, the Judas goat and the cuckoo. *Journal of the Royal College of General Practitioners* **28**, 199–206.

Marinker, M. (1984) The MRCGP revisited. *Journal of the Royal College of General Practitioners* **34**, 529–34.

Marks, M., Siddle, K., Warwick, C. and Kumar, C. (2000) A randomised controlled trial to assess the effect of specialised midwifery care on rates of postnatal depression in high risk women. Paper presented at the Biennial International Conference of the Marce Society Conference, Manchester, UK.

Markus, A.C., Murray Parkes, C., Tomson, P. and Johnston, M. (1989) *Psychological Problems in General Practice*. Oxford: Oxford University Press.

Marshall, M. and Lockwood, A. (1998) Assertive community treatment for people with severe mental disorders (Cochrane Review). *Cochrane Library* **3**, 2–25.

Matthews, K., Milne, S., Ashcroft, G.W. (1994) Role of doctors in the prevention of suicide: the final consultation. *British Journal of General Practice* **44**, 345–8.

Mayer, R. and Graham, H. (1998) Getting your Registrar to think families: *Education for General Practice* **9**, 234–7.

McCarthy, G. (1999) Attachment style and adult love relationships and friendships: a study of a group of women at risk of experiencing relationship difficulties. *British Journal of Medical Psychology* **72**, 305–21.

McDaniel, S., Campbell, T. and Seaburn, D. (1990) *Family-oriented Primary Care: a manual for medical providers*. New York: Springer-Verlag.

McDaniel, S., Hepworth, J. and Doherty, W. (1992) *Medical Family Therapy*. New York: Basic Books.

McGlashan, T. (1996) Early detection of schizophrenia: Research. *Schizophrenia Bulletin* **22**, 327 345.

McGlashan, T. (1998) Early detection and prevention of schizophrenia: rationale and research. *British Journal of Psychiatry* **172** (suppl. 33), 3-6.

McIntosh, J. (1993) Postpartum depression—womens help-seeking behavior and perceptions of cause. *Journal of Advanced Nursing* **18**(2), 178–84.

McLeary, G. (2000) Waiting with time. *British Medical Journal* **321**, 940.

McNeilly, C.L. and Howard, K.I. (1991) The effects of psychotherapy: a re-evaluation based on dosage. *Psychotherapy Research* **1**, 74–8.

McWhinney, I. (1996) The importance of being different. *British Journal of General Practice* **46**, 433–6.

McWhinney, I. (1997) *A Textbook of Family Medicine*, 2nd edn. Oxford: Oxford University Press.

McWhinney, I. (1999) The physician as healer: the legacy of Michael Balint. In: J. Salinsky (ed.) *Proceedings of the 11th International Balint Congress 1998*, pp. 63–71. Southport: Limited Edition Press.

McWilliams, M. and McKiernan, J. (1993) *Bringing It Out in the Open: domestic violence in Northern Ireland*. Belfast: HMSO.

Mellor-Clarke, J. (2000) Counselling in primary care in the context of the NHS quality agenda. British Association of Counselling and Psychotherapy.

Melzer, D., Hale, A.S., Malik, S.J., Hogman, G.A. and Wood, S. (1991) Community care for patients with schizophrenia one year after hospital discharge. *British Medical Journal* **303(6809)**, 1023–6.

Menage, J (1993) PTSD in women who have undergone obstetric and/or gynaecological procedures: a consecutive series of 30 cases. *Journal of Reproductive and Infant Psychology* **11**, 221–8.

Mental Health Act Commission (1991) $th Biennial Report, 1989-1991. The Stationery Office. Norwich.

Mental Health Act Commission (1997) *Guidance Note 3. Guidance on the Treatment of Anorexia Nervosa under the Mental Health Act 1983*. Nottingham: Mental Health Act Commission.

Merrill, J. and Ruben, S. (2000) Treating drug dependency in primary care: worthy ambition but flawed policy. *Drugs: Education Prevention and Policy* **7**, 203–13.

Mickelson, K.D., Kessler, R.C. and Shaver, P.R. (1997) Adult attachment in a nationally representative sample. *Journal of Personality and Social Psychology* **73**, 1092–106.

Midgley, S., Burns, T. and Garland, C. (1996) What do general practitioners and community mental health teams talk about? Descriptive analysis of liaison meetings in general practice. *British Journal of General Practice* **46(403)**, 69–71.

Miles, C.P. (1977) Conditions predisposing to suicide: a review. *Journal of Nervous Mental Disorders* **164(4)**, 231–46.

Millar, E., Garland, C., Ross, F., Kendrick, T. and Burns, T. (1999) Practice nurses and the care of patients receiving depot neuroleptic treatment: views on training, confidence and use of structured assessment. *Journal of Advanced Nursing* **29**, 1454–61.

MIND (1993) *MIND's Policy on Case Registers*. London: MIND.

Minuchin (1974) *Families and family therapy*. London: Tavistock.

Minuchin, S., Rosman, B.L. and Baker, L. (1978) *Psychosomatic Families*. Cambridge: Harvard University Press.

Møller-Madsen, S., Nystrup, J. and Nielsen, S. (1996) Mortality of anorexia nervosa in Denmark 1970–1987. *Acta Psychiatrica Scandinavica* **94**, 454–9.

Mooney, J. (1994) *The Hidden Figure: domestic violence in north London*. London: Islington Council.

Mullen, P. (1999) Dangerous people with severe personality disorder. *British Medical Journal* **319**, 1146–7.

Munk-Jørgensen, P., Møller-Madson, S., Nielsen, S. and Nystrup, J. (1995) Incidence of eating disorders in psychiatric hospitals and wards in Denmark 1970–1993. *Acta Psychiatrica Scandinavica* **92**, 91–6.

Murray, L. and Andrews, L. (2000) *The Social Baby*. Richmond: CP Publishing.

Murray, L. and Carothers, A.D. (1990) The validation of the Edinburgh Postnatal Depression Scale on a community sample. *British Journal of Psychiatry* **157**, 288–90.

Murray, L. and Cooper, P.J. (1997) Postpartum depression and child development. *Psychological Medicine* **27(2)**, 253–60.

Murray, L. and Cooper, P.J. (2000) A controlled trial of the long term effect of psychological treatment of postpartum depression: II impact on the mother child relationship and child outcome. *British Journal of Psychiatry*.

Murray, L., Stanley, C., Hooper, R., King, F. and FioriCowley, A. (1996) The role of infant factors in postnatal depression and mother- infant interactions. *Developmental Medicine and Child Neurology* **38(2)**, 109–19.

Murray, L., Sinclair, D., Cooper, P., Ducournau, P. and Turner, P. (1999) The socioemotional development of 5-year-old children of postnatally depressed mothers. *Journal of Child Psychology and Psychiatry and Allied Disciplines* **40**, 1259–71.

Murray, L., Woolgar, M., Murray, J. and Cooper, P.J. (2000) *Health Service Contacts and Women Vulnerable to Postnatal Depression*. Reading: Department of Health.

Murray, P., Brown, G.W. and Monck, E.M. (1962) The general practitioner and the schizophrenic patient. *British Medical Journal* pp. 972–976.

Mynors-Wallis, L.M., Gath, D.H., Day, A. and Baker, F. (2000) Randomised controlled trial of problem solving treatment, antidepressant medication, and combined treatment for major depression in primary care. *British Medical Journal* **320**, 26–30.

Nagel, T. (1979) *Mortal Questions*. Cambridge: Cambridge University Press.

Nathan, P.E. and Gorman, J.M. (1998) *A Guide to Treatments That Work*. Oxford: Oxford University Press.

Nazareth, I., King, M. and Davies, S. (1995) Care of schizophrenia in general practice: the general practitioner and the patient. *British Journal of General Practice* **45(396)**, 343–7.

Neely, C.T. (1991) 'Documents in madness': reading madness and gender in Shakespeare's tragedies and early modern culture. *Shakespeare Quarterly* **42(3)**, 315–38.

Neighbour, R.H. (1987) *The Inner Consultation*. Lancaster: MTP Press.

Nettleton, S. (1995) *The Sociology of Health and Illness*, Cambridge: Polity Press.

Newburn, M. and Singh, D.E. (2000) *Access to Maternity Information and Support. The Experiences and Needs of Women Before and After Giving Birth*. London: National Childbirth Trust.

Newton, T., Robinson, P. and Hartley, P. (1993) Treatment for eating disorders in the UK. Part 2. Experiences of treatment: a survey of members of the EDA. *Eating Disorders Review* **1**, 10–21.

Nielsen, D.A., Goldman, D., Virkunen, M., Tokola, R., Rawlings, R. and Linnoila, M (1994) Suicidality and 5-hydroxyindoleacetic acid concentration associated with a tryptophan hydroxylase polymorphism. *Archives of General Psychiatry* **51**, 34–8.

Nielsen, S., Møller-Madsen, S., Isager, T., Jorgensen, J., Pagsberg, K. and Theander, S. (1998) Standardised mortality in eating disorders—a quantitative summary of previously published and new evidence. *Journal of Psychosomatic Research* **44**, 413–34.

Noordenbos, G. (1998) Eating disorders in primary care: early identification and intervention by general practitioners. In: W. Vandereycken and G. Noordenbos (eds) *The Prevention of Eating Disorders*. London: Athlone Press.

Norman, R.M. and Malla, A.K. (1995) Prodromal symptoms of relapse in schizophrenia: a review. *Schizophrenia Bulletin* **21**, 527–39.

Norton, K. and Smith, S. (1994) *Problems with Patients*. Cambridge: Cambridge University Press.

Nutt, D.J. (1996) The psychopharmacology of anxiety. *British Journal of Hospital Medicine* **55(4)**, 187–90.

Nutt, D.J. and Bell, C. (1997) Practical pharmacotherapy for anxiety. *Advances in Psychiatric Treatment* **3**, 79–85.

O'Hara, M.W. and Swain, A.M. (1996) Rates and risk of postpartum depression—a meta-analysis. *International Review of Psychiatry* **8**, 37–54.

Obholzer, A. (ed.) (1994) *The Unconscious at Work: individual and organisational stress in the human services*. London: Routledge.

O'Dowd, T. (1988) Five years of heartsink patients in general practice. *British Medical Journal* **59**, 1–15.

Ogg, E.C., Millar, H.R., Pusztai, E.E. and Thom, A.S. (1997) General practice consultation patterns preceding diagnosis of eating disorders. *International Journal of Eating Disorders* **22**, 89–93.

Olds, D. and Korfmacher, J. (1998) The promise of home visitation: results of two randomised trials. *Journal of Community Psychology* **1**, 5–21.

Orona, C. (1990) Temporality and identity loss due to Alzheimer's disease. *Soc. Si. Med.* **30**, 1247–56.

Palazolli, M.S., Boscolo, L., Cecchin, G. and Prata, G. (1980) Hypothesizing circularity-neutrality: three guidelines for the conductor of the session. *Family Process* **19(1)**, 3-12.

Palmer, B.W., Heaton, R.K., Paulsen, J.S., Kuck, J., Braff, D., Harris, M.J. *et al.* (1997) Is it possible to be schizophrenic yet neuropsychologically normal? *Neuropsychology* **11**, 437–46.

Palmer, R.L. (1996) *Understanding Eating Disorders*. London: Family Doctor Publication.

Parker, I., Georgaca, E., Harper, D., McLaughlin, T. and Stowell-Smith, M. (1995) *Deconstructing Psychopathology*. London: Sage.

Parker, T., Leyland, L. and Paxton, R. (1997) Clinical psychology and counselling in primary care: where is the boundary? *Clinical Psychology Forum* **104**, 3–6.

Parkes, C.M (1972) *Bereavement: Studies of grief and loss in adult life*. London Tavistock Publications. 2nd edn. 1986.

Parry, G. (2000a) Developing treatment choice guidelines in psychotherapy. *Journal of Mental Health* **9**, 273–81.

Parry, G. (2000b) Evidence-based psychotherapy: an overview. In: N. Rowland and S. Goss (eds) *Evidence-based Counselling and Psychological Therapies*. London: Routledge.

Patten, B. (1996) *So Many Different Lengths of Time*. In: B. Patten (ed.) *Armada*, pp. 70–1. London: Flamingo.

Paxton, R., Shrubb, S., Griffiths, H., Cameron, L. and Maunder, L. (2000) Tiered approach: matching mental health services to needs. *Journal of Mental Health* **9**, 137–44.

Paykel, E. and Priest, R. (1992) Recognition and management of depression in general practice: consensus statement. *British Medical Journal* **305**, 1198–202.

Pedder, J. (1989) How can psychoanalysis influence psychiatry? *Psychoanalytic Psychotherapy* **4**, 43–54.

Pendleton, D., Schofield, T., Tate, P. and Havelock, P. (1984) *The Consultation: an approach to learning and teaching*. Oxford: Oxford University Press.

Pietroni, M. and Vaspe, A. (2000) *Understanding Counselling in Primary Care: inner voices from the city*. London: Churchill Livingstone

Plath, S. (2000) *Three Women* (Unpublished poem broadcast BBC Radio 4, 8 Jan).

Pokorny, A.D. (1983) Prediction of suicide in psychiatric patients. *Archives of General Psychiatry* **40**, 249–57.

Porter, D. (2000) The healthy body. In: R. Cooter and J. Pickstone (ed.) *Medicine in the 20th Century*, pp. 201–16. Amsterdam: Harwood Academic Publishers.

Porter, R. (1998) Can the stigma of mental illness be changed? *Lancet* **352**, 1049–50.

Preven, D., Katcher, E., Kupfer, R. and Walters J. (1986) Interviewing skills in first year medical students. *Journal of Medical Education* **61**, 842–4.

Prien, R.F. and Kupfer, D.J. (1986) Continuation drug therapy for major depressive episodes: how long should it be maintained? *American Journal of Psychiatry* **143**, 18–23.

Quitkin, F.M. (2000) Placebo effects and their non-specific factors. In: M. Gelder, G. Lopez-Ibor, Jr and C. Andreasen (eds) *The New Oxford Textbook of Psychiatry*. Oxford: Oxford University Press.

Ratnasuriya, R.H., Eisler, I., Szmukler, G.I. and Russell, G.F. (1991) Anorexia nervosa: outcome and prognostic factors after 20 years. *British Journal of Psychiatry* **158**, 495–502.

Resick, P. and Schnicke, C. (1993) *Cognitive Therapy for Rape Victims*. San Francisco: Sage.

Richardson, P.H. (1997) ABC in psychiatry: psychological treatments. *British Medical Journal* **315**, 733–5.

Ricoeur, P. (1984) *Time and Narrative*. Chicago: University of Chicago Press.

Rimmer-Yehudai, E. (2001) Hands on, hands off: handling the mind and its effect of the body. Unpublished paper presented at the Primary Care Section Conference of the Association of Psychoanalytic Psychotherapist in the NHS.

Rimmon-Kenan, S. (1983) *Narrative Fiction: contemporary poetics*. London: Routledge.

Robert, J.S. (2000) Schizophrenia epigenesis? *Theoretical Medicine and Bioethics* **21**, 191–215.

Roberts, G. (1999) The rehabilitation of rehabilitation: a narrative approach to psychosis. In: J Holmes and G. Roberts (eds) *Healing Stories. Narrative in Psychiatry and Psychotherapy*. Oxford: Oxford University Press.

Robin, A.L., Siegel, P.T., Moye, A.W., Gilroy, M., Dennis, A.B. and Sikand, A.A. (1999) Controlled comparison of family versus individual therapy for adolescents with anorexia nervosa. *Journal of the American Academy of Child and Adolescent Psychiatry* **38**, 1482–9.

Robinson, D., Woerner, M.G., Alvir, J.M. *et al.* (1999) Predictors of relapse following response from a first episode of schizophrenia or schizoaffective disorder. *Arch Gen Psychiatry*; 56: 241–247.

Rogers, A. and Pilgrim, D. (1996) *Mental Health Policy in Great Britain*, London: Polity Press.

Rosenbeck, R., Dunn, L., Peszke, M. *et al.* (1999) Impact of clozapine on negative symptoms and the deficit syndrome in refractory schizophrenia. *American Journal of Psychiatry* **156**, 88–93.

Roth, A. and Fonagy, P. (1996) *What Works for Whom? A Critical Review of Psychotherapy Research*. New York: Guilford Press.

Roth, S., Newman, E., Pelcovitz, D, van der Kolk, B and Mandel, F.S (1997) Complex PTSD in victims exposed to sexual and physical abuse: results from the DSM-IV Field Trial for PTSD. *Journal of Traumatic Stress* **10**, 539–55.

Rowland, N., Bower, P., Mellor-Clarke, J., Heywood, P., Hardy, G. and Godfrey, C. (2000) The effectiveness and cost effectiveness of counselling in primary care. *Cochrane Library*.

Royal College of General Practitioners (1972) *The Future General Practitioner*. London: British Medical Journal.

Royal College of Midwives (2000) *Life after Birth. Reflections on Postmatal Care*. London: Royal Colege of Midwifes.

Royal College of Psychiatrists (1991) The future of psychotherapy services. *Psychiatric Bulletin* **15**, 174–9.

Russell, G.F., Szmukler, G.I., Dare, C. and Eisler, I. (1987) An evaluation of family therapy in anorexia nervosa and bulimia nervosa. *Archives of General Psychiatry* **44**, 1047–56.

Rutt, G. and Batchelor, H. (1998) The doctor, the patient and the supervisor. *Education for General Practice* **9**, 508–11.

Rutz, W., von Knorring, L. and Walinder, J. (1989) Frequency of suicide on Gotland after systematic postgraduate education of general practitioners. *Acta Psychiatrica Scandinavica* **80**, 151–4.

Sackin, P. (1986) Value of case discussion groups in vocational training. *British Medical Journal* **293**, 1543–4.

Sackin, P., Barnett, M., Eastaugh, A. and Paxton, P. (1997) Peer-supported learning. *British Journal of General Practice* **47**, 67–8.

Sadowski, H., Ugarte, B., Kolvin, I., Kaplan, C. and Barnes, J. (1999) Early life family disadvantages and major depression in adulthood. *British Journal of Psychiatry* **174**, 112–20.

Said, E.W. (1985) *Beginnings: intention and method*. New York: Columbia University Press.

Salinsky, J. and Sackin, P. (2000) *What are you Feeling, Doctor? Identifying and Avoiding Defensive Patterns in the Consultation*. Oxford: Radcliffe Medical Press.

Salkovskis, P., Atha, C. and Storer, D. (1990) Cognitive-behavioural problem solving in the treatment of patients who repeatedly attempt suicide. A controlled trial. *British Journal of Psychiatry* **157**, 871–6.

Salzman, C. (1991) American Psychiatric Association Task Force report on benzodiazepine dependence, toxicity and abuse. *American Journal of Psychiatry* **148(2)**, 51–2.

Samson, A., Bensen, S., Beck, A., Price, D. and Nimmer, C. (1999) Post-traumatic stress disorder in primary care. *Journal of Family Practice* **48**, 222–7.

Sapolsky, R. (1994) *Why Zebras Don't Get Ulcers*. New York: W.H. Freeman and Co.

Scarry, E. (1985) *The Body in Pain*. Oxford: Oxford University Press.

Schmidt, U. and Treasure, J. (1993) *Getting Better Bit(e) by Bit(e). A Treatment Manual for Sufferers of Bulimia Nervosa*. Hove: Lawrence Erlbaum Associates.

Schmidtke, A., Bille-Brahe, U., Deleo, D. *et al.* (1996) Attempted suicide in Europe: rates, trends and sociodemographic characteristics of suicide attempters during the periods 1989–1992. Results of the WHO/EURO Multicentre Study on Parasuicide. *Acta Psychiatrica Scandinavica* **93**, 327–38.

Schrire, S. (1986) Frequent attenders – a review. *Family Practitioner* **3**, 272–5.

Seale, J.P., Amodei, N., Bedolla, M., Ortiz, E., Lane, P. and Gaspard, J. (1995) Evaluation of addiction training for psychiatric residents. *Substance Abuse* **16**, 1–18.

Seeley, S., Murray, L. and Cooper, C. (1996) The outcome for mothers and babies of health visitor intervention. *Health Visitor* **69(4)**, 135–8.

Selvini Palazzoli, M., Boscolo. L., Cecchin, G. and Prata, G. (1980a) The problem of the referring person. *Journal of Marital and Family Therapy* **6**, 3–9.

Selvini Palazzoli, M., Boscolo, L., Cecchin, G. and Prata, G. (1980b) Hypothesizing, circularity, neutrality: three guidelines for the conductor of the session. *Family Process* **19**, 2–12.

Sembi, S. *et al.* (1998) Does PTSD occur after strokes? *International Journal of Geriatric Psychiatry* **13**, 315–22.

Senior, R. (1994) Family therapy in general practice: 'We have a clinic here on a Friday afternoon'. *Journal of Family Therapy* **16**, 313–27.

Serfaty, M. and McCluskey, S. (1998) Compulsory treatment of anorexia nervosa and the moribund patient. *European Eating Disorders Review* **6**, 27–37.

Shapiro, D.A. and Shapiro, D. (1982) Meta-analysis of comparative therapy outcome studies: a replication and refinement. *Psychological Bulletin* **92**, 581–604.

Shapiro, D. (1996) Introduction. In: Roth, A. and Fonagy, P. (1996) *What works for whom? A critical review of psychotherapy research*. New York: Guildford Press.

Sharp, D., Hay, D.F., Pawlby, S., Schmucker, G., Allen, H. and Kumar, R. (1995) The impact of postnatal depression on boys' intellectual development. *Journal of Child Psychology and Psychiatry and Allied Disciplines* **36**, 1315–36.

Shepherd, G. *et al.* (1994) *Relative Values*. London: Sainsbury Centre for Mental Health.

Shepherd, M., Cooper, A.B., Brown, A.C. and Kalton, G.W. (1966) *Psychiatric Illness in General Practice*. Oxford: Oxford University Press.

Shoebridge, P. and Gowers, S. (2000) Parental high concern and adolescent-onset anorexia nervosa. *British Journal of Psychiatry* **176**, 132–7.

Sibbald, B., Addington Hall, J., Brenneman, D. and Freeling, P. (1993) Counsellors in English and Welsh general practice: their nature and distribution. *British Medical Journal* **306**, 29–33.

Sibbald, B., Addington Hall, J., Brenneman, D. and Freeling, P. (1996a) *The Role of Counsellors in General Practice: a qualitative study*, Occasional Paper 74. London: Royal College of General Practitioners.

Sibbald, B., Addington Hall, J., Brenneman, D. *et al.* (1996b) Investigation of whether on-site general practice counsellors have an impact on psychotropic drug prescribing rates and costs. *British Journal of General Practice* **46**, 63–7.

Simpson, S., Corney, R., Fitzgerald, P. and Beecham, J. (2000) A randomised controlled trial to evaluate the effectiveness and cost effectiveness of counselling patients with chronic depression. *National Coordinating Centre for Health Technology Assessment (NCCHTA) Health Technology Assessment* **4(36)**.

Sinclair, D. and Murray, L. (1998) Effects of postnatal depression on children's adjustment to school—teacher's reports. *British Journal of Psychiatry* **172**, 58–63.

Slinn, R.M., King, A.J. and Evans, J. (2001) A national survey of the hospital services for the management of adult deliberate self-harm. *Psychiatric Bulletin* **17**, 81–4.

Smith, C.W.L., Gross, V., Graham, H. and Reilly, J. (1983) The Health-Care meeting: eight years of collaborative work in general practice. *Group Analysis* **April**, 52–62.

Smith, M.L. and Glass, G.V. (1977) Meta-analysis of therapy outcome studies. *American Psychologist* **32**, 752–60.

Smith, S. (1998) Postmodernity and a hypertensive patient: rescuing value from nihilism. *Journal of Medical Ethics* **24**, 25-31.

Smith, S. (1999) Ethics and Postmodernity. In: Dowrick, C. and Frith, L. (eds) *General Practice and Ethics*. London: Routledge.

Smith, S. and Norton, K. (1999) *Counselling Skills for Doctors*. Buckingham: Open University Press.

Spiker, D.G., Weiss, J.C. and Dealy, R.S. (1985) The pharmacological treatment of delusional depression. *American Journal of Psychiatry* **142**, 430–6.

Sroufe, L.A., Carlson, E.A., Levy, A.K. and Egeland, B. (1999) Implications of attachment theory for developmental psychopathology. *Development and Psychopathology* **11**, 1–13.

St James-Roberts, I., Conroy, S. and Wilsher, K. (1998) Links between maternal care and persistent infant crying in the early months. *Child Care Health and Development* **24(5)**, 353–76.

Stamp, E.E., Williams, A.S. and Crowther, C.A. (1995) Evaluation of antenatal and postnatal support to overcome postnatal depression—a randomized, controlled trial. *Birth-Issues in Perinatal Care* **22(3)**, 138–43.

Stevens, J. (1974) Brief encounter. *Journal of the Royal College of General Practitioners* **24**, 5–22.

Strathdee, G. and Williams, P. (1984) A survey of psychiatrists in primary care: the silent growth of a new service. *Journal of the Royal College of General Practitioners* **34**, 615–18.

Strupp, H.H. (1978) Psychotherapy research and practice—an overview. In: A. E. Bergin and S. L. Garfield (eds) *Handbook of Psychotherapy and Behaviour Change*, 2nd edn. New York: Wiley.

Sullivan, P.F., Bulik, C.M., Fear, J.L. and Pickering, A. (1998) Outcome of anorexia nervosa: a case-control study. *American Journal of Psychiatry* **155**, 939–46.

Sutherby, K.G.D.M.A. (1992) *Developing a Strategy for a Primary Care Focus for Mental Health Services in South-east London*. London: Institute of Psychiatry.

Sutherland, V.J. and Cooper, C.L. (1993) Identifying distress among general practitioners: predictors of psychological ill-health and job dissatisfaction. *Social Science and Medicine* **37**, 575–81.

Tarrier, N., Sommerfield, C., Pilgrim, H. and Faragher, B (2000) factors associated with outcome of cognitive-behavioral treatment of chronic post-traumatic stress disorder. *Behaviour Research and Therapy* **38**, 191–202.

Tata, P., Eagle, A. and Green, J. (1996) Does providing more accessible primary care psychology services lower the clinical threshold for referrals? *British Journal of General Practice* 469–472.

Taylor, C. (1989) *Sources of the Self.* Cambridge: Cambridge University Press.

Taylor, D., McConnell, D., McConnell, H., Abel, K. and Kerwin R. (1999) *The Bethlem and Maudsley Prescribing Guidelines*, 5th edn. London: Martin Dunitz.

Telfer, I. and Clulow, C. (1990) Heroin misusers: what they think of their general practitioners. *British Journal of Addiction* **85**, 137–40.

Temperley, J. (1978) Psychotherapy in the setting of general medical practice. *British Journal of Medical Psychology* **51**, 139–45.

Thiels, C., Schmidt, U., Garthe, R., Treasure, J. and Troop, N. (1998) Guided self change for bulimia nervosa. *American Journal of Psychiatry* **155**, 947–53.

Thompson, C., Kinmouth, A.L., Stevens, L., Peveler, R.C., Stevens, A., Ostler, K.J. *et al.* (2000) Effects of a clinical-practice guideline and practice-based education on detection and outcome of depression in primary care: Hampshire Depression Project randomised controlled trial *Lancet* **355**, 185–91.

Thompson, M., Norris, F. and Ruback, R.B (1998) Comparative distress levels of inner city family members of homicide victims. *Journal of Traumatic Stress* **11**, 223–43.

Thornicroft, G. (1991) Social deprivation and rates of treated mental disorder—developing statistical models to predict psychiatric service utilisation. *British Journal of Psychiatry* **158**, 475–84.

Tomson, P.R.V. (1990) General practitioners and family therapy. *Journal of Family Therapy* **12**, 97–104.

Toombs, S.K. (1993) *The Meaning of Illness: a phenomenological account of the different perspectives of physician and patient.* Dordrecht: Kluwer Academic Publishers.

Treasure, J. (1998) *Anorexia Nervosa: a survival guide for families, friends and sufferers.* Sussex: Psychology Press, Hove.

Treasure, J., Murphy, T., Szmukler, G., Todd, G., Gavan, K. and Joyce, J. (2001) The experience of caregiving for severe mental illness: a comparison between anorexia nervosa and psychosis. *Soc Psychiatry Psychiatr Epidemiol* **36**, 343–7.

Treasure, J. and Ramsay, R. (1997) *Hard to Swallow: compulsory treatment in eating disorders,* Maudsley Discussion Paper No. 3.

Treasure, J. and Schmidt, U. (1997) *Clinicians Guide to Getting Better Bite by Bite.* Susses: Psychology Press.

Treasure, J., Schmidt, U., Troop, N. Tiller, J., Todd, G., Keilen, M. and Dodge, E. (1994) First step in managing bulimia nervosa: a controlled trial of a therapeutic manual. *British Medical Journal* **308**, 686–689.

Treasure, J., Schmidt, U., Troop, N., Tiller, J., Todd, G. and Turnbull, S. (1996) Sequential treatment for bulimia nervosa incorporating a self care manual. *British Journal of Psychiatry* **168**, 94–98.

Treasure, J.L., and Schmidt, U. (2000) Ready, willing and able to change: motivational aspects of the assessment and treatment of eating disorders. *European Eating Disorders Review* (in press).

Treasure, J.L. and Ward, A. (1997) A practical guide to the use of motivational interviewing in anorexia nervosa. *European Eating Disorder Review* **5**, 102–14.

Truax, C. and Carkhuff, R. (1967) *Towards Effective Counselling and Psychotherapy Training and Practice*. Chicago: Aldine.

Tuckett, D. (1999) Book review, Cassandra's Daughter: a history of psychoanalysis in Europe and America, by Joseph Schwartz. *International Journal of Psychoanalysis* **80**, 1249.

Turnbull, S., Ward, A., Treasure, J., Jick, H. and Derby, L. (1996) The demand for eating disorder care: a study using the general practice research data base. *British Journal of Psychiatry* **169**, 705–12.

Turner, S. (1999) Place of pharmocotherapy in post-traumatic stress disorder. *Lancet* **354**, 1404–5.

Tylee, A., Freeling, P., Kerry, S. and Burns, T. (1995) How does the content of consultations affect the recognition by general practitioners of major depression in women? *British Journal of General Practice* **45(400)**, 575–8.

UK Prospective Diabetes Study Group (1998a) Intensive blood-glucose control with sulphonylureas or insulin compared with conventional treatment and risk of complications in patients with type 2 diabetes (UKPDS 33). *Lancet,* **352**, 837–53.

UK Prospective Diabetes Study Group (1998b) Effect of intensive blood-glucose control with metformin in overweight patients with type 2 diabetes (UKPDS 34). *Lancet,* **352**, 854–65.

UK Prospective Diabetes Study Group. (1998c) Tight blood pressure control and risk of macrovascular and microvascular complications in type 2 diabetes: UKPDS 38. *British Journal of Medicine* **317**, 703–13.

Van Eijk, J. (1983) The family doctor and the prevention of somatic fixation. *Family Systems Medicine* **1**, 5–15.

van Furth, E.F. (1998) The treatment of anorexia nervosa. In: H. W. Hoek, J. L. Treasure and M. A. Katzman (eds) *Neurobiology in the Treatment of Eating Disorders*. Chichester: Wiley.

Vitousek, K., Watson, S. and Wilson, G.T. (1998) Enhancing motivation for change in treatment resistant eating disorders. *Clinical Psychology Review* **18**, 391–420.

Wallace, E.R. (1988) What is 'truth'? Some philosophical contributions to psychiatric issues. *American Journal of Psychiatry* **145**, 137–47.

Waller, D., Fairburn, C.G., McPherson, A., Kay, R., Lee, A. and Nowell, T. (1996) Treating bulimia nervosa in primary care: a pilot study. *International Journal of Eating Disorders* **19**, 99–103.

Wamoscher, Z. (1966) The returning patient. *Journal Royal College of General Practitioners* **11**, 166–72.

Ward, A., Ramsay, R., Turnbull, S., Steele, M., Steele, H. and Treasure, J. (2000a) The Adult Attachment Interview in inpatients with anorexia nervosa and their mothers. Submitted for publication.

Ward, E., King, M., Lloyd, M., Bower, P., Sibbald, B., Farrelly, S. *et al.* (2000b) Randomised controlled trial of non-directive counselling, cognitive-behaviour therapy, and usual general practitioner care for patients with depression: I Clinical effectiveness, Ibid II cost effectiveness. *British Medical Journal* **321**, 1383–8.

Waskett, C. (1999) Confidentiality in a team setting. In: R. Bor and D. McCann (eds) *The Practice of Counselling in Primary Care*. London: Sage.

Webb, E., Ashton, C.H., Kelley, P. and Kamali, F. (1996) Alcohol and drug use in UK university students. *Lancet* **348**, 922–5.

Weissman, M.M., Bland, R.C., Canino, G.J., Greenwald, S., Hwu, H.G., Joyce, P.R. *et al.* (1999) Prevalence of suicide ideation and suicide attempts in nine countries. *Psychological Medicine* **29**, 9–17.

Wessely, S. (1998) The medicalisation of distress. *RSM Journal*, **4**, 79–85.

Whiffen, V.E. and Gotlib, I.H. (1989) Infants of postpartum depressed mothers: temperament and cognitive status. *Journal of Abnormal Psychology* **98(3)**, 274–9.

White, M. and Epston, D. (1990) *Narrative Means to Therapeutic Ends*. New York: Norton.

Whitehouse, A.M., Cooper, P.J., Vize, C.V., Hill, C. and Vogel, L. (1992) Prevalence of eating disorders in three Cambridge general practices: hidden and conspicuous morbidity. *British Journal of General Practice* **42**, 57–60.

Whiteman, J. (2000) Interprofessional education—the perception of GP tutors in North West Thames Region. *Education for General Practice* **11**, 179–85.

Whitley, E., Gunnell, D., Dorling, D. and Davey Smith, G. (1999) Ecological fragmentation, poverty, and suicide. *British Medical Journal* **319**, 1034–7.

Whitton, A., Warner, R. and Appleby, L. (1996) The pathway to care in post-natal depression: women's attitudes to post-natal depression and its treatment. *British Journal of General Practice* **46(408)**, 427–8.

Wickberg, B. and Hwang, C.P. (1996) Counselling of postnatal depression: a controlled study on a population based Swedish sample. *Journal of Affective Disorders* **39(3)**, 209–16.

Wiener, J. (1996) Primary care and psychotherapy. *Psychoanalytic Psychotherapy, Conference Proceedings* **10**, Suppl.

Wiener, J. (2001) Confidentiality and paradox, the location of ethical space. *Journal of Analytical Psychology* **46(3)**, April 2001.

Wiener, J. and Sher, M. (1998a) *Counselling and Psychotherapy in Primary Health Care: a psychodynamic approach*. London: MacMillan.

Wiener, J. and Sher, M. (1998b) *Counselling and Psychotherapy in Primary Health Care*. London: MacMillan.

Wilder, T. (1972) *The Bridge of San Luis Rey*. Harmondsworth: Penguin.

Williams, B. (1981) *Moral Luck*. Cambridge: Cambridge University Press.

Williams, M. (1997) Helping people say goodbye. *British Medical Journal* **315**, 317–18.

Williamson, C. (1992) *Whose Standards?* Buckingham: Open University Press.

Wilson, S. and Nutt D.J. (1999) Treatment of sleep disorders in adults. *Advances in Psychiatric Treatment* **5**, 11–18.

Wing, J.K. (1990) Meeting the needs of people with psychiatric disorders. *Society of Psychiatry and Psychiatric Epidemiology* **25**, 2–8.

Winnicott, D. (1965) *The Maturational Processes and the Facilitating Environment*. London: Hogarth.

Wolff, K., Welch, S. and Strang, J. (1999) Specific laboratory investigation for assessments and management of drug problems. *Advances in Psychiatric Treatment* **5**, 180–91.

Wolff, K., Goldberg, D. P. and Fryers, T. (1988) The practice of community psychiatric nursing and mental health social work in Salford. Some implications for community care. *British Journal of Psychiatry* **152**, 783–92.

Yehuda, R. (1997) Sensitisation of the hypothalamo-pituitary-adrenal axis in post-traumatic stress disorder. In: R. Yehuda and A. McFarlane (eds) *Psychobiology of Post-traumatic Stress Disorder*. New York, *Annals of the New York Academy of Sciences*, **821**, pp. 57–75.

Zipfel, S., Löwe, B., Reas, D.L., Deter, H-C. and Herzog, W. (2000) Long term prognosis in anorexia nervosa a 21-year follow-up study. *Lancet* **355**, 721–2.

Index

Note: Entries in *italics* refer to tables. Those in **bold** refer to figures.